D1367047

EVER SINCE
I HAD MY BABY

UNDERSTANDING, TREATING, AND PREVENTING THE MOST COMMON PHYSICAL AFTEREFFECTS OF PREGNANCY AND CHILDBIRTH

ROGER P. GOLDBERG, M.D., M.P.H.

THREE RIVERS PRESS • NEW YORK

This book contains general information that may not be applicable to your specific situation. It should not be used as a substitute for the advice of a doctor or medical professional.

Published by Three Rivers Press, New York, New York.
Member of the Crown Publishing Group, a division of Random House, Inc.
www.randomhouse.com

THREE RIVERS PRESS and the Tugboat design are registered trademarks of Random House, Inc.

Printed in the United States of America

Design by Helene Berinsky

Library of Congress Cataloging-in-Publication Data
Goldberg, Roger P.
    Ever since I had my baby : understanding, treating, and preventing the most common physical aftereffects of pregnancy and childbirth / Roger P. Goldberg.
    1. Pregnancy—Complications.   2. Childbirth—Complications.   I. Title.
RG571 .G595 2003
618.3—dc21   2002155369

ISBN 0-609-80872-9

10   9   8   7   6   5   4   3   2   1

First Edition

In memory of Sara Distenfield

Acknowledgments

I first conceived of this book several years ago, during an early-evening drive through the Arizona desert, while on a short break from residency training in Boston. Having delivered a departmental grand-rounds lecture entitled "Childbirth and the Pelvic Floor" earlier that week, I was still feeling energized by the enthusiastic response of the doctors, nurses, and midwives in attendance. Yet as I drove, it came to me that women outside the medical community have had little or no exposure to the issues so essential to their physical well-being. Shouldn't *everyone* be familiar with these remarkably common postreproductive problems and their causes? Shouldn't women be better informed about making the most sensible decisions during pregnancy and delivery, and about the debates taking place over birthing choices? Aren't they entitled to know the best strategies for prevention and finding treatment for problems? Clearly, these were topics warranting debate not only among doctors but also among their patients. This was a book, I realized, truly waiting to be written. I pulled over at the next exit, pinned a napkin against the steering wheel, and scribbled my first few lines. Since then, the support and enthusiasm of numerous individuals have enabled those early ideas to reach the bookshelves.

I am grateful to have a truly remarkable publishing team. Dorian Karchmar, from Lowenstein Associates Literary Agency, embraced this book right from the start, shared my enthusiasm, and was invaluable in helping to shape my proposal with her sharp focus and skilled editing. I am indebted to Betsy Rapoport, who acquired the book for Three Rivers Press, recognized the importance of its subject matter, and understood its potential audience. I owe countless thanks to Caroline Sincerbeaux, my editor at Three Rivers Press, for her great talent and tireless efforts to create an accessible, user-friendly guide for women of all ages. Her editing skills were invaluable through the revision and shaping process. Lauren Shavell from Medical Imagery produced the book's vivid and original illustrations, and I thank her for providing a high level of artistic talent while approaching this project with energy and creativity. Thanks also to Brad Herzog, a good friend and great author, for reviewing the early manuscript and offering his valuable advice.

On the professional front, I would especially like to thank my colleague and mentor Dr. Peter Sand, a recognized leader in urogynecology and reconstructive pelvic surgery. The clinical material in the latter chapters of this book is in no small way a reflection of Dr. Sand's guidance and renowned teaching skills. Thanks are due also to Dr. Patrick Culligan, of the Urogynecology Associates of Louisville, for his valuable advice at several stages. I am indebted to all others with whom I have worked at the Evanston Continence Center, with special thanks to Karen Sasso and Dr. Sumana Koduri for their help during my first few years.

My mentors in the Department of Obstetrics and Gynecology at Beth Israel Deaconess Medical Center in Boston are too numerous to mention, but I owe special gratitude to Dr. Benjamin Sachs and Dr. Henry Klapholz for the direction and training they provided during my residency. Thanks, as well, to Dr. Toni Golen, an obstetrician-gynecologist also at Boston's Beth Israel, for a close and insightful reading of my early manuscript amid her busy schedule. I am deeply grateful to many other physicians and nurses at "The B.I." who imparted their high professional standards and their compassion for the patients.

Robert and Anita Goldberg, your influence on this project cannot be measured. Above and beyond your constant guidance and unwavering values, you made this book possible by instilling a few specific literary traits: a love for writing, a discipline for editing, and the desire to take creative chances. For all of that and much more, I love you both. To Anna and Tony Nocera, world's greatest in-laws: now that this book is finally on the shelves, we're overdue for a big, long Sunday feast.

Last and most important, to Elena, my wife, without whom this book simply could not have happened. Her patience and encouragement fueled the early mornings and weekends I devoted to this book. She shared my passion from the start and contributed to the end result in countless invaluable ways—as an editor, an adviser, and an inspiration. As in every other aspect of my life, our love has made it all worthwhile.

Contents

Preface

BEYOND THE LABOR ROOM AND AFTER THE PUSH:
INTRODUCING A LONG-OVERDUE CHAPTER
IN WOMEN'S HEALTH CARE

The decisions made during childbirth have consequences that can last a lifetime.

You'll find no mention of pelvic prolapse or urinary or fecal incontinence in prenatal classes, and little attention devoted to them in menopause guides. But ask a soccer mom or baby boomer about leaking, bulging, pads, and diapers in private, and you'll be likely to hear a personal story, see a surgical scar, or be asked the question "You mean that's not *normal* at my age?"

Not normal, but very common.

- Out of three million women who have vaginal deliveries each year in the U.S., between 5 and 30 percent will become incontinent of urine, a number that increases to over 60 percent by the time they reach menopause.
- Up to 65 percent will first notice their loss of bladder control during pregnancy or after childbirth.
- Roughly forty thousand of these three million individuals will eventually suffer anal incontinence—a loss of control over their bowels—although only a fraction of them will ever acknowledge the problem to a physician.
- Though it's difficult to imagine, by age seventy, 11 percent of the general female population will undergo major surgery for pelvic prolapse or incontinence—a number roughly equal to their lifetime risk of breast cancer.

• Although sexual dysfunction is reported by up to 43 percent of women when they are asked, many others quietly accept it, viewing diminished sexual satisfaction and pleasure as an inevitable aspect of a postreproductive body.

Finally, countless women notice that something else has changed during their postreproductive years—for some right after childbirth, for others not until decades later—around the pelvis, bladder, vagina, or bowel. Perhaps an episiotomy that never felt fully healed, pelvic pain, constipation, or an unruly bladder waking them at night. Incontinence, prolapse, urinary and sexual dysfunction—the major consequences of childbirth injury to the muscles, tissues, and nerves of the pelvic floor—have remained among the most common and costly medical disorders suffered by women, yet probably are the least discussed.

If you're among the many women affected by one of these problems, then you already know that the physical changes behind these astounding numbers are by no means cosmetic or trivial. They are conditions that can influence any woman's sense of control, self-esteem, independence, and sexuality. They can lead to social withdrawal of even the most vigorous women, and physical deconditioning of otherwise robust individuals who steadily abandon their exercise routines. They can represent the difference between staying home or exercising, attending the theater, and lifting children and grandchildren without hesitation.

We live in a world of women more physically fit and active than ever before, but perhaps you find yourself limited by the most basic concerns imaginable: control over your bladder or bowels. Perhaps you've noticed bulging and pressure symptoms "down there" and are wondering what exactly has gone wrong, or if it might get worse. Maybe you've been concerned about a change in your sexual satisfaction and about whether or not these changes are permanent, or how they might affect your relationship. If these issues sound familiar and you're seeking explanations and advice, then take a seat and read for a while. You've turned the first page of a long-neglected chapter in women's health care.

A Guidebook for Postreproductive Problems

This book is about improving your understanding and restoring control. You'll gain a new perspective on the female body and understand the effects of pregnancy and childbirth on its form and function. You'll learn what we know about preventing pelvic-floor disorders in the first place. If you're already coping with symptoms, you'll become familiar with countless ways to help yourself through lifestyle, exercise, diet, and healthy habits. The wide world of office therapy and surgical treatments—ranging from simple home tips to cutting-edge medical technology—will be covered in practical terms. And you'll have a reference for your decision making, office evaluation, and treatment, whether at home or in the operating room.

What about all of those robust middle-aged models promoting adult diapers and hygienic pads? You've probably come to realize that this approach is discouraging at best. It's time to familiarize yourself with a wellspring of far more satisfying alternatives. Did you know, for instance, that finding relief may be as simple as changing your diet, starting a new exercise routine, or using simple medications you may already have in your medicine cabinet? Are you aware that office collagen injections can cure many cases of urinary incontinence as effectively as they can plump a Hollywood starlet's lips? Or that tiny pacemakers and magnetic chairs might help you to restore control over your bladder, and that the latest operations for urinary incontinence can often be performed with local anesthesia and no hospital stay? Do you know how to maximize your chances for a successful surgery and optimize your recovery afterward? The chapters ahead will shed new light on female problems, but more importantly, they will teach you how to ameliorate, prevent, and cope with these conditions.

Preserving Wellness, Restoring Control: A Guide for Women of All Ages

Whether you're contemplating pregnancy, are in the midst of your childbearing years, or are looking back on those years to realize that they marked the beginning of problems that made life a bit less carefree, *this book is for you.* There are many ways to treat, reverse, and sometimes even prevent these conditions, beginning right in your own home. Promoting health for the most intimate areas of your body, maintaining control over your most basic physical functions, and preserving your sense of youth and sexuality: these goals deserve a place in your health planning at any age.

If you are an expectant mother or contemplating having a baby, did you know that pelvic exercises could lower your risk of incontinence after delivery? Are you aware of the risks and benefits of forceps delivery or episiotomy and what their proper role should be? What are the real effects of perineal massage, alternative pushing techniques, natural labor, or your choice of anesthesia? Though we have much to learn, a great deal is known about the long-term effects of childbirth on your body, including risk factors, treatment strategies, and prevention. You may be surprised to hear about all that can be done before, during, and after delivery to best maintain your gynecologic, urologic, and even sexual health—and you deserve a candid discussion. Indeed, choices made during childbirth have consequences that can last a lifetime. This book will enhance your ability to make informed decisions.

If you're already a mother and are considering having another child, you may be wondering if mild pelvic troubles will get worse or whether your obstetrical strategy should be different this time. Along with your family planning, these areas of personal planning should also be addressed. Now is the time to inform yourself and enhance your ability to discuss these topics with your doctor or midwife. Your daily habits and approach to future pregnancies may have major repercussions on the future physical well-being of the pelvic floor and the function of your postreproductive body.

If, as a baby boomer, you've convinced yourself that the problems your mother dealt with are inevitable milestones of growing older, read on. After all, you are part of the largest cohort of women ever to reach their postreproductive years, and the first to demand, with a unified voice, more state-of-the-art solutions than adult diapers and pad liners. As a group, you have higher expectations than ever before for remaining fully active and enjoying a high quality of life. For a surprising number of individuals, that means effectively treating physical changes that had long been ignored: incontinence, prolapse, sexual dysfunction, and other problems of comfort and control that affect the female body after childbirth. In the chapters ahead, you will become familiar with all the options for prevention and treatment—at home, in the office, and in the operating room.

Learning about what to expect while you're expecting is important, but you should also know what to expect over the years that follow. You should equip yourself with the basic tools you'll need to prevent problems and to cope with symptoms. Whatever your stage in life, you should be aware that normal life as a postchildbearing woman is *not* a daily routine of pads and liners, or a struggle with symptoms that diminish your enjoyment of life at home or work, at the gym or in the bedroom.

New Perspectives on Women's Health: Telescopes, Microscopes, and More

Childbirth is the most fascinating natural convergence of science, politics, economics, and miracle. There is no other biological event so intriguing, and so charged with personal, gender, and social issues. The vision of a natural delivery, deciding on a midwife or doctor, the choice over anesthesia, the idea of home birth—so many anxious issues surrounding a medical event that can never be fully anticipated or engineered. Its potential physical repercussions, likewise, encompass a great deal more than scientific facts and figures.

This book aims to provide a newly expanded perspective on your reproductive health by illuminating a number of often overlooked connections between obstetrical events and their gynecological repercussions, and by exploring how a wide array of nonmedical factors—including economics, health policy, even ethics—can influence your likelihood of facing these physical problems. Our journey toward understanding your postreproductive problems will lead us through worlds both big and small: from the tissue level of female pelvic anatomy and the function of your bladder and bowels to the societal level of health systems, gender politics, and your medical insurance. We'll need both microscopic and telescopic vision to see and understand the spectrum of childbirth's physical effects in its full context.

For starters, aim a telescope toward certain urban communities in Brazil, Colombia, and Peru, where cesarean rates approach a staggering 85 percent. Most of us would reflexively disregard these statistics as a product of technology-obsessed physicians, poorly informed patients, or societies preoccupied with youth and aesthetics. Perhaps, in the final analysis, these assumptions will be proven true; indeed, Brazil's minister of health described the childbirth trends in his nation as "a vicious circle of cultural phenomena and economic influences."

But consider for a moment the opposite end of the spectrum: our own medical culture and insurance environment allow women little power to choose their mode of delivery. Consider a 1996 survey of female obstetricians published in *The Lancet* in which over 30 percent stated that they would prefer cesarean section to vaginal delivery, with the vast majority citing pelvic injury as the main reason. Yet we've fostered medical systems within which doctors, midwives, and their departments and hospitals are actively encouraged to achieve the target rate of vaginal delivery for 85 percent of their patients.

Are women being held to guidelines and standards that their own physicians might not choose for themselves? Could the cultural phenomena, economic influences, and other nonmedical factors shaping our own childbirth trends be at odds with the best preventive medicine—or even be fueling a silent epidemic of pelvic-floor dysfunction?

As we explore the physical repercussions of childbirth, you'll learn that certain obstetrical practices and techniques should indeed be minimized whenever possible, and that vaginal delivery can increase the odds of various pelvic-floor disorders. But above all else, I want to be clear that my intent is *not* to advocate one method of delivery over another. Cesarean delivery carries potential risks that should never be trivialized, and for many women, those risks will far outweigh the potential advantages. For the majority of women, vaginal childbirth is not a problem. But you may be one of the countless women each year who cope with incontinence, prolapse, or another pelvic-floor disorder. You deserve better tools for understanding and treating these problems, as well as avoiding them in the first place, starting with an awareness of their possible obstetrical roots. You're entitled to a fresh assessment of traditional obstetrical practices, and to know that just because something has always been done that way, it might not represent the best science or what is best for you. You deserve the kind of informed consent one would expect before any major medical or surgical event. After all, childbirth is perhaps the single most dramatic physical experience of a woman's lifetime, and it should never be so politically charged that we hesitate to discuss its full effects, for better or worse. This book will help you find answers to your most intimate questions and tools to address them.

Out of the Shadows and into the Spotlight

At this moment in the evolution of women's health care, the physical repercussions of childbirth have finally been thrust directly into the medical spotlight. Women are at last openly discussing the dirty little secrets of incontinence, prolapse, and other postreproductive disorders. Their doctors have come to realize the overwhelming need for treatment, and researchers have shifted to full throttle in their search for solutions. As a public-health issue, postreproductive conditions represent a major burden, including billions of health-care dollars, and have assumed a high priority on the national women's-health agenda. They are the core problems addressed, medically and surgically, by one of medicine's most rapidly growing subspecialties: urogynecology. Today's medical marketplace is teeming with urogynecologists, female urologists, and other female pelvic medicine specialists rolling out the red carpet for this newly recognized patient: *you.*

Approaching the Crossroads

Women's health is approaching a crossroads as the process of childbirth is being evaluated from a new perspective: your body. It grows increasingly clear that obstetrics and gynecology—long treated as detached and distinct phases of women's health care—are intimately connected. The lifestyle and childbirth decisions of today's thirty-year-old may impact key aspects of her physical function at age forty, fifty, or sixty; and incontinence, prolapse, or sexual dysfunction in a fifty-year-old may relate to childbirth and lifestyle decisions she made years before. Knowledge is the most powerful compass with which to navigate your health most wisely. So whether you're looking forward to the wondrous experience of childbirth or looking back and seeking solutions, I hope that the chapters ahead provide you with a renewed freedom to enjoy life to the fullest.

PART 1

"WHAT'S HAPPENED TO ME DOWN THERE?"

THE PELVIC FLOOR, CHILDBIRTH, AND PROBLEMS THAT ARISE

~ 1 ~

Recognizing Your
Postreproductive Problem

INCONTINENCE, PROLAPSE, SEXUAL DYSFUNCTION, AND
OTHER COMMONLY OVERLOOKED CONDITIONS

*The reason why mothers are more devoted to their children than fathers:
it is that they suffer more in giving them birth.*

—Aristotle

Why didn't anyone tell me about this problem ten years ago?
—Linda, age forty-one, considering surgery

"What's happened down there?" you've asked yourself, as have so many other women from time immemorial. Ever since that wondrous day you gave birth—for the first time or the fifth—your body has never felt quite the same. Was it embarrassment over the loss of urine you first noticed while lifting your child, laughing with your friends, or making a run to the bathroom? Was it your growing self-consciousness about controlling your bowel movements or gas? Or maybe it was your worry that sex didn't feel the same as it once did, and that your partner's satisfaction might have changed also.

"I feel way too young for this!" you've told yourself while mothering, working, exercising, nurturing relationships, and striving for a full and active life. Yet more and more, you've found that these problems really *can't* be ignored, because they're making you less active, your life less complete. Never, at this stage in life, had you anticipated such challenges to your sense of control, intimacy, and self-image,

3

conditions that make you feel terribly alone and abnormal. What might the response be if you mentioned these problems to your peers?

More likely than not, their eyes would light up with interest and affirmation. Many of them have these problems, too. What's happened down there for you and many other women are the effects of pregnancy, labor, and delivery—of forceps, episiotomies, and a newborn's head, shoulders, arms, and legs—on your pelvic muscles, nerves, bladder, bowel, and vagina. They are long-term problems of the pelvic floor that modern obstetrics has overlooked in its efforts to make delivery safe and comfortable in the short term. Leaking, bulging, soiling, sexual dissatisfaction—women of past generations rarely complained about these "inevitable costs" of childbirth. After all, what could be done?

A New Chapter

Within the book of women's health, you've turned the first page of a new chapter whose time is overdue. Call it urogynecology, female pelvic medicine, or postreproductive women's health. By any name, it is finally centered on the female conditions that so often follow the most wonderful and dramatic physical event of your lifetime: childbirth. You've learned of the many ways to prevent and treat problems such as heart disease, breast cancer, and osteoporosis. But you've heard little about the countless ways to prevent and treat the physical effects of childbirth. From this chapter forward, you'll hear a great deal.

Along the winding road between childbirth and menopause, scores of women are affected by physical symptoms that often attest to the extraordinary physical demands of pregnancy, labor, and delivery. Some of these postreproductive changes are immediately apparent, affecting the quality of a woman's most vigorous years; other anatomic changes have no repercussions until decades later. Whether these physical transitions are subtle or severe, immediate or delayed, they are more common—and fortunately, more treatable—than you might think. Incontinence, prolapse, and pelvic and sexual problems are no longer the unspoken and inevitable costs of motherhood.

"Mom takes care of everyone, but who takes care of Mom?" The average working mother spends one and a half hours each day shuttling kids around, two hours preparing food and straightening the house, and what often seems like twenty-five hours listening to everybody else's problems! The time has arrived to better understand one of the most important physical events in *your* life, and learn how to treat the symptoms that are bothering you. Take a Calgon moment and read on. Doctor's orders.

Identifying Your Postreproductive Symptoms

URINARY INCONTINENCE AND LOSS OF BLADDER CONTROL

At least one of every three women will suffer significant loss of bladder control, and although incontinence affects many women without kids, up to 65 percent will notice this problem for the first time either during or after childbirth. Millions each year choose surgery for this debilitating condition, and millions more seek nonsurgical treatments; countless others silently endure their symptoms without ever seeking help. A loss of bladder control can make you feel lonely, ashamed, and antisocial, even unemployable. But what many women don't realize is that urinary incontinence, in most cases, boils down to a few common types—*all of them treatable.* Understanding your problem is your first step to reaching a cure.

STRESS INCONTINENCE

Allison

"I don't want to be Florence Henderson in diapers in a few years!"

"Excuse me?" I replied as I continued to jot down some notes on her medical history. It was her first office visit.

"I said, I don't want to become Florence Henderson!"

This was Allison, a thirty-three-year-old advertising executive, upbeat about everything except her four-year history of leaking urine. "Everything's felt different," she said, since the forceps-assisted vaginal delivery of her only child. During the months after delivery, she had begun to notice a few changes, a bit less control. Like a few of her friends, she'd wet her pants a bit when laughing or coughing hard. For security, she began wearing pads all month long. And for two years before coming to my office, she'd been doing occasional Kegel exercises at the recommendation of her internist. She hadn't noticed much improvement since starting with the exercises, although she couldn't swear that she'd been doing them correctly. I turned my chair toward Allison and, serving her up a bit of her own deadpan humor on that cold and rainy day, reassured her that in my medical opinion, her risk of becoming Florence Henderson was very, very small.

Allison's comment resonated in my mind as we continued her office visit, reviewed the testing plan, and discussed her most likely treatment options. Though I wasn't sure Mrs. Henderson ever advertised adult diapers or spoke publicly about incontinence, I understood the message loud and clear. Lurking behind Allison's campy quip was a great deal of anxiety—about youthfulness and aging, about losing control. She was facing a problem that, in her mind, belonged to the "Golden Girls," the Brady Bunch mom—not a young, working city slicker just starting her family life.

Should she worry? Research suggests that even a completely problem-free vaginal childbirth would leave her with a significant risk of incontinence. And though forceps may have been used with good reason, they further increased the likelihood that she would develop bladder problems; she stood at several times the usual risk of severe stress incontinence by age forty, as compared to women with no previous forceps delivery. Furthermore, there is compelling evidence to suggest that her current symptoms would not improve over time but rather would progress to needing treatment. One study concluded that when certain types of urinary incontinence persist three months after delivery, the risk of long-term leakage approaches 94 percent.

The questions arise: how can Allison help herself, at this early stage, to feel better and prevent her problem from getting worse? How can she avoid joining the fifty thousand women undergoing surgery for stress incontinence each year? And how could we have helped her to avoid this scenario in the first place?

Stress incontinence refers to the sudden accidental leakage of urine when you cough, sneeze, laugh, lift a heavy object, hit a tennis or golf ball, or quickly change your position—in other words, during any activity that creates pressure or stress in your pelvic area. Does this sound familiar? If so, it should come as no surprise—stress incontinence is the most common type of urine leakage in women aged thirty to fifty. Up to a third of women in their thirties report significant loss of urine during exercise. If you're a gymnast, tennis player, or aerobics enthusiast, in particular, maybe you've noticed leakage with sudden straining. More bothersome urinary incontinence, which can mean leakage during simple walking or light lifting, becomes a problem for around 15 percent of women under sixty-five, and closer to a third of women above that age. If you're severely stress-incontinent, you may even leak silently—in other words, when you're hardly exerting yourself at all, such as during a bumpy car ride or while bending down to tie your shoes.

Stress incontinence results from a urethra that lacks enough strength to hold back urine when the bladder pressure rises during physical exertion. As you'll learn in chapter 8, it is a condition whose roots begin with pregnancy and childbirth in many but not all cases. Most importantly, you'll become familiar with a broad range of strategies—including exercise, lifestyle tips, office procedures, and minimally invasive surgical options—allowing you to toss those pads and enjoy an active life without concern over keeping dry.

THE COST OF LEAKING

Can you believe there are more than fifty thousand hospital admissions each year for the treatment of stress incontinence? In the United States alone, over $1.14 billion is spent on stress-incontinence operations, and that doesn't include the cost of nonsurgical treatments. For each woman seeking treatment, a silent handful just lives with the problem.

URGE INCONTINENCE AND THE OVERACTIVE BLADDER

Linda

"Who's the kid here?" Linda asked me on her first visit to my office. "Here I am trying to toilet-train my daughter, wearing pads myself, and wetting them each time I run after her." A thirty-nine-year-old occupational therapist and mother of two girls aged two and a half and six, Linda was simply too busy to be bothered with these problems.

She'd been waking two or three times each night with a strong urge to urinate, and reaching the bathroom in time had become a serious challenge. During the workday, tired from her poor night's sleep, she found it increasingly difficult to make it through her patients' thirty-minute occupational-therapy sessions, and several times each week, she actually leaked urine on the way to the ladies' room. Linda began emptying her bladder every half hour to minimize her chances of an accident, and she routinely mapped the nearest bathroom wherever she was. She even started to wear dark, baggy clothes, just in case. "My husband hates to travel with me! He gets frustrated when we're on the highway and we have to pull over...I know every bathroom in the city! It's taking the spontaneity out of my life." The problem also affected their relationship in the bedroom, as Linda's fear of leaking during intercourse was making it more and more difficult for her to relax and enjoy.

For two years, she had thought about finding a doctor to discuss the problem with. But somewhere between her older daughter's soccer practices and her younger daughter's preschool, she hadn't managed to act on that thought until now. Three weeks before our visit, Linda had been at her nephew's wedding. "There I am in this beautiful dress, and as I'm standing up from my chair, I have a huge accident. Thank goodness the dress was long and wide, and I was wearing a pad. But right then and there, I said to myself: 'Enough of this!' "

Across the top of her medical questionnaire, Linda had written, "I'm here because I need a bladder operation." Surprised by her assumption that these symptoms would require surgery, and curious to know whether that was the reason for her avoiding help all this time, I posed a few questions. Had she ever considered that she might not have a surgical problem at all? Was she aware that diet and exercise might be enough to control her symptoms, or perhaps physical therapy or a simple medication? Did she know how many other women were facing the same problem? As we continued that first office visit, Linda's expression spelled surprise, then relief, as she realized that one way or another, she might be feeling better soon.

Have you ever lost urine for no apparent reason, under stressless circumstances? Do you find yourself running to the bathroom with a strong urge that you sometimes can't control before reaching the toilet? Ever feel a sudden need to void when you hear running water, wash the dishes, or simply enter the house? Do you think of your bladder as undersized?

If so, you've probably experienced the other major type of urinary incontinence commonly affecting postreproductive women: *urge incontinence, or the overactive bladder.* An overactive bladder can occur at any age, even among women without any children. But it's more common after childbirth, following the loss of vaginal and pelvic supports, so it's a key concept to understand if you're coping with postreproductive pelvic symptoms. The overactive bladder can mean accidental leakage of urine for women who wet themselves during strong bladder urges; for others, the problem is urgency, frequency, and waking at night to void, as if the bladder were too small. In any of its forms, it can lead to a slow but steady withdrawal from an active daily life. According to a survey called the National Overactive Bladder Screening Initiative, sponsored by Pharmacoa & Upjohn, 26 percent of women with overactive bladder symptoms reported that they regularly avoided places and situations due to the concern that a bathroom may not be nearby.

Do these overactive-bladder symptoms sound familiar to you? The good news is that normal adult bladder behavior can be relearned, and urge incontinence can be controlled. In chapter 8, you'll learn all about the impact of simple habits and behavioral techniques, diet and medication, special exercises, electrical stimulators, magnetic chairs, implantable pacemakers, and more.

THE KEY-IN-THE-DOOR ("LATCHKEY") URGE

Ever notice that you have a strong sudden urge to urinate when returning home from work or play and fumbling with your front door? You're not alone. An overactive bladder muscle, and the bundle of nerves surrounding it, often begin to sense that a bathroom is nearby. In chapter 8, you'll learn how to retrain your bladder for better behavior.

MIXED INCONTINENCE

Stress incontinence, urge incontinence—how many different causes can there be for one *very* annoying symptom?

Actually, there are more. It's surprisingly common for postreproductive women to have more than one incontinence type occurring in tandem, or *mixed incontinence*. By some estimates, more than half of all women visiting a specialist's office for leakage will be diagnosed with mixed incontinence, usually defined by the presence of both stress and urge incontinence. If you've found yourself leaking urine with a cough, and also while running to the toilet, you just might have mixed incontinence. If you wake during the night with a strong urge and also lose control while lifting your child during the day, that's likely to be mixed incontinence. The overall prevalence of mixed incontinence among women has been estimated at 36 to 38 percent. In chapter 8, we'll discuss the way your doctor determines whether you have mixed incontinence or other problems with bladder function, and how this might influence your road to relief.

PELVIC PROLAPSE: BULGING, DROPPING, AND FALLING DOWN BELOW

Joanne

"I'm falling apart . . . literally!" said Joanne, a sixty-one-year-old fourth-grade teacher, tossing her hands up the air.

Joanne was a mother of three grown children, two delivered vaginally and the third by cesarean as a result of her baby's slow heartbeat during labor. Joanne's vaginal deliveries had been induced after their due dates, and both babies weighed over eight pounds at birth. During her first labor, she contracted for fifteen hours and pushed for over three. Her second labor and delivery were a breeze, under three hours from start to finish. She hadn't noticed any incontinence problems in the first several years after childbirth, though she struggled with constipation, and her urinary stream seemed weaker. At age forty-three, she underwent a total hysterectomy for small fibroids (benign tumors) of the uterus, which had been causing very heavy and painful periods. Nine months later, the real problems began. She began noticing heaviness in her pelvis and lower back, and vaginal pressure after a long workday. Before long, the feeling became more constant. Though she'd never had bowel troubles before, now she needed to strain on the toilet, with a feeling that she could never fully evacuate her stool. Even more disturbing was the fact that she was soiling her underwear, despite all her efforts to keep herself meticulously clean. "It feels," she told me, "like everything's gone loose down there. I don't even feel much during intercourse anymore."

Six months before our visit, while she and her husband were seeing their youngest son off to college and helping him to move boxes and furniture into the dormitory room, she had first noticed a bulging of tissue at the vaginal opening, "like a ball." Somewhat panicked, Joanne told nobody but quietly started to withdraw from her social routine. She had given up her regular early-morning walk and Saturday golf game for half a year by the time she walked into my office one October afternoon. The only reason she'd finally come was that during her annual checkup, her internist had told her that her vagina or bladder had dropped, and had sent her to our office for further evaluation. "That sounds pretty bad," she said, with a look that made it clear she'd been agonizing over the meaning of this change, and assuming the worst about her prognosis. "I'm a healthy person. Why did this happen to me?"

Pelvic prolapse (genital prolapse) refers to loss of support within one or more of the key pelvic structures, including the uterus, vagina, bladder, and rectum. Prolapse can lead to a wide spectrum of potential symptoms, sometimes right after childbirth but more often several years later. For some women, it starts with simple difficulty retaining a tampon; for others, it's gradually increasing discomfort in the vagina, pelvis, abdomen, or lower back. Perhaps you've noticed some vaginal pressure at the day's end, or increasing difficulty moving your bowels despite a healthy diet and stool softeners. You may have felt pain or uncomfortable pressure during intercourse, or diminished sexual pleasure that you'd assumed was a cooling of your previously torrid sex drive but in fact was due to a specific anatomical change. Urinary symptoms accompanying prolapse may include incontinence, a weakened stream, or a sense of bladder fullness even after you've finished voiding. Perhaps you've noticed what is often the most alarming symptom: a bulge of tissue seen or felt at the vaginal opening, anywhere from the size of a plum to an orange, or even much larger. Unfortunately, it's often not until reaching this advanced stage of prolapse that many women finally acknowledge they have a problem and seek advice.

If all of this sounds surprisingly familiar, you're not alone—this problem is shared by many of your otherwise healthy friends. After learning a bit about the nature of pelvic prolapse in chapter 9, you'll feel relieved to understand that no, you're not falling apart at the seams, and yes, there are many ways for you to start feeling better and prevent your problem from getting worse. But right now let's briefly review the most common prolapse types.

CYSTOCELE: THE BULGING BLADDER

A *cystocele* is often referred to as a dropped bladder, and it is one of the most common prolapse bulges among postreproductive women. A cystocele forms when the normally flat upper vaginal wall loses its support and sinks downward. This allows the bladder, which is located right above the upper vaginal wall, to drop right along with it. When a cystocele becomes advanced, the bulge may become visible outside the vaginal opening. The visible tissue is the weakened vaginal wall; the bladder is right behind this skin but cannot be seen.

The symptoms caused by cystoceles can include vaginal bulging or pressure, slowing of the urinary stream, overactive-bladder symptoms, and an inability to fully empty the bladder.

RECTOCELE: THE BULGING RECTUM

A *rectocele* is the mirror image of a cystocele. Cystoceles result from a weak upper vaginal wall, allowing the bladder to bulge downward, while rectoceles result from a weak *lower* vaginal wall, allowing the *rectum* to bulge *upward*. This creates an extra pouch in the normally straight rectal tube.

Rectoceles cause symptoms related to incomplete emptying of the rectum, just like cystoceles cause incomplete emptying of the bladder. But unlike cystoceles, which tend to cause few symptoms until they become quite large, rectoceles often cause symptoms in their early stages. Even a rectocele bulge that cannot be visualized at the vaginal opening may cause difficulty with bowel movements—including the need to strain more forcefully, a feeling of rectal fullness even after a bowel movement, increased fecal soiling, and in some cases, incontinence of stool or gas. Those symptoms result from stool and air remaining within the rectocele pouch even after defecation, in contrast to the normal rectum, which fully empties. Larger rectoceles can bulge right through the vaginal opening and look like a cystocele, although this time it is the lower vaginal wall accounting for the bulge.

UTERINE PROLAPSE

Uterine prolapse, or a dropped womb, occurs when the uterus and cervix fall into the vagina after their supporting pelvic ligaments have weakened. If the uterus drops only slightly, it may cause mild pressure in the vagina or rectum, or even lower back pain. If the uterus drops a lot, you may see the cervix itself outside the vaginal opening, or feel discomfort with intercourse. Sometimes recognizing uterine prolapse is easy—you see the cervix protruding, or feel a firm bulge of tissue inside while inserting a tampon. But most of the time, your doctor makes the diagnosis during the office exam. As we'll discuss in chapter 9, uterine prolapse is a common reason for needing a hysterectomy, usually performed through a vaginal incision. You'll also learn about simple devices called pessaries, which can relieve some cases of uterine prolapse without any operation at all.

VAGINAL VAULT PROLAPSE

If you've already had a hysterectomy, the top of the vagina (called the *vault* or *apex*) should be attached to supportive ligaments on either side of the pelvis. These attachments prevent the top of the vagina from bulging outward beneath the constant pressure of the abdominal contents. However, if these attachments weaken and the vaginal apex drops, a bulge may form near the vaginal opening. This is called *vaginal vault prolapse,* a condition that happens only to women who have had a hysterectomy, and one that can cause severe pressure and bulging symptoms. Similar to cystoceles, rectoceles, and uterine prolapse, some cases of vaginal vault prolapse can be managed with simple devices; surgical repair is also common and can be performed by a number of vaginal, abdominal, and even laparoscopic techniques. In chapter 9, you'll become an expert on all of your options, including the different ways a vaginal vault suspension can be performed, and what this operation will mean for your recovery and long-term results.

ENTEROCELE: THE FEMALE HERNIA

When the intestines bulge downward into the upper vagina, then you have an *enterocele.* It's the last of the postreproductive pelvic bulges you should know about, and the most difficult to conceptualize. Among all types of female prolapse, enteroceles share the most similarity with the hernias that can develop in the abdominal and groin areas of both women and men: both involve bulging of the intestines into weakened supports nearby. In a man, hernias bulge through the abdominal wall; in a woman, enteroceles bulge into the top of the vagina. The symptoms are often vague, including a bearing-down pressure in the pelvis and vagina, and perhaps a lower backache. They often exist alongside vaginal vault prolapse in women who have had a hysterectomy.

"BUT I NEVER HAD A VAGINAL DELIVERY!"

Significant numbers of women with prolapse, incontinence, and other pelvic-floor problems have never delivered vaginally. How could this be? First, the weight of a pregnant uterus may itself cause important changes over the course of nine months, even without a vaginal birth. Second, everyone's tissues vary in strength and resiliency. You'll find women who've had eight deliveries and no loss of bladder control, and others with major incontinence and prolapse after only one tiny baby. A recent survey of more than three thousand South Australians found that having a cesarean did not offer full protection against the silent epidemic of prolapse and incontinence. Each woman's body responds differently to the stresses of pregnancy and delivery.

ANAL INCONTINENCE: LOSS OF BOWEL CONTROL

If you've been bothered by some loss of control over your stool or gas, chances are you've never mentioned it to your doctor. Neglected by physicians who rarely address this issue with their patients, and endured by patients feeling too embarrassed to mention it, anal incontinence remains underdiagnosed. In a world where almost all of our other problems are now openly discussed, including urinary incontinence, anal incontinence has been left behind as perhaps the most stigmatized postreproductive disorder, still an unspeakable problem. But the problem *does* exist among otherwise healthy women after childbirth—it's reported in some form by 20 to 59 percent—

though sometimes not arising until many years later. At any age, it can be among the most disabling of all disorders to cope with; accidents are difficult to mask and, of course, humiliating. Few conditions in gynecology cause as much personal and social distress.

What is anal incontinence? For many women, it means the inability to avoid passing gas in public. For other women, it means the accidental loss of stools. And for others, it's soiling of underwear despite careful hygiene. Not all cases of anal incontinence are caused in the labor room, but childbirth injury is the most common factor. In chapter 10, you'll learn about the obstetrical events that can lead to anal incontinence, along with a handful of tips for prevention and a host of effective treatments if you're already affected.

Your risk for anal injury and incontinence is influenced by a number of specific obstetrical events and procedures, including forceps and vacuum delivery, episiotomies, and pushing style. Later on, you'll learn about all that can be done inside the labor room to reduce your risk. If you're already coping with symptoms of anal incontinence, you'll learn about how to find relief through diet, medication, and simple healthy habits.

POSTREPRODUCTIVE SEXUAL CHANGES

A 2001 Harvard study found that six months after childbirth, roughly one quarter of women experience diminished sexual function after a first vaginal birth. Other studies have indicated higher rates following forceps or vacuum delivery.

When these changes occur right after childbirth and then resolve, the reasons are most often perfectly normal. Even the most routine changes—such as weight gain, changes to your body shape, and stretch marks—can give rise to self-image issues, which in turn can affect intimacy between partners. Normal breast-feeding can cause dryness and irritability of the vaginal skin because of decreased estrogen levels, which leads to sexual discomfort that fully reverses later on. Normal perineal healing, be it after an episiotomy or spontaneous laceration, can cause tenderness for weeks and sensitivity for months. And the normal transition to parenthood can drastically reduce the time and effort that two partners will devote to keeping the flame of their romance aglow.

But sometimes postreproductive sexual problems are *not* part of a normal transition and don't go away after the postpartum period ends. Too often, women shrug them off as an inevitable aspect of their new body, unaware of not only the physical changes accounting for the problem but also of the preventive strategies and effective treatments. In chapter 11, we'll explore these conditions and their solutions in depth.

- *Changes to the vagina or perineum.* Perineal injuries can increase the risk of sexual pain after childbirth but can be preventable. Widening of the vaginal entrance, due to stretch and separation of the perineal muscles and supports, is actually a very common anatomic change after childbirth. For most women, it poses no problem. But for some, the vagina becomes extremely lax, and intercourse is simply not enjoyable in the same way for either partner. Many women who have noticed this problem are reluctant to tell their doctor, but there are effective solutions.

- *Sexual effects of incontinence and prolapse.* Advanced prolapse, urinary incontinence, and anal incontinence can each have a negative impact on sexual identity and functioning. Prolapse bulges can interfere with penetration. Pressure of the penis against a large cystocele can cause bladder discomfort and urgency, and bumping against a rectocele can cause rectal discomfort or an urge to defecate. *Coital incontinence* refers to the leakage of either urine or stool during sexual intercourse or orgasm. A recent British analysis found that among more than 4,100 women evaluated at a single urogynecology center, coital urinary incontinence was reported by 21 percent, with 72 percent reporting an adverse effect on sexual function. It's an embarrassing problem that patients don't usually like to discuss, so it's more common than even most physicians would suspect. Although it can deep-freeze sexual relations between even the most solid partners, it's almost always remediable.

- *Hormonal changes, decreased libido, and diminished sensation.* Hormones change wildly during pregnancy and afterward. During the postreproductive years, hormones and their impact on sexual function often take on central importance. Loss of libido, diminished sensation, disorders of arousal—all may impact postreproductive sexual function, and in most cases, the problem can be alleviated.

"OBSTETRICS, THEREFORE GYNECOLOGY": EXPLORING THE ROOTS OF YOUR POSTREPRODUCTIVE PROBLEM

The *way* you deliver your babies may be just as important to your postreproductive health as the number you choose to have. Countless decisions made in the labor room—from preparing your pelvic floor and perineum during pregnancy to your choice of position during labor and when and how you should push—can affect your comfort and control afterward. Did you know, for instance, that the length of time you push might relate to your risk of incontinence later on? If avoiding labor and vaginal delivery altogether can prevent these changes to some degree, when is choosing a cesarean a reasonable option? In Part 2, you'll learn that although some aspects of labor and delivery can't be controlled or predicted, many others can. We'll revisit labor-room strategies that are usually taken for granted yet probably shouldn't be. You'll learn the basics of preventive obstetrics to protect these areas of your body, from the first week of pregnancy right up to the final push. Whether you gave birth three years or three decades ago, or are still in the planning stages, exploring these connections will allow you to understand your postreproductive body in a whole new way.

OTHER CHANGES "DOWN THERE"

Finally, we'll address other problems that can occur around the pelvis, bladder, vagina, or bowel in the years after childbirth. Some might not have existed before childbearing, such as an episiotomy that never felt fully healed, worsened constipation, or pelvic pain. Or a problem may have preceded childbirth but became more bothersome, such as vaginal irritation, bladder infections, or hemorrhoids. If you're postmenopausal, you should understand how natural hormonal changes might be affecting any problems down there, as well as your options for treatment and prevention. In the chapters ahead, you'll gain a new understanding of how to find the most effective relief for a number of gynecological problems and general ailments that are often overlooked.

What Caused All This?

So there you are. You've identified some of the issues that seem to have come with the territory of your postreproductive body. You've learned that they aren't nearly as unusual as you thought. But how did it all sneak up on you? Whether you're preparing for childbirth or looking back on its aftermath, you've probably never stopped to consider how this defining life event might affect your body and physical function long afterward.

Let's aim our microscope at pregnancy and childbirth and make the connection between these postreproductive problems and the physical events of pregnancy and labor that first triggered them, sometimes many years earlier. As you begin to better understand the cause of your postreproductive problems, you'll be closer to the cure.

2

Introducing the Pelvic Floor

ANATOMY, FUNCTION, AND PHYSICAL CHALLENGES

I thought this was something that only happened to old people!
—Jan, first visit to the office, three
years after the birth of her twins

I like to work and travel. I want to improve my quality of life!
—Marian, forty-nine-year-old, eldest
daughter just left for college; seen
for incontinence

Fateful Moments on the Stage

Across cultures, continents, and generations, the birth of a newborn is a human moment that elevates us and provides our single clearest glimpse into the divine. What other experience throughout the human life cycle so universally suspends our cynicism and rekindles the possibilities of wonder and miracle? Childbirth is a timeless drama centered on the strength and determination of a heroine, supported by a cast of secondary players. Building its intensity with wailing, screaming, and puffing, it climaxes with a cry, collective awe, and lives forever changed. Labor is truly our most primal and natural act upon life's stage.

On a less majestic plane, labor and delivery for our species represent a monumental physical strain. Whereas most physical degeneration in our bodies accumulates gradually across the years and decades of adulthood, during childbirth, we witness immediate and often irreversible injury occurring right before our eyes. At no other time would doctors and family members passively observe physical injury to a loved one without intervening—in a hospital room, no less! The blinding intensity of the labor drama, and our overwhelming fixation on the safe journey of the fetus, allow little opportunity for other concerns—even those concerning potential long-term problems for Mom. "Just give us a healthy baby," the young and the restless pray, "and we'll deal with all the rest later on."

A mother's fate is often sealed in different ways. From that moment in time, for significant proportions of childbearing women, the die has been cast; they are destined to suffer urinary incontinence, anal incontinence, and pelvic-organ prolapse later in life. Through stretching, tearing, detachment, and compression, childbirth remains the major risk factor for these pelvic disorders. Within months or years, some of these women will be quizzing their peers and scanning the Internet, researching the various causes and latest treatments. Years later, greater numbers will stream into a doctor's office in need of medication, a device, or surgery, expressing amazement that so many of their female friends seem to be suffering the same symptoms.

WHY ALL THE STRUGGLE?

Why have humans, for all our innocent efforts to procreate, been dealt such a complicated hand in the labor room? Let's consider, from the standpoint of obstetrics and gynecology, the impact of the past several million years of evolution on the human race. It's been a mixed blessing, to say the least.

First, to accommodate an enlarging brain, the size of our cranium gradually increased well out of proportion to the rest of our body. While this change immensely improved the quality of cocktail conversations and university lectures, it wreaked havoc on the act of childbirth, leaving us with an extraordinarily large fetal head in comparison with the usual maternal pelvis. Look at polar-bear mothers: weighing over five hundred pounds, they deliver babies with heads smaller than humans'. In human obstetrics, there is *very* little room to spare!

Problem number two: we stood upright. While this earned us the ability to walk along the beach holding hands, and dramatically improved the aesthetics of ballroom dancing, we were unfortunately left with a pelvis much narrower from front to back, and a bit wider from side to side, in comparison to our knuckle-walking ancestors. This standing bipedal posture also shifted the opening of our bony pelvis directly underneath all of the weighty contents of the abdomen and pelvis. All of our organs were stacked right over a wide-open space, so the pelvis needed to devise enough strength and support to resist the forces of gravity pushing the bladder, uterus, vagina, and bowel downward through this bony pelvic opening. The vagina, in particular, was faced with the seemingly impossible task of supporting the weight of the uterus, bladder, rectum, and bowels all its life, then allowing a full-term baby to pass through—and afterward resuming function as a sexual organ while providing enough strength within its walls to continue holding back the bladder and rectum.

To make this new anatomy all the more challenging, the disproportion between baby and pelvis increased further as improving nutrition resulted in larger offspring over the centuries. For women who have multiple vaginal births, any supports covering this bony opening are stretched wider and wider with the delivery of each newborn.

The Pelvic Floor

What would happen over the millennia as a result of the remarkable physical stresses involved in childbirth? For every evolutionary challenge, the human body always seemed to devise a clever adaptation. But was this evolutionary mismatch, and the stress of human childbirth, too much of a challenge for the female body to surmount? No chance! On the contrary, the human species devised a remarkably clever solution: the pelvic floor.

The first priority of the pelvic floor would have to be providing support for the various organs lying above, including the uterus, bladder, and bowel. On the other hand, the floor couldn't be a solid surface: through it, a few key hollow structures must pass, including the urethra, vagina, and rectum. While providing strength, the pelvic floor would need to allow these structures to function properly, keeping them closed most of the time but allowing them to open when needed. A seemingly impossible compromise between competing demands: *strong* enough to withstand the constant pressure of internal organs, *supportive* enough to allow the vaginal, rectal, and urinary tubes to maintain control over bodily wastes, and *flexible* enough to allow a full-term baby to pass through. Quite an engineering challenge!

Introducing your pelvic floor. It consists of several layers of muscular support stretching like a hammock across your pelvic opening. Intertwined within these layers are broad, overlapping muscles and connective tissue that surround your organs and secure them to your pelvic bones and spine. Muscles flexing, nerves firing, and bodily wastes being held at bay only inches from the outside world: could you have guessed that so much drama was taking place in this hidden area of your body?

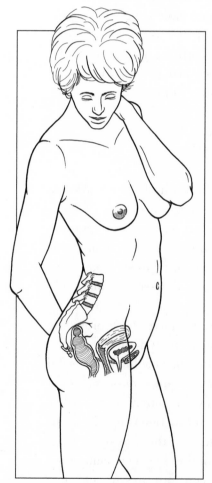

Let's draw a map of your pelvic anatomy in the most practical terms, for those of you trying to understand your own bulging, dropping, or leaking, and for those looking ahead to childbirth. Aim your microscope at the basic components of the pelvic floor, so we can explore the physical act of childbirth from a new point of view.

"Normal anatomy": female pelvic organs and the pelvic floor

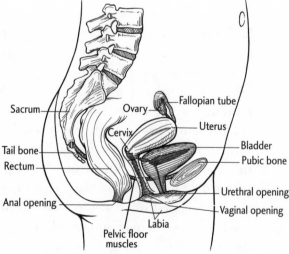

THE PERINEUM

The illustration here shows the *perineum,* the bridge of tissue between the opening of the vagina and the anus. It's actually the connection point for several muscles that form the opening of the vulva and vagina. The perineum is a relatively easy anatomic structure to orient yourself to, because it's external and visible, and also because it is the tissue intentionally cut during an episiotomy. So, let's start our map of the pelvis right at the perineum, and use it as our first landmark of your pelvic floor.

Finding the perineum on your own body is easy. Looking in the mirror, identify your anal and vaginal openings; in between, you'll see the span of tissue that is the perineum. It can vary in size from the width of a finger to several inches.

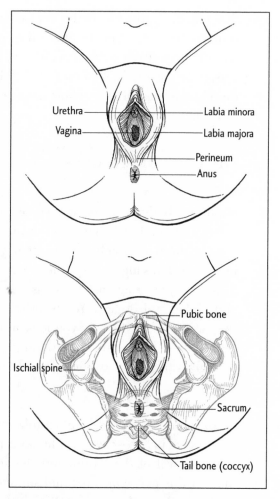

(*Above*) The outer genitals and perineum
(*Below*) "Deeper view" of pelvic bones

In its normal prechildbirth form, the perineum joins several muscles (*bulbocavernosus* and *transverse perineal*) that form a solid muscular rim around the vaginal opening.

Now take a look at the anatomy surrounding your perineum. Above and to the sides, you'll see the outer lips of the vagina, their outer surface covered with hair. When these *labia majora* are separated, you'll see the *labia minora,* which look like thinner, hairless folds. At their top margin, they come together in the middle, near the *clitoris.* At their lowest point, they meet in the middle to form the *fourchette,* a sensitive area that can be a source of vaginal irritation.

Beneath the perineum is the anal opening, surrounded by the anal sphincter muscles. Finally, above the perineum and the vaginal opening, orient yourself to the *urethra*. Notice how the urethra sits right above the vagina. In chapter 8, you'll learn about the importance of this close relationship and how changes to the area during childbirth can lead to problems.

THE LEVATOR MUSCLES

Let's move to a deeper layer of the pelvis to reach perhaps the most important body parts when it comes to the physical effects of pregnancy and childbirth. The *levator muscles* are the true foundation of your pelvic floor. Each day, whether you're running, coughing, lifting, or just taking it easy, they're the bedrock that provides your insurance policy against the constant downward force of the pelvic and abdominal organs. You'll never see or touch the levators, and they won't affect the way you look in a swimsuit. But make no mistake—the health and conditioning of your levator muscles can strongly affect the way you feel and function.

A Shelf

Remember the wide, vulnerable opening right at the bottom of your bony pelvis—that problematic product of evolution? Like a shelf, several of the levator muscles form a sturdy barrier covering most of this pelvic opening and supporting the uterus, vagina, bladder, and other pelvic organs. When it's functioning properly during a strong cough or sneeze, these organs and their supports bounce against the muscular floor like a trampoline, rather than bulging through the open space toward the outside of the body. The levator shelf provides your critical first-line pelvic-floor support and best protection against prolapse and other types of pelvic-floor dysfunction. Like any quality trampoline, the levator shelf can remain strong and resilient—bounce after bounce, year after year—unless it's overly stressed, stretched, or abused.

A Sling

Other parts of the levator muscles function like slings, wrapping around the anal and urethral sphincters and keeping them tight when you're not yet ready to void. These sling muscles play a major role in keeping you continent of urine, gas, and stool. The *pubococcygeus* and *puborectalis* are two of the most vital, encircling the rectum, urethra, and vagina. When you cough, bend, or swing a five-iron on the golf course, these muscles tighten almost instantaneously, contributing a burst of pressure at each sphincter to hold back the various waste products inside your body.

The levator muscles: a supportive "floor" for the pelvic organs

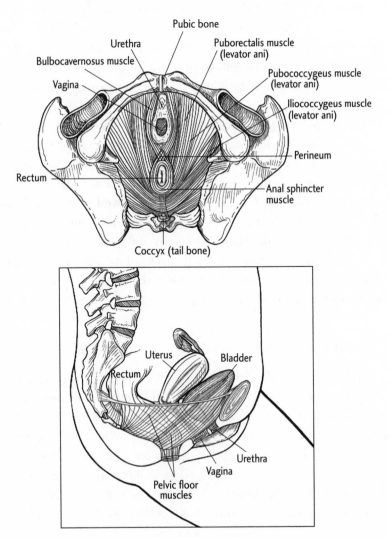

Confused? Actually, you can locate your levator muscles by performing a pelvic-floor or Kegel exercise. Kegels represent a willful contraction of the levator shelf and sling muscles, causing a tightening and lifting of the pelvic supports. In Appendix A, you'll learn tips on doing the perfect Kegel exercise.

PELVIC NERVES

The big, strong levator muscles of the pelvis, like all other muscles, depend on a healthy nerve supply to maintain their strength, position, and tone. One nerve in particular—the *pudendal*—is actually a pair of nerves, one on either side of your pelvis, and is a major power source. These nerves originate in your lower spine and divide into branches that nourish the vaginal area, perineum, and most other pelvic structures crucial to continence and support.

Healthy pelvic nerves are responsible for maintaining pelvic-floor strength, keeping the shelf and sling of the levator muscles (the foundation of your pelvic floor) well toned and healthy. The pudendals are also responsible for providing sensation to the pelvic area, including around the bladder and bowel as well as sexual. Unfortunately, the anatomical positions of the pudendal nerves—right near the birth canal—make them especially vulnerable to wear and tear in the labor room. Later on, we'll discuss how injury to the pudendal and other nerves might represent the initial trigger eventually leading to incontinence, prolapse, and other pelvic-floor problems.

PELVIC CONNECTIVE TISSUES AND LIGAMENTS

Connective tissue, also called *fascia*, is a dense, firm, light-colored material encasing the pelvic organs and vagina and helping secure them to the bony walls of your pelvis. Most of the so-called ligaments in your pelvis are thicker areas of this same material. Compared with the levator muscles, which provide the strongest foundation of your pelvic supports, the connective tissues play only a secondary role. Think of your pelvic connective tissues like carpenter's glue for your pelvis, helping to secure your pelvic organs as glue would beams of wood, whereas the organs are really held together by the nails and screws of the levator muscles and their nerves. Despite their secondary status, certain connective tissues do help to keep the pelvic organs in their proper places.

- *Between the rectum and vagina.* A thick layer called the *recto-vaginal septum* separates these two structures, preventing the rectum from bulging up into the vagina. When this layer becomes weak or thin, a rectocele may form.
- *Within the upper vaginal wall and around the bladder.* Connective tissues within the upper vaginal wall provide solid support for the bladder and urethra. When these connective tissues have torn or weakened after pregnancy and childbirth, dropping of the bladder and urethra may occur.
- *Uterosacral ligaments.* These ligaments attach the upper vagina and the lower part of the uterus to the pelvis. When they weaken, prolapse of the uterus and upper vagina can occur.

CONNECTIVE TISSUES: KEY INGREDIENTS FOR PELVIC SURGERY

Despite some amazing innovations in the surgical treatment of prolapse, incontinence, and other pelvic-floor problems, even the best surgeon's ability to re-create your normal pelvic anatomy—and prechildbirth foundation of levator muscle support—remains limited. Connective tissues and ligaments are the anatomic structures most often used for surgically repairing prolapse and incontinence, simply because the levator muscles and their accompanying nerves can't be surgically rebuilt. If, during surgery, your pelvic connective tissue and ligaments are found to be weak or thin, then your surgeon may recommend using mesh or natural-tissue grafts to take their place. Sound like a hernia repair? As you'll see in chapter 9, it is.

PELVIC BONES: THE IMPORTANCE OF CHILDBEARING HIPS

Last but not least, your pelvic shape. What could be more basic to the way a baby travels through your pelvis? The width, depth, and space between your pelvic bones have important effects not only on how fast labor progresses but also on what types and how much pelvic injury might occur during childbirth. Yet you've probably heard very little about this aspect of your body and how it can influence childbirth decisions.

Through your obstetrician's eyes, your pelvis has an inlet, an outlet, and in between, a midpelvis. Though every woman has her own unique pelvic shape, four classic shapes identified in the 1930s are still used to describe your bony pelvic shape, and to predict—though not always very reliably—the way it might affect the course of your childbirth. Your doctor can determine your pelvic shape by taking a series of measurements during a regular pelvic examination (called *pelvimetry*). Unfortunately, it's not possible to guess your pelvic shape based on outward appearance.

Gynecoid

This is the most common female pelvic shape, found in around 30 percent of women. Fortunately, it is the one most suited for a successful childbirth. The gynecoid pelvis has relatively plentiful space in all areas—front, back, and sides. Its front pubic bones are fairly open and wide, and the spines of the pelvis (a knob of bone located on either side of the pelvis's inner wall) don't protrude very far into the birth canal. So if you have a gynecoid pelvis, take a moment to thank your parents: they've handed down some good childbearing genes!

Android

This pelvic shape with the *Star Wars* name can present problems for vaginal delivery. Much like the typical male pelvis (*andro* means *man*), the front arch of the pubic bones is narrower than the gynecoid shape, and the spines on the pelvic sides tend to jut into the birth canal, shrinking the passageway for the fetal head. In the rear, the tailbone and lower spine (*sacrum*) also protrude forward, closing off precious space. Overall, these features create a narrow heart shape, relatively small at both the inlet and outlet, making a difficult delivery more likely. Although fewer than 5 percent of women are thought to have a pure android shape, many women have mixed pelvic shapes, including both android and gynecoid features.

Anthropoid

This pelvic shape, seen in fewer than 15 percent of women, is a thin oval. The spines on the pelvic walls are often large, leaving relatively little side-to-side space for the fetus during delivery.

Platypelloid

This is the least common pelvic shape, resembling an oval tipped on its side. Some experts claim that women with a platypelloid pelvis are at significantly higher risk for incontinence and prolapse, as well as recurrent prolapse after surgery has been performed, due to the pelvic organs and supports being more exposed and vulnerable to the trauma of childbirth and also the forces of gravity. An interesting hypothesis, but one that has yet to be scientifically tested.

Female pelvic shapes: four "classic" types

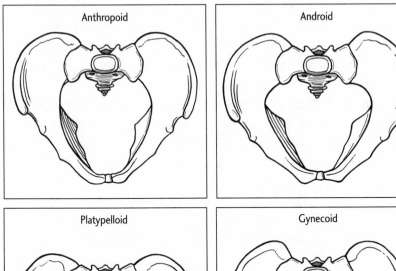
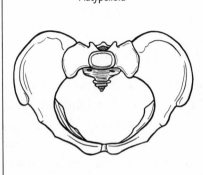
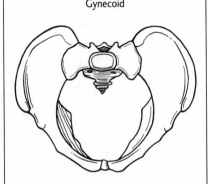

What's Your Pelvic Shape?

Whatever the shape of your pelvic bones, they're important to your postreproductive health. They can impact childbirth's physical ease or difficulty, the way your baby travels through the birth canal, and the amount of pressure, stretch, and potential injury to each area along the way. That, in turn, has an impact on the problems you're at risk for afterward.

Consider the shape of your *pubic arch*, formed by the bones that you can feel for yourself at the front of your pelvis, below your pubic hairline. If the pubic arch is narrow (android or anthropoid), that means less room for the fetus in the front of your pelvis. As a result, a large fetal head or wide shoulders may be more likely to stretch and tear downward, into the perineum and rectum, during delivery. If, on the other hand, you have a wide pubic arch (gynecoid, platypelloid), or a tailbone that angles forward, the fetal head might tend to be pushed up toward the pubic bone, directly into the bladder and urethra. What if the bones are narrow along the sides of your pelvis, creating pressure points between the fetal head and the pudendal nerve running along each pelvic side wall? Consider how much more force might be applied to those nerves in a narrow anthropoid pelvis, compared with a wide gynecoid one.

A great deal remains to be learned about how pelvic shape may influence the effects of vaginal delivery on your postreproductive body. In chapter 4, you'll learn how your doctor or midwife might evaluate your pelvic shape during a pelvic examination.

Physical Challenges:
Your Pelvis During Pregnancy and Delivery

PREPARING AND ADAPTING: BABY AND MOM

Nobody ever said that life would be easy or worry-free. But could there be any match for the emotional stress a fetus might feel, lying in the womb the night before beginning its journey through the pelvis? Our in utero friends face a struggle of epic proportion on their way out—the equivalent of a slow train ride through a tunnel that's narrower than the train itself. But fetuses are equipped with several

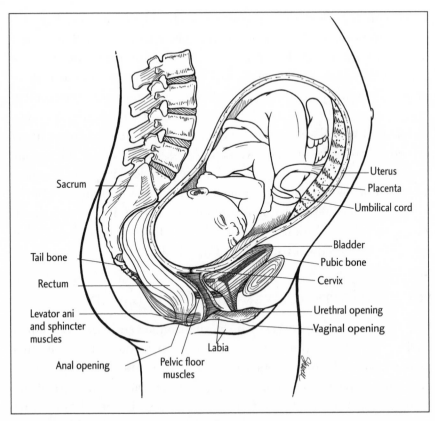

Sacrum

Tail bone

Rectum

Levator ani
and sphincter
muscles

Anal opening

Labia

Pelvic floor
muscles

Uterus

Placenta

Umbilical cord

Bladder

Pubic bone

Cervix

Urethral opening

Vaginal opening

The pelvic organs and pelvic floor during pregnancy

remarkable features that ease their journey, including soft spots between skull bones that actually bend and overlap (*molding*), naturally lubricated skin, and that well-known cone-head shape that narrows the width of the baby's cranium. Like a good Boy Scout or Brownie, a fetus arrives in the labor room prepared.

The changes that occur within Mom's pelvis are equally impressive. Throughout the nine months of pregnancy, the lower half of your body takes a number of steps in an effort to prepare itself for the big task ahead.

First, changes occur to the soft tissues of your pelvis. The vaginal walls become significantly thicker as the stretchy smooth muscle enlarges and the usually firm connective tissue layer softens. While these changes cause the vagina to become longer and thicker, there is also a steady increase in vaginal secretions and natural lubrication, which enables your soft tissues to stretch out of the way. Perhaps more surprising are the changes taking place with your pelvic bones. A special hormone produced by the ovary during pregnancy, appropriately named *relaxin,* appears to cause relaxation and some expansion at the pelvic joints. The *pubic symphysis,* which is the connective tissue connecting the bones right at the front of your pelvis, becomes mobile and wider—these pubic bones can separate (*diastasis*) up to several centimeters in some women! Also, the *sacroiliac* joint, connecting the side bones of your pelvis to your lower spine, becomes more mobile. When your hormone levels return to normal after birth, the pelvic bones return to their original rigid state. But as your body anticipates the evolutionary mismatch of a lifetime, these changes are taking place to reduce your odds of physical harm.

YOUR DUE DATE ARRIVES—ARE YOU ENGAGED?

"Has the head dropped yet?" It's a question asked by many women during their last month or two of pregnancy. But what does this question actually mean? As your due date nears, the baby's head often lowers itself into the bony pelvis. When the widest part of the fetal head secures itself within the pelvic cavity, the fetus has become *engaged,* in obstetrical terms. Some women may suddenly feel they're able to breathe more easily, since they've begun to carry lower. Others notice increased urinary frequency and constipation as the fetal head creates more pressure in the pelvis. Engagement does not always occur before your first labor begins; one recent study conducted by midwives found engagement in only 31 percent of first-time mothers-to-be, though most other estimates have been higher. Nevertheless, when engagement does occur in a first pregnancy, many practitioners consider it a sign that a good fit exists between mother and baby, perhaps reflecting an easier labor and delivery ahead. In subsequent pregnancies, when the pelvic tissues are more lax, an unengaged fetus at the onset of labor is not considered a prognostic sign.

But what if you're past the due date of your first pregnancy and the baby's head is still floating up above the pelvic bones, unengaged? According to some obstetricians, this might represent the first warning that your pelvic shape and your baby's head aren't the world's most ideal fit; there is data to show that you might be at higher risk for a labor that fails to progress to a successful vaginal delivery. One recent Johns Hopkins study of more than twelve hundred women carrying their first pregnancy showed the risk of cesarean section nearly tripled if the baby's head was not engaged when active labor began. Another study found that a floating fetal head conferred a longer second stage of labor (the time from being fully dilated until delivery) and increased the risk of cesarean from 6.9 to 27 percent. Other studies have contradicted these findings, concluding that engagement might not be a very reliable predictor of a successful vaginal birth. Many practitioners disregard the issue of engagement, claiming equal success at achieving vaginal delivery even if the fetal head is floating.

What does all this have to do with your pelvic floor and postreproductive body? It's a matter of what efforts are required to achieve vaginal delivery and how these efforts might impact your body. Delivery of an unengaged fetus might take considerable extra effort and reduce your odds of an easy vaginal birth. But deciding whether this extra time and effort creates more risk of physical injury to you is not usually clear. Engagement is just one measure of maternal-pelvic fit, which has prognostic value only during your first pregnancy and can't flawlessly forecast an easy versus a traumatic delivery. The significance of fetal engagement remains a question that future research will hopefully help to resolve.

LABOR—THE PELVIS UNDER PRESSURE

Finally, labor begins. Obstetricians and midwives divide labor and delivery into a few stages, and acquainting yourself with them can help you to understand how childbirth might affect your body.

Labor's first stage begins when your uterine contractions become painful and frequent, and the cervix begins to dilate—that is, to open. It ends when the cervix is fully dilated at ten centimeters. The first stage of labor requires patience—during your first pregnancy, reaching just four to five centimeters can take up to twenty hours from the time your labor contractions first begin. Most women remain at home during the early part of this stage; after arriving at the maternity unit, some may rest with the help of pain medication, while others walk the hallways or even lie in a warm bath. But however they're laboring, most are focused on one central question: "Am I ten centimeters yet?"

When you do reach ten centimeters—or, more precisely, when the cervix is fully dilated—you've entered the second stage of labor. This stage ends with delivery of your infant. Its duration ranges from around two hours for a first delivery to only twenty minutes for women who have had previous vaginal births.

When the second stage begins, one of the first things you'll notice is more intensive monitoring by the doctors and nurses of both your labor progress and your baby's well-being. The beginning of the second stage is usually when you're instructed to start pushing, the most physically stressful part of labor for both baby and mom. *Fully dilated* might accurately describe the cervix as the second stage begins, but it's not true for the rest of your pelvis. A tremendous amount of dilation throughout the pelvis has yet to occur, and the majority of fetal descent still lies ahead. Along the way, as this dilation and descent take place, stretch and compression affect the vagina, bladder, urethra, muscles, and nerves. When you push, all of these forces are magnified. Pressures generated between the fetal head and vaginal wall can average 100mmHg and reach peaks of 230mmHg. For those of you without an engineering or physics background, rest assured that this a remarkable force in biological terms. A force of only 20 to 80mmHg will stop the flow of blood in most human tissues, and can damage them beyond repair if applied for a prolonged period. As you can imagine, forces up to three times that intensity, within the narrow confines of the pelvis, might change nearby structures.

Aim your telescope at childbirth drama during labor's second stage, and you'll observe a true irony within modern women's health care: a monitored fetus and a sometimes overlooked mom. You'll see most eyes in the modern delivery suite—including those of the health-care team, the mother, and her partner—trained on the squiggly lines of the fetal monitor from the start of the pushing, squatting, and "hut-hut-hooing" to the baby's first cry. All the while, the maternal pelvic changes, which can affect some women for a lifetime, may escape the gaze of all the players on childbirth's stage.

Arguably, the potential effects of labor on the maternal body are among the most neglected topics in women's health. In chapters 4 through 7, you'll learn about the ways you can help yourself—through prenatal preparation, pushing techniques, avoidance of risky procedures, and so on—making it less an event of chance and more a process of choice.

MAKE YOURSELF A REAL MAGICIAN

Childbirth is a magical experience for women and their partners. Unfortunately, doctors and midwives are *not* magicians! Guiding a baby through your pelvis is far trickier than pulling a rabbit out of a hat, and the problems that you can be left with are not entertaining. Once you understand your postreproductive body, you're on track to improving your heath, relieving your symptoms, and possibly even preventing future ones. Knowledge works like real magic, and the upcoming chapters will provide you with countless tricks of the trade.

NEW PERSPECTIVES ON YOUR POSTREPRODUCTIVE BODY

You've become aware of the pelvic floor, an important area of your body that you may not have known before. You've learned that it looks a certain way before childbirth and another way afterward. With this new "pelvic perspective" in mind, let's examine how various obstetrical events and procedures can affect your function afterward, and what to do when things go awry.

☙ 3 ❧

The Pelvic Floor After *Childbirth*

INJURIES AND ANATOMIC CHANGES
AND THE OBSTETRICAL EVENTS THAT CAN CAUSE THEM

Between the oceans of pain, there stretched continents of fear; fear of death and dread of suffering beyond bearing.

—Woman, 1885, on childbirth

Can I get my epidural, please?

—Woman, circa 1995, on childbirth

Whether childbirth is easy or difficult, long or short, natural or operative, one fact remains constant: *a woman's body will never be exactly the same after pregnancy, labor, and delivery, as it was beforehand.* The good news? For the vast majority of women, these physical changes are subtle and inconsequential, visible to the doctor during a pelvic exam but creating no problems for the woman herself. The other side of the story? If you've reached for this book, it's likely that you *have* noticed some sort of change, and you're looking for relief. As the next step, now that you're familiar with your pelvic area, it's time to learn about the most common and significant changes that can arise.

Perineal Injuries and Episiotomies

Dr. David Chapin, an esteemed vaginal surgeon at Harvard Medical School, has been known to occasionally quip to the resident physicians he's instructing: "The obstetrician-gynecologist spends the first half of

36

his career *supporting* the perineum, and the second half of his career *being supported by* the perineum." Dr. Chapin makes this point with a lighthearted touch, but it has stuck in my mind and always rings true. The same women who keep young obstetricians busy in the labor suite tend to keep them busy again in the operating room years later, reconstructing those pelvic supports that were lost during childbirth. For countless women, the specialty called obstetrics and gynecology could be more accurately dubbed obstetrics, *therefore* gynecology.

YOUR PERINEUM DURING AND AFTER CHILDBIRTH

During childbirth, as the fetal head or shoulders are delivered, the perineum can tear spontaneously or be cut intentionally with an episiotomy. Perineal tears can be partial, extending only through the vaginal skin; or they can be complete, extending all the way through the perineal muscles and even into the rectum. If the perineum is torn during childbirth and not adequately repaired, any or all of the perineal muscles (including the bulbocavernosus and transverse perineal) can become permanently separated, creating a gaping appearance to the vaginal opening.

When childbirth widens the perineum, you may later begin to notice a bulging sensation near the vagina and rectum, or a loss of sensation or vaginal fullness during intercourse. When the anal area is involved, it can lead to incontinence of both gas and stool. If, on the other hand, the perineum becomes too tight or scarred, intercourse may be painful. Even with a proper repair, the perineal muscles and tissues may not properly heal. In chapter 7, you'll learn more about alleviating the problems that can accompany healing of your perineum. You'll also learn how to help prevent these injuries from occurring in the first place.

DID YOU KNOW . . . ?

Even in the absence of an episiotomy, between 35 and 75 percent of women suffer some degree of perineal injury while giving birth. For those who have a perineal injury during their first delivery, the risk of a spontaneous perineal tear during the next delivery is more than tripled.

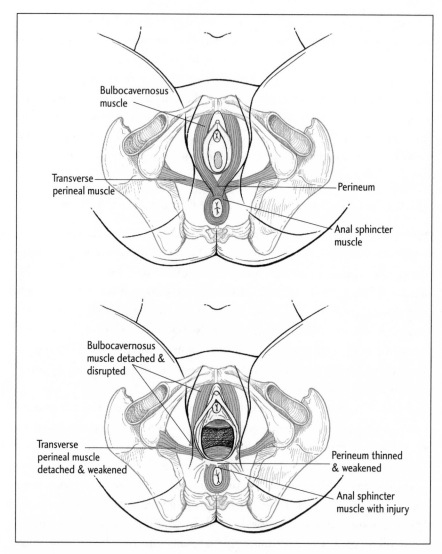

(Above) Perineal anatomy before delivery. (Below) Common changes after childbirth, affecting the perineum and nearby structures

EPISIOTOMY: THE "LITTLE CUT"

For some women, the decision over episiotomy—to cut or not to cut—symbolizes whether her delivery is smooth or traumatic, natural or medicalized, and whether she considers herself injured or intact afterward. The procedure is performed with a snip of the perineum, that bridge of tissue between the vaginal and anal openings. By creating more space at the vaginal opening, episiotomies hasten delivery of the newborn. Did you know that aside from cutting the umbilical cord, episiotomies are the most common obstetrical operations (1.2 million per year) performed in our country and also across the world?

First utilized in Europe, episiotomies were imported to the United States and brought into widespread use during the early 1900s. For decades thereafter, many doctors performed them routinely, claiming they resulted in a wide variety of benefits: speeding labor, protecting pelvic muscle tone, preserving sexual function, aiding maternal healing, sparing compression of the fetal head, and reducing the risk of anal sphincter injury. To this day, some practitioners argue that it's better to cut and neatly repair the perineum and vagina than to allow these tissues to spontaneously stretch and lose their virginal tone altogether.

But among the majority of physicians, there has been close to a 180-degree reversal in these beliefs. The strategy of routine episiotomy simply has not withstood the scrutiny of modern research, and it is no longer mainstream. At least five studies have shown that episiotomies seem *not* to protect against the development of urinary incontinence. In fact, there is plenty of evidence to suggest that episiotomies increase the overall risk of harm to your pelvic function.

INJURIES FROM EPISIOTOMIES: ANAL SPHINCTER, PELVIC MUSCLES, HEALING, AND PAIN

It's unfortunate but perhaps not all that surprising how few high-quality research studies have been performed to understand the physical effects of episiotomy. After all, this procedure involves a highly intimate area of the female body charged with a rich supply of nerve endings, making it a complex area to study and master. Beyond that, episiotomies have always been highly politicized—representing, for many women, a symbol of invasive delivery, and making physicians and patients equally reluctant to test different strategies at the time of birth. Despite the fact that our understanding of this procedure has evolved at a shamefully slow pace, a fairly clear picture has begun to emerge. It's perhaps best summarized by the Cochrane Group, a team of analysts that draws scientific conclusions based on the best research for a given topic. Their report concluded that routine episiotomy *increases* the overall risk of trauma and complications during vaginal delivery, and therefore should be used selectively. But what are the specific benefits of avoiding episiotomy that led to this overarching conclusion?

- *To improve healing and preserve muscle strength.* One study from several years ago involved more than two thousand Argentinean women who were randomly assigned to receive either routine episiotomy or selective episiotomy based on need—in other words, performed only if their obstetrician felt that a significant perineal injury was about to occur. Overall, pain and healing complications were found to be more common among women who received routine episiotomy. Other studies indicate that over the long term, women who undergo episiotomy tend to be left with weaker vaginal muscle strength than those with an intact perineum after delivery, or those who tear spontaneously. Eventually, this weakening of vaginal muscle might tip the balance of continence or pelvic support for a good number of women.

- *To spare lacerations.* During first deliveries, episiotomies in general appear to increase the risk of a torn anal sphincter. Midline episiotomy (a straight-down incision from the opening of the vagina toward the anus) in particular has been associated with up to twenty times the usual risk of lacerations involving the rectum; one large Canadian study found that nearly all tears extending into the anal sphincter muscle followed an episiotomy. With second, third, or later deliveries, the overwhelming majority of severe perineal injuries originate with episiotomies. In Sweden, a decline in episiotomy rate from 28 to 10 percent was associated with a slightly decreased rate of anal sphincter injury.

These obstetrical injuries to the anal sphincter increase the risk of anal incontinence during a woman's postreproductive years. It's been reported that just over 40 percent of women with anal sphincter disruption during childbirth will have temporary anal incontinence after delivery, and that 7 percent will experience permanent loss of anal control to some degree.

- *To safeguard sexual function.* What about the bedroom? While the long-term impact of episiotomy on sexual function is unknown, a 1994 study found sexual satisfaction at three months postpartum to be greatest among women without perineal injury. Satisfaction was lowest among women with an episiotomy that had extended, or torn further, during delivery.

TWO TYPES OF EPISIOTOMY: WHICH ONE IS BEST?

There are two basic types of episiotomies.

- A *median* episiotomy is cut right down the center of the perineum, between the vagina and the rectum.
- A *mediolateral* episiotomy is angled off to the side, into either the right or the left labial area.

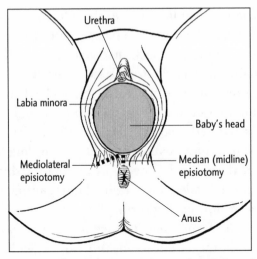

Two types of episiotomy—median and mediolateral

Which type of episiotomy is preferable if you have to choose? Median episiotomies have been associated with less postpartum and sexual pain, less blood loss, and a lower risk of infection. However, because it's positioned right down the middle, the median approach confers a very substantial risk of tearing into the anal opening or rectum, somewhere between 11 and 12 percent. Mediolateral episiotomies are associated with more postpartum and sexual pain and possibly more muscle weakness, but they generally decrease the risk of anal or rectal injury to around 1 to 2 percent.

There are pros and cons to both types, and there is no obvious right choice that applies to all women. For women with a short perineum—meaning the distance between vagina and rectum is very small—a mediolateral might best help to avoid extension of the episiotomy into the anal sphincter. With a long perineum, a median episiotomy might help to avoid tearing into the labia. Median episiotomies are more popular in North America, whereas mediolateral episiotomies have remained more popular in Europe, and doctors from both sides of the ocean have long debated which method is less traumatic. Unfortunately, despite the fact that these procedures involve their most intimate parts, women have rarely been invited to join the debate.

"Wait a second," I can hear you asking, "aren't episiotomies, and all of these associated injuries, repaired before leaving the labor room?" Isn't everything put back into place after delivery, allowing you to eventually heal back to full strength? Though you might assume so, the data argues otherwise. First of all, it's been found using ultrasound that even after repair of a torn anal sphincter right after delivery, separated anal muscles are still seen in up to 40 percent of these women postpartum. Secondly, according to a survey of obstetricians in the United Kingdom, less than a third of doctors reported that they felt adequately trained in repairing anal sphincter injuries that occur during childbirth.

As the problem of anal incontinence has begun to earn its long-overdue place on the women's health-care agenda, debate has increased regarding the best techniques for repairing perineal and anal injuries in the delivery room. Some expert surgeons specializing in obstetrical anal sphincter injury have recently begun to advocate a more meticulous surgical approach in the labor room, using overlapping repair techniques that attach the torn muscles more strongly. In the short term, this method has been reported to lower the risk of anal incontinence, but overlapping sphincter repair is not yet included in most general obstetrical training; nor has it been proven to be the best technique over the long run. As the problem of anal incontinence continues to be addressed, you'll undoubtedly see greater efforts being made to prevent and repair these injuries in the delivery room, whether with the overlapping repair or other innovations. For now, reducing the number of unnecessary episiotomies in our obstetrical world would probably do the most good.

When an episiotomy is avoidable, *avoid it!*

WHEN SHOULD YOU HAVE AN EPISIOTOMY?

Physicians trained in recent years tend to favor a relatively hands-off approach when it comes to episiotomies, compared to their predecessors, who tended to intervene with less hesitation. But even today, there are a handful of absolutely, positively justified reasons for your doctor or midwife to cut an episiotomy. For instance:

- In cases of fetal distress or an abnormal fetal heart rate close to delivery, a well-timed episiotomy can shorten the time to delivery by critical minutes.

- If the baby becomes stuck during delivery—particularly if the shoulders are wedged behind the pubic bone (*shoulder dystocia*)—an immediate episiotomy is warranted to help prevent asphyxiation of the newborn.

- Sometimes an obstetrician will notice a particularly severe injury occurring in some place other than the perineum—for example, the labia, urethra, or clitoral area—and perform an episiotomy to relieve pressure and spare extensive injury that can be both painful and difficult to repair.

- Clinicians would routinely include an episiotomy with each forceps or vacuum (a soft suction device used to gently pull the fetal head toward the vaginal opening) delivery, creating more room for inserting these devices. However, most physicians have abandoned the routine use of episiotomy even during these operative deliveries, using them on a more selective basis.

If you have an episiotomy, the overwhelming odds predict that you'll do absolutely fine. But if your doctor or midwife recommends *planning* an episiotomy with the intent of protecting your body from injury, then it's time to ask some questions and perhaps explore your provider's style. According to some specialists in obstetrical injury, the most appropriate episiotomy rate should be no higher than around 20 to 30 percent for uncomplicated pregnancies. Recent trends are encouraging in this regard; one review of more than thirty-four thousand vaginal deliveries found a decline in episiotomy rate from 69.6 percent of all vaginal births in 1983 to 19.4 percent in 2000. Episiotomies will always have an important place in the labor room, but today's research says there's little basis for routinely cutting one in order to preserve your pelvic floor.

EPISIOTOMY: JUST THE TIP OF THE ICEBERG OF PELVIC CHANGE

In the end, episiotomies probably carry as much symbolic and emotional weight as actual medical importance. Injury to the perineum is just the tip of the iceberg of pelvic injury that can result from childbirth—the surface damage that, however significant, is often small compared with the more extensive, deeper changes that occur at its base. Before reaching the perineum, the fetus has traversed the foundation of your pelvic supports and a number of structures that will determine your postreproductive function and control. Sometimes the most important damage has already been inflicted, completely unseen.

It's time for you, the central person in the labor room, to familiarize yourself with the parts of your body hidden beneath the iceberg's tip. Let's continue unfolding the anatomy of labor and take a look at the unseen structures that are essential to your health, independence, and intimacy beyond the labor room. A little knowledge can empower you to prevent future problems and alleviate those you might already have.

Muscle and Nerve Injury: Changes to the Iceberg's Base

THE LEVATOR MUSCLES AFTER CHILDBIRTH

If you developed prolapse or incontinence any time during your postreproductive years—even decades later—it's likely that the seeds of your problem were silently planted when the levator muscles (remember, the foundation of your pelvic-floor supports) stretched, separated, or weakened at the time of vaginal delivery. Injury to the levator muscles and their accompanying nerves may be one of the most problematic changes that can occur to your lower body during childbirth.

Levator changes after childbirth may take a few different forms. The levator muscle shelf may start to drop, leaving the pelvic organs supported only by the much weaker connective tissues, which often begin to stretch beneath the burden. With levator injury, the iceberg of pelvic support weakens at its base, and the chain of events leading to prolapse and other pelvic-floor problems begins.

If the sling portions of the levator muscles encircling the urethral and anal areas are torn during delivery, the sphincters may fail to instantly tighten during a cough or sneeze. This may spell incontinence over time.

You can improve the strength and function of your levator muscles using exercises and a variety of pelvic-floor treatments. Even if you don't rebuild the full strength of your pelvic-floor foundation, you can often make enough progress to restore your control and relieve your postreproductive symptoms. In Appendix A, you'll learn the best techniques for rehabilitating your pelvic floor.

The *levator ani* muscles are the elevator for the pelvis, keeping the female pelvic organs lifted and preventing prolapse and incontinence. Improving these muscles' strength and function is a major strategy for treating a number of postreproductive problems.

The Importance of Nerve Injury During Childbirth

Time for the million-dollar question: can you name the type of nerve injury you're most likely to experience during your lifetime? Here's a quick clue—it's not a pinched nerve in your neck, and it's not carpal tunnel syndrome in the wrist. No, it's injury to the pelvic nerves during pregnancy and childbirth, which may represent the most likely instance of nerve damage during a woman's lifetime; it's seen in up to

15 percent of women after delivery. Though many women will never feel any symptoms, others will experience incontinence, prolapse, or other pelvic-floor disorders later on.

But why all the fuss over nerve injury if we just learned that changes to the *muscles* are the cause of prolapse and incontinence? The reason is that injuries to nerves and muscle are closely related. Have you ever crossed your legs for too long to find your foot has fallen asleep? Or have you watched a movie with your spouse lying across your arm, then stood to find that the muscles in your arm felt completely dead for a minute or two? In both cases, you've compressed a major nerve where it was exposed and vulnerable to external pressure—behind the knee and inside the upper arm. What you've felt temporarily are the effects of this nerve compression on neighboring muscles. Fortunately, in both of these cases, the nerve compression was mild and brief, so its effect on the nearby muscles lasted only a short time.

When a nerve is injured for longer periods of time, however, the muscle groups at its end begin a more permanent process of weakening, or *atrophy*. Examples of muscle atrophy following nerve injury can be found all over the body—for instance, in the facial droop of a stroke patient or in the thinned legs of a paraplegic. In these cases, damage to a nerve supply acts like snipping the roots of a plant: the nearby muscles, like flowers, begin to wilt.

THE PELVIC NERVES, FROM A BRAND-NEW, FEMALE POINT OF VIEW

Surprised that you've never heard about nerve injury as an important feature of childbirth? You should be. After all, urologists counsel their male patients at length regarding the risks of nerve injury and erectile dysfunction accompanying prostate surgery. Shouldn't women understand, in a basic way, how certain choices surrounding childbirth might influence the long-term health of their pelvic nerves? Although childbirth is a natural life-cycle event, not a disease, you're no less entitled to be informed of the effects of obstetrical procedures.

PUDENDAL NERVE INJURY AND LEVATOR ATROPHY

As previously mentioned, you'll find your most important pelvic nerves—the pudendals—on either side of your pelvis's inside walls. Stretching and compression of the pudendal can occur as the fetus passes through the pelvis. But how and when? The nerves may be most exposed and vulnerable to injury where they pass a prominent protuberance of bone called the *ischial spine*, located on either side of your inner pelvis. There, the pudendal can be directly compressed by anything trying to squeeze its way through. Imagine those remarkable forces generated between the fetal head and maternal pelvis during maternal pushing, applied right onto a nerve that's roughly the size and strength of a spaghetti noodle cooked al dente. Then imagine the same nerve getting caught between the metal edge of a forceps blade and the solid bone of the pelvic wall.

Nearly 20 percent of normal vaginal deliveries are associated with pudendal injury afterward, and a significant number persist over the long term; forceps deliveries increase your risk of pelvic nerve injury by 40 to 60 percent. Long labors, large babies, and multiple deliveries have also been linked to diminished nerve function. Remarkably, two separate studies showed that cesarean delivery—when performed before labor begins—tends to preserve normal nerve function.

What are the consequences of pudendal nerve injury? Injury to the pudendal nerve might be the common-denominator obstetrical event leading to some of the more typical postreproductive problems after vaginal childbirth. Compression and stretching of this key nerve begin the process of muscle weakness, leading to wilting of the shelf and sling levator supports. If pelvic-nerve injury occurs—even if you have no symptoms right after childbirth—you still may be at significant risk for developing prolapse, urinary and anal incontinence, and other pelvic symptoms over time.

Now you can see why labor and delivery might be the most likely cause of nerve damage in women, and how nerve injury in the pelvis is a crucial and often overlooked aspect of your postreproductive health and control. Whether it's the pudendal nerve or other nearby pelvic nerves that are most vital for your future function remains an ongoing scientific question. Regardless, the rather unsettling reality

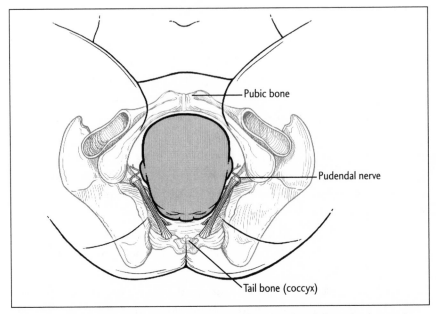

Compression of the pudendal nerve between the fetal head and the pelvic bones during labor

remains the same: many pelvic nerve and muscle injuries occur relatively early in labor, long before the events commanding most of our attention, episiotomies and perineal injuries.

Connective-Tissue Injuries

After childbirth virtually every woman has some degree of injury to her pelvic connective tissues—that fibrous support layer surrounding the pelvic organs and helping attach them to the bony pelvis. Why is that? First of all, their location leaves them vulnerable to injury during childbirth. The pelvic connective tissues are a major component of the vagina, enveloping its walls and attaching the vaginal tube to the pelvic sidewalls. As a result, when the vagina stretches, the connective tissues are placed under tremendous strain. Second, the pelvic connective tissues are prone to permanent injury, rather than temporary strain, because they are not very elastic. They're less able than muscle to stretch and then return to their original shape, so they do poorly with the physical stress of childbirth and afterward, when the physical strain of daily activity and exertion creates further wear and tear.

What is the significance of connective-tissue injury? As mentioned in chapter 2, the connective tissues do not provide the main foundation for the pelvic organs, but they do play an important secondary role. Particularly for women whose levator muscles (the nails and screws of pelvic support) weaken after childbirth, the connective tissues (the carpenter's glue of the pelvis) help to maintain the positions of the bladder, bowel, and vagina. If these connective-tissue supports of the pelvis also give way, there's nothing left to prevent pelvic prolapse and incontinence in their various forms.

Weakening of the connective tissues:

- Between the bladder and vagina causes a cystocele.
- Between the rectum and vagina causes a rectocele.
- Between the uterus and pelvis causes uterine prolapse.
- At the top of vagina causes an enterocele.
- Around the urethra can lead to urinary stress incontinence.

Your Bladder During Pregnancy

A landmark 1960 study showed that while around 18 percent of women experienced some incontinence before pregnancy, over 50 percent had complaints by their third trimester. Since then, other studies have confirmed that incontinence symptoms reach a peak around thirty-eight weeks. So even if you've never leaked, or have never given birth, pregnancy alone can be enough to cause urinary stress incontinence. If you've had some stress incontinence before pregnancy, the odds are that your symptoms will get worse during those nine months. But why?

First, the uterus is located right next to the bladder and urethra. As your baby grows and the uterus expands during pregnancy, pressure on these nearby structures slowly but surely increases. The most obvious symptom resulting from this pelvic space crunch is the frequent need to urinate, as your bladder, with limited room to expand, begins to feel full with less and less fluid inside. Eventually, as the fetal head drops into the pelvis, your bladder's capacity becomes just a fraction of what it was before pregnancy. That's one reason, along with an overall increase in urine produced, why most women are constantly running to the women's room during those last few months before delivery.

But beyond this inconvenience, could permanent problems result from this constant pressure on the urethra, bladder, and nearby vaginal supports? For some of you, the answer is yes. Through stretching and injury to the nearby muscles, connective tissues, and pelvic nerves the prolonged force of a pregnant uterus can cause a number of lasting changes to bladder function, including the floppy urethra and the thin-walled urethra.

Second, hormones can have a major effect on the way your bladder behaves during pregnancy and beyond. Progesterone is a hormone of pregnancy that acts like a muscle relaxant in various locations all over your body. That's why so many women become constipated even early in pregnancy, as high progesterone levels slow down the bowel muscles. On the plus side, it's one reason why the uterus (another smooth-muscle organ) is able to relax and stretch from the size of a pear to the size of a watermelon over the course of nine months. Because smooth muscle also happens to be a major ingredient of the bladder, urethra, and vaginal wall, high levels of progesterone during pregnancy can cause the supports of these areas to relax and stretch along with the uterus. Sometimes this relaxation is enough to tip your tenuous balance of continence, allowing leakage to occur when you cough, sneeze, or bend over to lift a can of pink or powder-blue paint while decorating the baby's room.

So even before delivery, several pelvic-floor changes may have already occurred—enough, in many cases, to cause stress incontinence. One survey of more than fifteen hundred women experiencing stress incontinence after childbearing found that nearly 63 percent said their incontinence began during pregnancy. Other data indicates that up to 80 percent of such women will recall that their leakage began before delivery. These physical changes help to explain why even women delivering by cesarean at full term may be left with stress incontinence up to 9 percent of the time. Later on, you'll learn a handful of tips to help minimize the effects of pelvic-floor injury during pregnancy—just as important to your prenatal routine as vitamins, hospital tours, and Lamaze.

Your Bladder During Labor and Delivery

There's a great deal of scientific interest these days in the effects of labor and delivery on your pelvic area, including your bladder—and for good reason. A fetus compressing against your pelvis, then stretching its way through and past almost all of your pelvic muscles, nerves, ligaments, and supports can cause a number of physical problems, with stress incontinence at the top of the list. Strong as the odds for pelvic injury during vaginal delivery may be, you'd be surprised how rarely the risk of pelvic damage is factored into obstetrical decision making, and how infrequently it's discussed with the person it actually involves: you. It's time to become your own expert on your body during childbirth.

WILL INCONTINENCE GET WORSE
IF I HAVE ANOTHER BABY?

Several studies have suggested that your first pregnancy and delivery will have a greater impact on your risk of urinary incontinence than any that follow—as if the first baby clears the way for later siblings, slowly dilating and stretching the pelvic tissues. Based on these results, even if you started to leak after your first delivery, it probably wouldn't make sense to request a cesarean for later ones in hopes of preventing the problem from worsening. But some researchers have concluded differently. One study of more than seven thousand Irish women indicated that the risk of incontinence does indeed seem to increase with each delivery; other investigators have estimated this additional risk to be as high as 10 percent per vaginal birth. Until more conclusive research is done, we don't know the safest and most reasonable way to prevent incremental injury from one childbirth to the next.

Big Babies and Multiple Pregnancy: Effects on Your Body

MACROSOMIA: PHYSICAL EFFECTS OF A BIG BABY

It's been long recognized that very large fetuses (called *macrosomia*) face their own increased risks in the labor room, including birth trauma, shoulder dystocia (when the baby's shoulders become stuck after delivery of the head), and even low fetal Apgar scores, used for rating each newborn's level of alertness and activity. But delivering a very large baby can also present risks to your body. Macrosomia is associated with a higher occurrence of spontaneous perineal injury and episiotomies, nearly two and a half times the usual risk of rectal injury during childbirth, and a higher risk of pudendal nerve injury after childbirth. A Danish study of eight thousand women showed that delivery of a newborn weighing over 8.8 pounds resulted in twice the usual risk of urinary incontinence later on, and a slightly higher chance of later surgery to correct the problem. A study from Boston showed macrosomia to be associated with a 60 percent increase in the risk of episiotomy. Another study discovered that a larger newborn head circumference is an independent risk factor for perineal injury during childbirth, raising hope that in the future, more accurate ultrasound measurements of a baby's size might allow us to predict each woman's risk for perineal injuries. More studies are needed, however, to fully understand the postreproductive experience of mothers delivering large newborns.

TOUGH ON THE BODY, ALL OVER THE WORLD

For women carrying a large baby, looking ahead to vaginal delivery can be a nerve-wracking process. What's the right birthing plan for both baby and you? Following a handful of tips for pregnancy and labor—such as pelvic-floor exercises and perineal massage—might help. In Part 2, you'll learn the ways to begin.

TWINS, TRIPLETS, AND HIGHER-ORDER PREGNANCIES:
WHAT ARE THE PHYSICAL EFFECTS?

Multiple pregnancy and delivery are major features of today's obstetrical landscape, due in large part to assisted reproductive techniques used for the treatment of infertility, which often result in multiple births. The number of twin deliveries has doubled over the last ten years alone. The first study of postreproductive pelvic-floor problems among mothers of multiples recently found that among 733 mothers of multiples—their average age at the time of the study only thirty-seven—rates of pelvic-floor symptoms appear to be remarkably high.

- *Urinary stress incontinence.* Forty-five percent of these women reported accidental leakage of urine with coughing, sneezing, lifting, or straining. Remarkably, women who delivered by cesarean had a 50 percent reduction in their risk of urinary stress incontinence.
- *Overactive bladder symptoms.* Urge incontinence was reported by 27 percent of the group.
- *Anal incontinence.* An inability to hold back gas in public was reported by 25 percent, some degree of fecal incontinence (loss of stool) by 10 percent, and fecal soiling by 10 percent.
- *Other pelvic-floor symptoms.* A number of other symptoms relating to the pelvic floor were also present, including painful intercourse (20 percent) and vaginal bulging or pressure (21 percent).
- *Quality of life.* The presence of pelvic-floor symptoms was strongly associated with diminished quality of life among these women.

These high rates of pelvic-floor symptoms among women with previous multiple childbirths need to be better understood. Is it multiple pregnancy and birth placing these women at risk, or simply their greater number of children? What aspect of multiple gestation is most high-risk when it comes to Mom's body—carrying the weight of the pregnancy or childbirth itself? Are mothers of multiples at this level of risk simply because they're more likely to undergo certain obstetrical procedures? Is there a best way to deliver twins, triplets, or higher? Finding better ways to prevent these postreproductive problems will benefit an ever-increasing number of women. After all, raising multiples is quite enough for these supermoms to worry about, without the pelvic-floor problems to contend with.

TURNING CHANCES INTO CHOICES: NEW PERSPECTIVES ON LABOR AND DELIVERY

Many aspects of childbirth can impact your postreproductive health. Despite the tendency to feel that your role is merely to react by reflex and accept the inevitabilities of the birthing process as they unfold, many events and outcomes are *not* inevitable. A number of decisions are being made, and if you're not helping to make them, they're being made for you. If you're concerned with avoiding the postreproductive problems you might have seen your mother deal with, what are the right questions to ask?

- When it comes to pushing, how long is too long?
- Is resting rather than pushing (passive laboring) less or more of a strain on your body?
- What's the best position for your body—lying faceup or facedown, sitting, or squatting?
- Can perineal massage during labor reduce your risk of second-stage trauma?
- What risks are posed by forceps or vacuum delivery?
- How about big babies or even twins?

There is a great deal not yet understood about the physical effects of pregnancy, childbirth, and their various stages. Familiarizing yourself with a handful of preventive tips, based on what *is* known today, might help you to prevent problems later on. In the next chapter, you'll learn how to start turning chance into choice.

"But I Never Had a Baby!"

Pelvic-floor problems, including incontinence and prolapse, can occur even if you've never had a baby. Any urogynecologist can attest to this reality and recall plenty of patients with a loss of bladder control or prolapse bulging, despite never having given birth. One recent survey of nuns, interestingly, showed that up to 47 percent of them reported some degree of incontinence, with 29 percent reporting stress incontinence at an average age of sixty-eight. And in the Women's Health Initiative—a large study of hormone use in postmenopausal women (see chapter 12)—although previous childbirth was strongly associated with increased rates of pelvic prolapse later on, 19 percent of women with no previous delivery also had prolapse.

How could this be?

- Weakening of the pelvic floor can, in some cases, result from chronic physical straining unrelated to pregnancy and childbirth: in the form of routine physical exertion and exercise, a long-standing cough, or chronic constipation. Even the wear and tear of normal daily activities can be enough to cause symptomatic weakening of the pelvic supports.

- As the strength of pelvic tissues decreases after menopause, due to a decline in estrogen supply, the effects are more likely to become apparent in the form of pelvic-floor symptoms.

- Other women may be predisposed to a loss of pelvic support due to an innate weakness of their connective tissues—in other words, one that was present at birth. Over time, this generalized weakness may lead to problems in the pelvic area. Connective-tissue disorders run in families but are fortunately very rare.

As you learn about these postreproductive problems, remember that although they often stem from pregnancy and childbirth, this is not always the case.

From Problems and Evolution to Cures and Solutions

For humans, as with all other species, reproduction always has and will forever be our biological purpose in life. But along the evolutionary road, childbirth became more and more of a stress test for each mother's body—painful and often life-threatening in the short term, sometimes debilitating in the long run. Modern medicine met the challenge of the short-term problems during the twentieth century: today you can take for granted that childbirth is rarely life-threatening, and its pain can be quite easily managed. But only in the past few years have the long-term physical repercussions to your body been raised for discussion. Preventing incontinence, prolapse, sexual and other pelvic dysfunction remains a challenge for the twenty-first century to confront.

Let's start today.

PART 2

PREVENTIVE OBSTETRICS

A NEW OUTLOOK ON PREGNANCY AND CHILDBIRTH TO PROTECT THE PELVIC FLOOR AND AVOID PROBLEMS BEFORE THEY ARISE

🐟 4 🐟

Preparing for Your Due Date

WHAT YOU CAN DO DURING PREGNANCY
TO MINIMIZE PELVIC STRAIN

Forethought spares afterthought.

—Amelia E. Barr

When it comes to the future, there are three kinds of people: those who let it happen, those who make it happen, and those who wonder what happened.

—John M. Richardson, Jr.

We all hope to chart a more healthful course through middle age than did generations past. We want to wrinkle less, exercise more, stay hipper longer, and somehow preserve our full physical functioning in ways that our parents and grandparents weren't always able to do. Despite the reality that many age-related transitions still remain inevitable, there is a great deal we are able to prevent in this modern age of tummy tucks, lid lifts, estrogen replacement, and Viagra. Prevention has evolved from the realm of late-night-TV public-service announcements to a core crusade in mainstream society and medical practice. Dermatologists these days stress the importance of avoiding sun exposure; after all, avoiding sunburns will easily outperform the latest antiwrinkle cream or even Botox. Primary-care doctors watch your blood pressure and preach smoking cessation, since preventing hypertension will leave you healthier than treating hypertensive strokes after they've occurred; and quitting smoking is far more successful than cutting out a cancerous tumor from the lung.

Seat belts, sunscreen, blood-pressure monitoring, and the multi-billion-dollar industry of vitamins and herbal remedies all reflect our expectation for an increasingly long and full postreproductive life, and our willingness to plan ahead and ensure it. Today's medical mind-set goes beyond reversing disease processes that are already in motion. It strives to keep us out of harm's way in the first place.

Women's health continues to undergo its own major transformation toward prevention, and as a result, today's forty-and-up women are healthier overall than their mothers were at the same age. Deaths from heart disease have declined by more than 50 percent since the 1970s, in part because these women are more likely to exercise and less likely to smoke and drink. As menopause approaches, women are inundated with information and recommendations centering on hormone-replacement therapy and its substitutes; and though the absolute right hormonal strategy remains unknown, at least there's a sophisticated debate taking place.

At the time of childbirth, it's easy to take for granted the many forms of obstetrical prevention that steer a fetus from harm. Early ultrasounds can detect physical abnormalities, amniocentesis can raise a red flag for genetic problems, and a daily folic-acid tablet from the start of pregnancy can prevent birth defects. But what's happening from the maternal standpoint?

Numerous conditions that devastated the lives of countless women only a few generations ago are now fully preventable, and maternal and fetal death are, thankfully, a rarity. Consider the obstetrical fistula—an abnormal connection or hole that forms between either the bladder and vagina or the bowel and vagina, leading to constant urinary or anal incontinence. This postreproductive disorder once left substantial numbers of women socially isolated for the remainder of their lives after vaginal delivery. By learning that fistulas were a direct consequence of prolonged and obstructed labor, we learned prevention, and today the problem is virtually nonexistent in the developed world. But what about prevention of the other physical risks of childbirth today, and the life-changing conditions that can sometimes follow years or several decades later?

❧

Sunscreen for the Pelvis

A popular pregnancy guide compares the loss of pelvic function after vaginal childbirth to getting a sunburn while on vacation in the Hawaiian tropics. The book's gist: just as you wouldn't skip the opportunity for a spectacular vacation because you feared a sunburn, you should accept the physical changes that follow childbirth as part of an unforgettable delivery. In one respect, the "sunburn in Hawaii" analogy was right on target: given the information most women are provided with today, they will gladly accept the entire package of childbirth and take their chances with the "sunburn" of pelvic injury. But the comparison fails to consider one major item that you'd find packed in any suitcase headed for the tropics: *sunscreen.* Whether boarding a flight to Hawaii or looking ahead to a first pregnancy, every woman deserves the best available prevention, if not a full shield from the strongest rays, then at least a partial block. After all, changes to the pelvic floor are a natural consequence of labor, like skin cancer is a natural consequence of sun exposure. Both are real, both can greatly affect quality of life, and both, in many cases, are preventable.

Unfortunately, obstetricians haven't discovered an ideal sunscreen for the pelvis. Thus far, many more dollars have been devoted to diapers and pads than to prevention. But this will change—not through luck but through science. At this moment, the National Institutes of Health is devoting millions to the study of postreproductive pelvic-floor disorders, and women in the future will undoubtedly reap the fruits of these investments. In the same way that few dermatologists would neglect to mention the dangers of sun exposure today, it will be routine for tomorrow's obstetrician to outline each woman's best strategy for protecting her pelvic floor during pregnancy and childbirth.

How can you practice preventive obstetrics in the meantime? Some basic tips may help, before, during, and after pregnancy. For a generation of women increasingly determined to prevent disease, and to maintain vigor rather than quietly accept the physical marks of aging, the notion of preventive obstetrical care is long overdue.

The Early Stages of Pregnancy

SELECTING THE RIGHT PROVIDER FOR YOU: DOCTOR OR MIDWIFE?

Obstetrics is partly art and partly science and can be practiced in many different ways. When you choose an obstetrician or midwife, discuss his or her philosophy regarding episiotomy, pushing styles, forceps, and cesarean. If you're already dealing with postreproductive symptoms from a prior pregnancy, discuss what might be the best strategy to prevent them from getting worse. The beginning of labor is *not* a good time to discover that your provider has a 90 percent episiotomy rate or recommends the use of forceps for most normal deliveries. It'll be difficult, not to mention untimely, to voice your concern between the contractions!

The best time to start practicing prevention is during your first pregnancy. As we've discussed, evidence suggests that the first pregnancy and delivery has the most potential for damage and is the one during which you can probably do the most good. So think prevention right from the start, because you may never have as good an opportunity again.

If your first pregnancy is behind you, don't be discouraged. Several pelvic-floor problems have the potential to worsen from baby to baby, and you should be aware of all you can do to minimize this risk.

Finally, remember that professional stereotypes are most often based on at least a kernel of truth but go only so far. The stereotypical doctor, for instance, is committed to the goal of preventing catastrophe, even at the expense of more monitoring and medical intervention than necessary. The quintessential midwife stands by, encouraging her own style of nonintervention while pushing hard to achieve vaginal birth, even if it entails a prolonged struggle for all involved.

Across the decades of modern childbirth, individuals on either side of this timeless rivalry have not hesitated to portray an epic struggle of us versus them, nature versus technology, for the sake of their own particular views. William Tyler Smith, president of the Obstetrical Society of London, pleaded in the late 1800s for the science of obstetrics to be distinguished from the art of midwifery—reflecting a mutual intolerance between the two camps during a time when their differences were stark. Midwives waited too willingly through long, protracted labors, which too often ended badly for Mom; and obstetricians, eager to expedite the process, reached for the forceps far too often. But these days, the differences between skilled and upstanding providers on each side are far more subtle. You're fortunate to live in an era when most doctors and midwives have learned from each other and have learned to get along. Some of the finest obstetricians take pride in standing by, intervening with forceps, cesarean section, or episiotomy only when necessary. And a competent nurse-midwife will not hesitate to intervene or call upon her backup for intervention when the situation calls for it. Each profession has brought a valuable perspective to the modern labor room.

That being said, the differences that still exist between doctors and midwives may be of interest to you. Overall, according to a 1997 study from the University of Washington, women who choose midwives are ultimately the recipients of 12 percent fewer resources, ranging from electronic fetal monitoring to cesarean birth. Whether "fewer resources" ultimately represents an overall advantage or a disadvantage is a complex debate that lies well beyond the scope of this book. Likewise, a 1995 Public Citizen Research Group survey reported an 11.6 percent average cesarean rate among midwives, lower than the 23.3 percent national average at the time. Again, which of these represents the most accurate cesarean rate is not clear.

Whatever your outlook, be sure that whomever you choose brings experience and provides first and foremost a safe birthing environment. Look past the timeworn stereotypes, listen to the attitudes and beliefs of the provider, and consider whether *your* body is receiving the attention it deserves throughout the process.

THE DOULA EFFECT

Doulas are female birth assistants, experienced in childbirth, whose coaching, reassurance, and continuous support throughout labor and delivery have been shown to help some women cope with pain, push more effectively, and perhaps deliver more quickly. One 1991 study from Case Western Reserve University randomly assigned 412 woman to receive either doula assistance or no doula assistance. Was there a "doula effect"? Substantially lower rates of epidurals, forceps deliveries, and cesarean sections were seen among women with doulas; and labors were, on average, two hours shorter. A recent metaanalysis of eleven clinical trials concluded that continuous doula support—when compared with no doula support—is linked to shorter labors, decreased use of pain medication and oxytocin (for stimulating contractions), and lower odds of both forceps and cesareans. Maybe the lesson is that moral support, whether from doula, friend, relative, or partner—can have physical consequences.

PREDICTING PROBLEMS: SKIN LINES, PELVIC SHAPES, AND BEYOND

Each baby descends through the pelvis by twists and turns, during hours of stretching and compressing past the key pelvic supports. But predicting the ease or difficulty of its journey, and forecasting whether any physical problems will be left in its wake, has stumped medical science for centuries. How smoothly will your labor and delivery progress? How likely are you to experience a pelvic injury to your muscles, ligaments, fascia, or nerves? Even today, answers to these questions remain for the most part a medical mystery.

For generations, obstetricians have searched for links between outer physical traits and inner pelvic-floor vulnerability. Some of these traits are downright quirky: double-jointed fingers and stretchy skin have each, in the past, been identified as red flags signaling a higher risk for developing incontinence and/or prolapse, perhaps due to those individuals' relatively weak connective tissues. Whether these research findings can help us to predict or prevent injuries remains unclear. In the 1940s, some obstetricians were even convinced that *striae*—those colored lines that appear on the abdomen as the pregnancy hormones surge—could predict the risk of pelvic injury. "When the striae are broad and coarse, laceration of the perineum is likely, and early episiotomy is indicated," they claimed, yet "when there are no or fewer striae, there may be little risk." Again, an interesting theory, but its reliability has never been proven.

Since those days, the search for maternal risk factors has continued. A recent study of 131 women found that a perineum shorter than three centimeters increased the risk of rectal injury from 4 to 40 percent, and a risk of forceps or vacuum delivery increased from 9 to 28 percent. A study from Great Britain indicated that when bladder ultrasound showed a high degree of mobility within the urethra and bladder before delivery, it foretold a greater risk of incontinence afterward. Abnormal spinal curvature has been associated with over three times the usual risk of pelvic prolapse, according to one recent study. Among African mothers, those shorter than 150 centimeters (just under five feet) were found to be at increased risk for disproportion between baby and pelvis, leading to failed labor. African mothers shorter than the tenth percentile had double the risk of cesarean delivery and fifteen times the average risk of needing forceps or vacuum assistance. And a report from the University of Miami of more than fifty thousand women found that even age might relate to susceptibility of the pelvic floor. During a first delivery, severe lacerations involving the anal sphincter or rectum were less likely among younger moms.

Despite these scattered insights into the relationship between each woman's outward appearance and her risk of pelvic-floor problems, a clear and reliable picture of the woman at risk has yet to emerge.

PELVIMETRY: MEASURING YOUR PELVIC PROFILE

Few obstetricians or midwives will be likely to count your striae or check whether you're double-jointed during a prenatal office visit. But *pelvimetry* is a technique that could play a role in your care. Pelvimetry measures the distance between specific bones of your pelvis during a regular pelvic examination. How much space is present within the pelvis? Where is it narrow, and where is it wide? How does the baby fit into your pelvic bones? Remember those classic pelvic shapes described in chapter 2? Obstetricians and midwives can use pelvimetry during pregnancy or labor to determine which category you fit into. High-tech variations include the use of X rays, CT scans, and MRI.

PELVIMETRY: A WORK IN PROGRESS

Forecasting pelvic-floor injuries and postreproductive problems based on pelvic shape poses more questions than answers. If you have a short anthropoid pelvis, what's the risk of injury to the bladder or rectum? If your pelvic walls are very narrow, will a forceps delivery put you at high risk for pudendal nerve injury or a severe vaginal tear? Might a narrow pelvic arch force the fetal head away from the front of the pelvis and toward the rear, leaving you at greater risk for anal injury? Unfortunately, neither regular nor high-tech pelvimetry is a perfect predictor for the course of labor and delivery, or for identifying a pelvic shape that can accurately foretell a rough time in the labor room. But for pelvic shapes that are markedly abnormal, pelvimetry may help by warning the obstetrician that she needs to be on the lookout for trouble. Along with more accurate technology and more research, our ability to predict will hopefully improve.

Later in Pregnancy: Your Due Date Approaches

"My sister had an eight-pound, six-ounce baby and wound up with big problems. Is there anything I can do differently?"

As your due date approaches and you're surrounded by the commotion over painting the nursery, planning the baby shower, or tying up loose ends at work, it's easy to overlook one of the most central issues: your body. After all, it's undergoing rapid changes, preparing in some basic biological ways for a monumental physical event. As we've discussed, it's not just delivery but pregnancy itself that sets the stage for postreproductive problems. There's no better time than pregnancy to pause and focus a bit of careful planning on yourself. Would you enter into any other major physical challenge without stretching, working out, and getting yourself in shape?

EXERCISING YOUR PELVIC FLOOR

Kegel exercises are the basic workout for the pelvic floor, which you'll learn all about in Appendix A. Your first pregnancy is one of the best times in your life to learn pelvic-floor exercises. Not only because the need is so great—up to 70 percent of women will have some degree of urinary stress incontinence during or after pregnancy—but also because your pelvic muscles and nerves are still at their greatest potential. These muscles will be easier for you to identify before delivery than afterward. If you're on your second, third, or fourth pregnancy, you should still take time to focus on your pelvic-floor muscles. Building their strength will benefit your postreproductive body in several ways.

- *Builds a healthy reserve before childbirth.* The reserves you build up before delivery may make the muscles less injury-prone and will help to accelerate your healing afterward.

- *Provides a useful tool* during *labor.* Locating these muscles and developing their tone before your due date will help you to focus on relaxing them during labor and delivery.

- *Improves muscle strength* after-ward. Evaluation at six weeks postpartum has shown that women performing Kegel exer-cises during pregnancy prevent a loss of muscle strength and tend to emerge with pelvic muscles stronger than their prepregnancy baseline. Nonexercisers usually lose strength during pregnancy and childbirth.

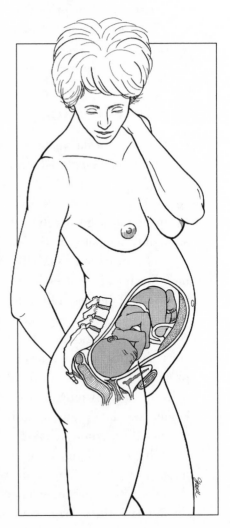

- *Reduces the odds of symptoms.* The greater your pelvic-floor muscle strength, the lower your risk for developing postreproduc-tive pelvic symptoms. One recent study showed that starting a Kegel routine before pregnancy reduced the risk of bladder, bowel, and vaginal symptoms after a first vaginal delivery from 69 percent to around 30 percent. Of four randomized trials on the preventive use of pelvic-floor rou-tines during pregnancy, three have shown the exercises to be beneficial, including a 1998 study showing significantly less urinary incontinence for the first six months after delivery. You'll also preserve your ability to brace the pelvic floor during moments of stress (see Appendix A).

ANOTHER LESSON FROM THE FAR EAST

In some Eastern cultures, pelvic-floor exercises are taught during young women's transition to adulthood—a female rite of passage. Unfortunately, pelvic-floor exercises haven't found that sort of niche in the Western world. One Australian survey showed that only 6 percent of pregnant women had their pelvic-floor muscles assessed before childbirth. As you've seen, learning the exercises afterward is a much steeper hill to climb.

PERINEAL MASSAGE

The hard and still will be broken.
The soft and supple will prevail.
                              —Tao Te Ching

Perineal massage involves gentle stretching of the perineum, that span of tissue between the vagina and rectum, using your fingers and a bit of lubrication (K-Y jelly, Astroglide, or even a few drops of olive oil). The idea is to stretch, soften, and prepare this area with the hope that it will be less likely to tear during delivery. Using a rolling motion, gently massage and squeeze the lubricated perineal body. Nothing should be inserted into the vagina itself. Women commonly start perineal massage at around thirty-four to thirty-five weeks of pregnancy and perform it for ten to fifteen minutes each day until delivery. Other women massage for the first time only after labor has begun, as a late preparation for crowning—when the newborn's head reaches the vaginal opening and perineum.

Will perineal massage really protect your body? Two studies have shown that it may decrease the risk of perineal injury. One demonstrated that in women thirty or older, massage performed during the third trimester of pregnancy and also during labor increased the chances of an intact perineum by 12 percent. A larger study, from Canada in 1999, involved over fifteen hundred women and found that for those without a previous vaginal birth, three weeks of perineal massage increased the odds of an intact perineum by 9 percent. A follow-up study of the same group found that among those with a previous vaginal birth, perineal massage was associated with slightly less perineal pain at three months postpartum. However, a 2001 study involving more than thirteen hundred Australian women showed no benefit to women performing massage in the labor room only.

At the very least, most women who perform perineal massage during pregnancy and/or labor view it as a positive experience. Up to 80 percent of women reported in one study that they would do it during subsequent pregnancies. Give it a try—it certainly can't hurt. One of the simplest means of prevention may literally be right at your fingertips.

EXERCISING THE REST OF YOUR BODY AND OPTIMIZING YOUR WEIGHT

Pregnancy is a great time for exercise, for many good reasons. First, a regular mild workout routine can dramatically improve your sense of well-being and physical control at a time when uncontrollable physical events seem to be occurring all around you. Second, beyond the obvious cardiovascular health benefits, epidemiological data shows that regular exercise may help to prevent gestational diabetes. Third—and most important with respect to this book's focus—keeping close to your optimal weight throughout pregnancy may help to reduce your odds of developing postreproductive problems.

WEIGHT

Both your prepregnancy weight and weight gain during pregnancy may be linked to your risk of pelvic-floor injury. Avoiding excess pounds means less stress on the pelvic-floor muscles and nerves during pregnancy and the months of healing afterward. One recent study showed that although women of all shapes and sizes may experience urinary incontinence during pregnancy that improves postpartum, *persistent* leakage is more likely among those who gain a lot of weight before delivery. A 1997 study from Denmark demonstrated that being overweight prepregnancy is a potential risk factor for urinary stress incontinence and urgency after delivery. Automatic formulas for calculating your body mass index (based on height and weight) can be found on the Internet; a body mass index above thirty has been associated with a higher risk of stress incontinence after delivery.

A reasonable target for weight gain is two to four pounds during the first three months of pregnancy, and around a pound each week thereafter; this means roughly twenty-five to thirty-five pounds for a full-term pregnancy. If you're overweight before pregnancy, significantly less weight gain (fifteen to twenty pounds) is acceptable. Weight loss, however, should never be your goal. Always check with your obstetrician or midwife about how much weight gain is ideal for you.

Diet, of course, plays an important role in this area. One rule of thumb is that most pregnant women require an extra three hundred calories beyond their usual diet to maintain proper nutrition. For a woman of average size, twenty-five hundred calories per day should suffice. If you exercise a lot, you may need more. Avoid empty-calorie junk food, and consult your doctor or prenatal guide on the intake of protein, calcium, and other nutrients.

Exercise

What exercise routine is best during pregnancy? Your body will feel different—changes in coordination, posture and balance, breathing patterns, softer ligaments, and a vulnerable pelvic floor mean you should give some thought to your routine before heading to the gym.

Warm Up, Stretch Out, and Cool Down

Five to ten minutes of stretching before and after will help to prevent injury and will be more important than ever, given the excess weight your body is carrying. Try pelvic tilts while lying on the floor, feet flat and knees bent. Inhale and tilt your pelvis upward while tightening your abdomen and buttocks and avoiding any arching of the back. Hold for a count of five to ten seconds and keep breathing, then slowly lower your body to the floor. Try fifteen repetitions a day. The same exercise can also be done while standing, with your hands on your hips. Also try gentle ankle and leg stretches, since your legs will be bearing more weight than during your nonpregnancy workout.

Aerobic Exercise

Aim to do a whole-body aerobic activity for twenty to thirty minutes, two to three times each week, along with your stretch. Walking, swimming (no diving), cycling, and exercise machines should be fine, with your doctor's permission. Alternate with resistance or strength training (use isometric techniques or light weights only), and keep your peak heart rate at moderate intensity—under 140 beats per minute, for most healthy women of reproductive age. If you're already a runner, you should be able to continue a modified routine, but discuss a plan with your doctor. Don't work to the point of complete exhaustion; you should be able to hold a conversation while exercising without being short of breath.

Start slowly, especially if you had no regular prepregnancy exercise routine. Consider a prenatal exercise group if one exists in your area, even if you already consider yourself a fitness expert.

Water Exercise

Water aerobics provide a good workout, nonstressful to the pelvic floor and also the joints and spine, all of which are particularly vulnerable beneath the extra weight of pregnancy. Water's antigravity effect can provide true relief to your overworked body, especially during the last few months before delivery.

Prenatal Yoga

Yoga improves blood circulation, relaxes the body, strengthens muscles, and makes you feel great. In addition, it may help to prepare you for different laboring and birthing positions, to improve the flexibility of your joints, and to develop pain-coping strategies. A variety of poses designed to tone and open the pelvic area, and strengthen the pelvic-floor musculature, are safe for a low-risk pregnancy. Be sure to find a prenatal yoga class, or at least an instructor who is familiar with safe poses for pregnancy.

Posture and Lifting

As the uterus enlarges during pregnancy, changes in posture naturally occur. Perhaps most visibly, women may tilt their pelvis forward and throw their shoulders back as the abdomen protrudes. The result is often a poorly aligned spine, increased strain on the muscles and ligaments, and most importantly from our perspective, pressure on the pelvic floor. You've already learned one strategy to counteract these changes: the pelvic tilt. In the standing position, tuck the pelvis back into a position more in line with the spine, by activating the buttocks and abdominal muscles while straightening the upper back: this will improve your posture and help to protect your lower back and pelvic floor. With developed abdominal muscles, this posture will

Changing postures during pregnancy

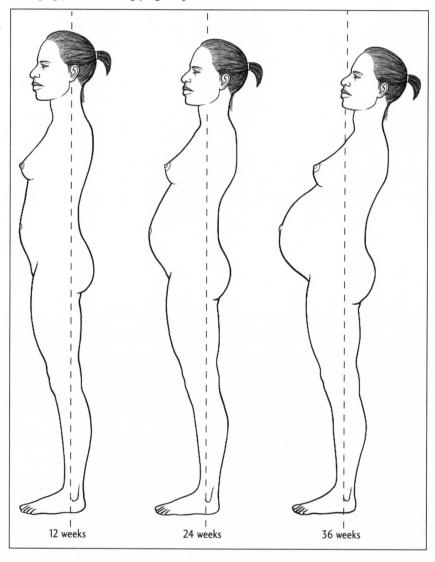

12 weeks   24 weeks   36 weeks

be easier to maintain. Remember when lifting to brace the pelvic floor with an inward Kegel squeeze, rather than bearing down as you would during a bowel movement; this will prevent undue stress against the pelvic floor when it is most vulnerable (see Appendix A).

What to Avoid

Steer clear of jumping and jolting exercises. The hormone relaxin makes your joints stretchier, so be sure *not* to force them beyond their normal range of motion, or to overstretch to the point of pain.

When starting your exercise routine during pregnancy, keep in mind some basic guidelines recommended by the American College of Obstetricians and Gynecologists:

- During pregnancy, you can continue to exercise and derive health benefits even from mild to moderate exercise routines. Regular exercise (at least three times a week) is preferable to intermittent activity.

- After the first trimester, avoid exercise in the supine position (on the back). This position is associated with decreased cardiac output. Prolonged periods of motionless standing should also be avoided.

- Since oxygen availability is decreased during exercise, modify the intensity of exercise according to your symptoms. Stop exercising when fatigued, and don't exercise to exhaustion.

- Any exercise that involves a potential threat of abdominal trauma or loss of balance and risk to mother or infant should be avoided.

- Since pregnancy requires an additional three hundred calories per day, make sure you're eating adequately if you're exercising.

- Adequate hydration, appropriate clothing, and optimal environmental surroundings are important for body-temperature regulation during exercise.

- Anytime you experience an unexplained discomfort or concern, stop and call your doctor. Warning signs include, among others: pain, vaginal leakage or bleeding, abdominal cramps, difficulty breathing, pain in the chest or legs, increased swelling, headaches, or decreased fetal movement.

- Before starting any new exercise program, review the plan with your obstetrician. If you are in a high-risk pregnancy category, or have a medical condition, the exercises recommended in this chapter may not be appropriate for you.

Sources: American College of Obstetricians and Gynecologists Jan. 2002 technical bulletin; *The Official YMCA Prenatal Exercise Guide.*

PREVENTING CONSTIPATION

Pregnancy makes you constipated—largely an effect of the pregnancy hormone progesterone on the bowels, sometimes heightened by oral iron tablets. Avoiding constipation is important not only for your comfort but also to prevent straining on the toilet and stressing the pelvic-floor supports. You'll also help to prevent hemorrhoids and varicosities (swollen veins) in the vulva and perineum, which can cause aching, heaviness, or heavy bleeding during labor and delivery. Winning the battle of the bowels may take several strategies, including lots of fiber and fluids, regular exercise, stool softeners, and occasional laxatives. Make a habit of bran, fruits, raw veggies, and plenty of hydration. Consult with your doctor or midwife before starting any laxatives during pregnancy. See chapter 10 for more tips.

EXERCISING YOUR MIND: THE PRENATAL SELF-HELP YOU SEEK

Countless classes and groups are available these days, ranging from mind-body exercises to full-fledged medical-review courses. The majority of these programs orient women and their partners to natural birthing techniques, controlled breathing, and relaxation: great preparation for the uncertain journey ahead, during which "mind over matter" can go a long, long way. Unfortunately, their focus on your lower body often begins and ends with the perineum and strategies to avoid episiotomy. The scope of concern needs to extend much wider to have a real impact on your postreproductive body. Still, these techniques can help prepare you mentally and provide you with a better ability to relax your pelvic floor during labor and delivery.

༠ 5 ༠

Learning How to Labor

EXPLORING YOUR OPTIONS FOR STYLES, POSITIONS, AND TECHNIQUES

So, I ended up going overdue and being induced . . . laboring for over thirteen hours and no progress. I ended up with a C-section. My OB came out to talk to me while I was in recovery and said there would have been no way I could ever have (vaginally) delivered my son.

—T.F., chat-room contributor,
www.gocesarean.com

I told the doctor I wanted to avoid a C-section if possible, if he thought the baby would be OK. He told me, "Well, the head is coming down, but I'm not sure if you're going to be able to push this baby out." I was very sure I could, and I wanted this baby out. I had no drugs and was very, very tired. I looked at my husband, and I told him I was going to prove this doctor wrong—I was going to push this baby out. I started pushing with all my might.

—Entry on www.birthstories.com

It is seldom in life that one knows that a coming event is to be of crucial importance.

—Anya Seton

*F*inally, your due date arrives. The mounting flurry of plans, emotions, decisions, and preparations all start to revolve increasingly around one simple question: when will labor begin? But other questions, in the midst of it all, may have been overlooked: how have you prepared for delivery? Have you discussed your thoughts regarding forceps, vacuum deliveries, and episiotomy, and have you learned about your pelvic shape and baby's size? After the final push, when the feedings and diaper changes begin, what will you do to ensure the most complete healing for your body? Events in the labor room may seem predestined or inevitable, but they are in fact choices and decisions—and in preparing for labor, you must understand and influence all that you can. Though your obstetrician or midwife is the driver, you should be an educated passenger.

IN THE AGE OF DESIGNER CHILDBIRTH, REMEMBER SUBSTANCE AMID THE STYLE

Childbirth today is not just a biological event, it's a boutique industry. The traditional labor room has given way to birthing suites filled with music and massage, acupuncture and armoires, whirlpools and yoga as women and their partners are invited to participate in a well-planned drama orchestrated according to taste. Few would disagree that atmosphere and aesthetics go a long way; what a great improvement today's labor room is over yesterday's stark walls mounted with monitors, and metal stirrups extending like claws from an antiseptic examining table. But even today, behind all of the window dressing lies the physical reality of childbirth—which, as you've learned, is still no day at the spa. Be sure your labor planning reflects as much substance as it does style. Long after you've forgotten the aromatherapy, fancy furniture, and parquet floors, you'll have no regrets if you choose to make the basic principles of preventive obstetrics—rather than hospital aesthetics—your highest priority.

Coping with Early Labor

RELAXATION TECHNIQUES

Tension within the pelvic-floor muscles, due to pain or anxiety, can slow your progress during early labor. In theory, flexing or guarding the pelvic floor with contraction of the levator muscles may increase the amount of resistance against the descending fetus, as well as the degree of physical strain on a number of vaginal supports and pelvic-floor attachments. Meditation, visualization, breathing exercises, and yoga can help to keep the pelvic floor and the entire body relaxed as dilation of the cervix and descent of the fetus occur. If you've already found your levator muscles during pregnancy and built their strength with Kegel exercises, you should be better able to relax them.

EARLY-LABOR STRATEGIES

Especially for your first delivery, if your pregnancy was uncomplicated and your water hasn't broken, then staying home through early labor will not only keep you in a comfortable and familiar environment it will also allow you to do a great deal of dilating before reaching the hospital. If your doctor or midwife permits, take a bath, walk, or just rest. Walking, whether it's at home or around the maternity ward, may help to keep your uterine contractions regular and to direct the fetal head against the cervix and surrounding tissues that are in the process of dilating. It has not been scientifically proven which early-labor strategies offer the best protection for the pelvic floor.

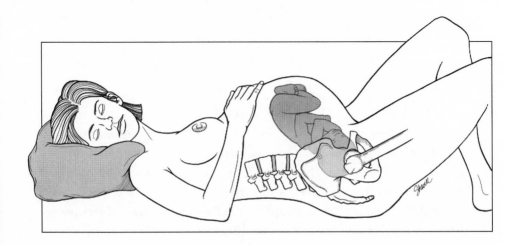

Pushing Smart: When to Start, When to Stop, and Which Technique

Pushing during childbirth represents a few critical hours of your lifetime. A variety of positions is often mentioned, from squatting to standing. Some women are instructed to push immediately after reaching the goal of full dilation, others are encouraged to wait until the baby's head is low, and still others are coached to avoid pushing until the urge becomes unbearable. You should understand the potential effects of these various techniques on your body.

PUSHING POSITIONS

Mothers of previous generations were invited to deliver only while lying on their backs—especially those choosing to give birth in a hospital. Nowadays, you may have the opportunity to push out your baby while lying down, sitting on a chair or stool, standing upright, or even soaking in a pool of warm water. Exploring and finding the positions that feel best can have a major influence on each woman's comfort and sense of control in the labor room; alternating positions may even help you to better cope with labor pain. Sometimes one position becomes preferable for medical reasons: for instance, lying on your side to improve blood flow to the baby when it shows signs of strain or fatigue. But when all is well, and your delivery position is simply a matter of choice, what might the effects be on your postreproductive body?

ON YOUR BACK

The lying-down position (*lithotomy*) is probably the one you're most familiar with, and is used mostly with an epidural (since numbness in the legs often occurs). Typically, the mother's legs are held in a fully flexed and upward position during each contraction, and the chin is curled into the chest during the push. Critics argue that by working opposite the direction of gravity, lithotomy makes delivery more difficult, like pushing uphill. The more frequent objection to lithotomy is simply that some mothers feel overly exposed, more restricted in their movement, and less in control. Other women prefer lithotomy, feeling that it allows them to maximize their rest between contractions. Whether lithotomy translates into longer labor or any added risk of pelvic-floor stress is uncertain.

SQUATTING

Many nurses, midwives, and doctors swear by this more gravity-friendly, woman-centered pushing position. You should be well supported, with the knees separated and the back arched open, not hunched over. Your arms should be grasping something higher than waist level; a squatting bar is sometimes fastened to the bed to help Mom maintain her stability. According to some practitioners, squatting can increase the diameter of the pelvic outlet by up to 30 percent, compared with the lying-down position, and helps to shift the tailbone out of the baby's way during birth. One 1993 study of three hundred women showed the squatting position to be associated with a greater likelihood of finishing labor with an intact perineum, lower risk of episiotomy, and fewer injuries to the anal sphincter (1 percent versus 14 percent). Other studies have reported conflicting results. One Indian study found that women randomly assigned to squatting rather than lying flat were more likely to deliver quickly but were also more likely to experience maternal injury (presumably to the perineum). An Australian study recently found squatting to be associated with perineal injury in 58 percent of women, higher than any other birth position assessed. The effects of squatting on the deeper pelvic floor, for better or worse, are entirely unknown.

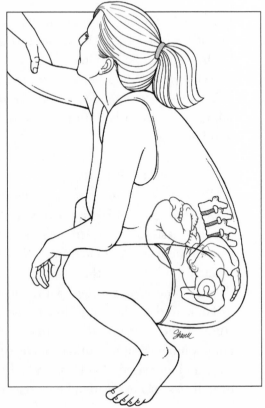

Squatting position

THE SITTING POSITION

Some women choose to labor while sitting upright in either a specialized chair or on a toilet seat. Advocates of birthing chairs once claimed that they led to quicker deliveries; however, the few studies performed indicate that swelling of the perineum may be more likely, and blood loss may be increased. Labial tears may also be more common. Birthing chairs are rarely used nowadays, but some women will use a toilet seat for the same purpose. An oversize birthing ball (just like those large rubber workout balls at the gym) can be used to help maintain a comfortable, wide, sitting or squatting position during certain parts of labor, but not the delivery itself.

SIDE LYING

For the woman who has had a vaginal childbirth, the side position may improve control over the speed of her next delivery, as well as helping to prevent injury in some cases. As the fetal head crowns at the vaginal opening, Mom may have a greater ability to ensure slow expulsion of the fetal head past the vaginal opening, potentially reducing her odds of a perineal injury from a precipitous delivery. A recent analysis of 2,891 vaginal births in Australia found that of all birth positions, side lying was associated with the best odds (66.6 percent) of avoiding perineal injury. The side-lying position is also sometimes recommended when the baby's heart rate slows during labor, since it can help to increase the flow of blood to the placenta and baby.

THE UPRIGHT POSITION

Proponents of the stand-and-deliver approach have claimed that it can result in a quicker delivery and a reduced need for forceps or vacuum assistance, and there's been at least one study supporting each of these claims. One from 1997 involved more than five hundred women and found that upright laboring was associated with decreased perineal trauma, pain, and risk of receiving an episiotomy as compared to the lying-down position. On the downside, a 1994 study found that upright birth was associated with higher rates of anal sphincter injury; others have suggested higher rates of labial tears and increased blood loss. Whether upright delivery carries more overall risk or benefit remains unclear; at present, it appears to be a reasonable alternative for some women. However, as with the sitting or squatting positions, if your perineum begins to swell in this position, it's probably time to make a change.

HANDS AND KNEES

This facedown position can provide relief from a backache, and it may help the baby to rotate from an abnormal position—including *occiput posterior* (baby facing the front of your body, rather than back), which has been linked to higher rates of anal sphincter injury. It's also possible, but not proven, that if the perineum appears headed for imminent injury, the hands-and-knees position may help to shift pressure away from that area and toward the front of the pelvic outlet.

IF IT FLOATS YOUR BOAT: WATER DELIVERY

According to some enthusiasts of water birth, the hydrostatic pressure of water against the body may benefit Mom's lower body by massaging blood away from the skin and possibly reducing edema (swelling) of the perineum, vulvar area, and lower body. These maternal benefits have not been scientifically proven, but water delivery appears to be a reasonably safe alternative for those interested. Keep in mind that it's not always safe to be sitting in water. If your doctor is concerned about fetal exhaustion or suspects a difficult delivery, a regular birthing technique may be necessary.

PUSHING TECHNIQUES

DIRECTED VALSALVA PUSHING

Valsalva is the "close your mouth and push like there's no tomorrow" style, and the one that you're probably most familiar with: a deep breath at the start of each contraction, blowing out, then inhaling for another ten-second push until the contraction ends. Advocates of pushing early and often maintain that without a constant effort on Mom's behalf, labor lasts too long, creating more stress for the baby, and also for your pelvis. Critics of active pushing argue that pushing shortens labor less than you might think, while at the same time exhausting Mom, stressing her pelvic supports, and perhaps even increasing the risk for pelvic injury. According to at least one long-standing textbook on vaginal surgery, aggressive pushing before the cervix is fully dilated may severely stress the pelvic floor by pushing the cervix and its attachments ahead of the baby's skull. Most providers recommend active valsalva pushing simply because it's most familiar to them. In other cases, aggressive pushing becomes necessary to speed the delivery process; if the baby has an abnormal heart rate or a fever, it's not an option to sit back and wait.

DELAYED PUSHING

Most laboring women are actively coached to push, push, push! But could there be some instances when it's best to relax, relax, relax? Delayed pushing means resisting the urge to push while allowing the fetus to passively descend past the pelvic supports. Waiting for fetal descent is also sometimes called *laboring down*. Medical literature dating back to the 1950s suggested that normal first deliveries require no encouragement to push, and that non-pushers appeared to have a lower risk of forceps delivery and injury to the perineum. After years of attracting little research interest, the issue of labor pushing has been recently readdressed. One multicenter study was performed at twelve locations throughout Canada, Switzerland, and the United States to investigate whether a delayed pushing strategy could benefit mothers during the first birth. A total of 1,862 women agreed to be randomized to either immediate pushing once fully dilated, or to wait for two hours before pushing if possible. The women were, on average, twenty-eight years old, and all received epidural pain control. Difficult deliveries were less likely among women in the delayed pushing group, and forceps assistance was necessary less often.

The benefits of delayed pushing appeared to be greatest for women whose fetus was still relatively high in the pelvis, or not yet turned to the facedown position, at the time of full cervical dilation. Slightly higher rates of maternal fever were associated with the delayed strategy, but no increased maternal or neonatal complications were seen. A 2002 study reported that women randomly assigned to delayed pushing benefited from a decreased overall average pushing time, less maternal fatigue, and fewer cases of a slowed fetal heart rate.

In each of these studies, all participants received epidurals. No research to date has assessed the strategy of delayed pushing in patients without pain control. Without an epidural, the natural urge to start pushing—and the difficulty in keeping the pelvic muscles relaxed—would make this labor approach infinitely more difficult. However, based on the evidence, delayed pushing may well be a worthwhile labor-room option for women choosing an epidural. A few tips might increase your odds of success.

- *Breathing exercises and relaxation techniques.* Delayed pushing works best when you're relaxed, mentally and physically. Try slow, focused breathing in between contractions. Rapid and deep breathing (huffing and puffing) and shallow panting may help you cope with contractions while resisting the urge to push. Punctuate these with long, deep breaths at each contraction's end. If you've learned Lamaze, or an alternative relaxation/breathing technique, give it a try.

- *Pain control.* Severe pain can completely prevent relaxation of the pelvic floor, slowing the progress of labor and making it impossible to labor down. An epidural can allow you to remain fully alert while laboring down more comfortably. Although the risks of an epidural are relatively small, always discuss them with the anesthesiologist and make an informed choice.

- *Positions.* Alternating between the labor positions discussed earlier in the chapter may provide distraction and help the baby to navigate the pelvic anatomy most effectively. Labor nurses, doctors, and midwives are almost always open to Mom's preferences unless specific safety issues arise.

PHYSIOLOGIC (SPONTANEOUS) PUSHING

The *physiologic*, or spontaneous, approach is a type of delayed pushing that entails waiting to push until you feel the natural overwhelming urge to do so, following the lead of your physical sensations rather than the direction of a coach or a predetermined schedule. One 1984 study suggested that perineal injury was less likely if women pushed only in response to strong involuntary urges (spontaneous pushing) rather than when they were coached to do so. A 1999 University of Michigan survey compared spontaneous to directed pushing and found that spontaneous pushers were less likely to have advanced perineal lacerations and more likely to have an intact perineum after delivery. Another study concluded that active pushing for over an hour caused more injury to the pudendal nerve, whereas extended periods of passive laboring after full dilation (relaxation during contractions rather than pushing) seemed to avoid this risk. Interestingly, spontaneous pushing does not seem to prolong the overall duration of the second stage. At the very least, it may decrease your level of exhaustion throughout the delivery process.

OPEN-GLOTTIS PUSHING

This involves breathing or making noise while pushing, rather than keeping quiet, holding your breath, and bearing down. Although most women in the United States bear down silently, *open glottis* is the standard custom within many other cultures. The mellifluous ululation and high-pitched chants of Haitian and Caribbean women are well known to most labor-room nurses and always leave medical students amazed when hearing them for the first time. Because it's virtually impossible to bear down as strongly while laboring with the open-glottis technique (try straining while holding your breath, then again while allowing it to escape), it seems quite possible that the pelvic floor might be exposed to less stress over the course of a long labor. Whether this could ultimately reduce the odds of pelvic-floor injury and subsequent symptoms remains unknown. More research is needed to understand the pros and cons of the technique.

FACTORING FETAL POSITION

The position of the baby relative to your pelvic bones is a major determinant of how difficult a delivery might be. Although few specifics regarding the effect of fetal position on the maternal pelvic floor are known, the basics of normal and abnormal positions are useful to understand.

- *Occiput anterior.* Most babies deliver in this facedown position, with the baby facing the mother's backside. It is the easiest and most biologically correct way in terms of delivery.

- *Occiput posterior.* In this position, the baby comes out faceup, or "sunny-side up," as some labor nurses are known to say. It's been long observed that these deliveries may be more prolonged, with increased discomfort and pain focused in the lower back. A recent study from Ireland documented these observations by analyzing a large number of deliveries and comparing babies who descended in the occiput posterior and occiput anterior positions. Posterior deliveries were associated with markedly different outcomes, including a sevenfold increase in anal sphincter injuries, and higher rates of delivery by cesarean and forceps. Fewer than half of them achieved spontaneous vaginal birth. As mentioned earlier in this chapter, certain labor positions (for example, hands and knees) may help the baby to turn from the posterior position before maternal pushing begins.

- *Transverse.* When the baby fails to complete even its first requisite turn in Mom's pelvis, it becomes stuck in the *transverse* (side-facing) position. Forceps were often used to rotate the baby's head in this situation, allowing its descent; today that approach is less common, since the overall risks associated with forceps are more widely appreciated. If the second stage of labor begins with a fetus in the transverse position, cesarean may be the best choice, since for some women, the odds of a long and difficult push, or needing operative assistance (forceps or vacuum) are quite high.

- *Breech.* When the baby's feet or buttocks come out first. To deliver vaginally, the fetus must be fairly small compared with Mom's pelvic opening. Certain types of breech presentations are far more likely than others to succeed with a vaginal birth. Unless forceps assistance is used, vaginal breech in itself poses no known increased risk to the pelvic floor. But the overall risks of attempting a breech delivery are complex and far beyond the scope of this book.

- *Brow and face.* The *brow* position, in which the baby's forehead presents first, is uncommon. It often requires a cesarean, because the broadest part of the baby's head may have trouble clearing the pelvic bones. The *face* position looks like it sounds—the baby's face, rather than the top of its head, presents itself first. Certain types of face positions are compatible with vaginal birth, and others are not. Neither the brow nor the face position poses any specific risk of injury to the pelvic floor.

LENGTH OF PUSHING: HOW LONG IS TOO LONG?

There was once a time when prolonged labor meant a truly epic and dangerous struggle for Mom, often lasting for several days. That period of time, we came to understand, was too long, since truly obstructed labors caused a handful of problems, including, on the maternal end, fistulas—abnormal openings between the vagina and bladder, urethra, or bowel after prolonged compression against the fetal head. But even today, the true limits of normal labor remain unclear. A first stage (from the beginning of regular contractions to full dilation) longer than fifteen hours may begin to raise valid suspicion about successful delivery. For the second stage (from full dilation to delivery), the American College of Obstetricians and Gynecologists defines the normal limits as not exceeding three hours for a woman's first delivery, and two hours for those who have previously given birth. Yet in actual practice, some women—especially those who are comfortable with epidurals—will be encouraged to persevere through second stages lasting many hours more. After all, large studies have shown that with vigilance and modern obstetrical monitoring, long labors pose no specific risk to the newborn. But aside from the fetal perspective, other questions are less commonly addressed: could the length of your labor influence the function of your postreproductive body later on?

- *Nerve function.* Several studies have suggested that a longer pushing stage is associated with diminished pudendal nerve function afterward. As we've discussed, this type of injury may represent the first step toward postreproductive pelvic-floor disorders, including prolapse.

- *Anal function.* A recent German study compared women whose second stage during their first delivery lasted less than two hours, to those with a second stage over three and a half hours. The long-labor group had a significantly higher rate of new-onset flatal incontinence (inability to control gas).

- *Bladder control.* One study demonstrated that every additional twenty minutes of pushing time resulted in a 20 percent rise in the risk of bladder dysfunction. Other small studies have failed to demonstrate that a longer duration of pushing leads to a higher risk of incontinence. Definitive research on this question has yet to be done.

- *Operative deliveries.* A very prolonged second stage of labor, especially with early and sustained bearing-down efforts, tends to exhaust Mom. In some cases, this may lead to a greater likelihood of forceps or vacuum assistance. These interventions, as you've already learned, substantially raise the risk of a pelvic-floor injury.

How long is too long for *your* lower body? The question may not have a simple answer, but it's worth discussing with your provider. As future research unravels the questions surrounding labor's second stage, the right approach will hopefully become clear.

WHEN CROWNING FINALLY OCCURS: THE FINAL PUSH

Crowning refers to that long-awaited final stage of labor when the baby's head reaches the perineum and becomes visible through the vaginal opening. The perineal tissues stretch and bulge forward, and Mom usually experiences an overwhelming urge to push hard and finish the job. What's your best strategy when this moment of truth for the perineum finally arrives?

- *Arrive prepared.* Hopefully, perineal massage and pelvic-floor exercises during pregnancy have left you well toned and flexible, inside and out.

- *Relax and breathe.* Rather than bearing down strongly, women are sometimes coached during the crowning stage to "puff out the birthday candles." These short, shallow breaths allow the force of the uterine contraction alone to ease the baby's head slowly past the perineal opening.

- *Control the speed of delivery.* Doctors and midwives usually apply a bit of counterpressure against the fetal head to prevent it from delivering too quickly. Moms are sometimes shown how to help guide the baby out, and to control the speed of delivery, using their own hands. These maneuvers are meant to decrease the risk of perineal laceration.

- *Avoid traumatic positions.* According to some physicians, pulling back the legs too much (*hyperflexing*) may increase the risk of a sudden laceration due to the baby's head quickly popping past the perineum. As a result, it should be avoided during that final push. However, in certain emergency situations, this maneuver may become necessary.

- *Avoid fundal pressure. Fundal pressure* refers to a simple push of the hand across the top of Mom's uterus in an effort to push the baby down and expedite delivery. In some countries, this practice is common, but in most settings, it is reserved for emergency situations, specifically to help dislodge the baby's shoulder when it becomes stuck behind the pubic bone. Although the physical effects of fundal pressure on Mom's pelvis have not been studied, it's probably safe to assume that stretching the uterine and pelvic supports when they are soft and vulnerable to injury may cause harm. It should be done only when it's a necessity, and not as a routine procedure.

PUSHING FOR ANSWERS:
CHALLENGING OUR CHILDBIRTH TRADITIONS

In 1997 a report from the University of British Columbia examined all of the existing studies on pushing styles and arrived at a few conclusions:

> First, too few high-quality research studies have addressed this women's-health issue. "The way physicians and midwives manage labour and delivery today," the study concluded, "is based on opinion rather than scientific evidence." Second, based on the few studies that do exist, the second stage of labor appears not to be prolonged by the relatively gentle open-glottis or physiologic pushing styles, even for a first pregnancy. Finally, less forceful pushing appears to be associated with lower risk of perineal injury.
>
> This is an interesting set of conclusions, and a stark contrast to the obstetrical styles you'll find advocated in many labor rooms. Even more remarkable is the fact that such basic women's health questions

remain unanswered. Do you think if men were faced with the biological task of expelling a tennis ball through their urethra that the least harmful strategy wouldn't have been thoroughly researched? It's time the physical efforts of motherhood are acknowledged, not as an inevitable sacrifice but as a challenge to be solved.

6

Cesareans, Forceps, Epidurals, Etc.

KEY OBSTETRICAL CHOICES AND THEIR POTENTIAL PHYSICAL EFFECTS

*R*egardless of the technology, engineering, and modern conveniences that have entered today's labor room, one simple fact remains: there are just two ways for a baby to be delivered—vaginally or by cesarean, from below or from above. Even a perfectly routine natural vaginal delivery, as we've discussed, can have detrimental implications for future pelvic-floor function, even when the birth itself appears uneventful.

But what about when the birth becomes more interventional?

In some cases, operative techniques, such as cesarean delivery, forceps, or vacuum devices, may be used to achieve vaginal delivery. Do these interventions increase or decrease the risk of future pelvic trouble? Or do they affect that risk at all? Let's take a look at a few of the most important obstetrical interventions and choices you might face in the labor room.

Forceps and Vacuum and the Pelvic Floor

Forceps look something like oversize salad spoons, and they are used for two basic purposes—either to help the baby pass through the vaginal canal, or to rotate its head and enable vaginal delivery. Two basic types of forceps deliveries are in use today. *Outlet*, or *low*, forceps refers to their use after the baby's head has reached the pelvic floor and is visible at the vaginal opening; *midforceps* refers to applying the device to a fetal head higher in the pelvis.

Before addressing the rather strained relationship between forceps and your body, let's make one historical point clear: forceps have probably saved more lives, maternal and fetal, than any other obstetrical device. Back when obstructed labors commonly led to maternal death, these instruments were often the only way out. Vacuum and forceps procedures still play a truly valuable role in obstetrical care, under a number of circumstances. For instance, when the baby is close to delivery and develops an abnormal heartbeat, or when Mom is simply too exhausted to keep pushing, these two devices can facilitate the safest birth for both you and your baby.

But it's equally safe to say that forceps have been the most overutilized devices in the labor room. As the pendulum of medicalized childbirth took a rather wide swing around eighty years ago, women were commonly sedated, then etherized, during the second stage of labor. An episiotomy was then cut, and forceps were used to deliver the fetus. Many obstetricians believed that this liberal use of forceps could reduce the risk of pelvic injury by resulting in a more controlled delivery, with less pressure against perineum as the fetal head was lifted out. Forceps and episiotomy together, it was felt, offered the best protection against pelvic injury for some women.

But that was then, and this is now. What is known today about the pros and cons of this procedure when it comes to your postreproductive body? And how about the pros and cons of the vacuum—a suction-cup device applied to the baby's head, an increasingly common alternative to forceps.

FORCEPS AND VACUUMS TODAY

There's no question that both forceps delivery and, to a lesser degree, vacuum devices, increase the risk of injury to your perineum. Episiotomies are often cut to make room for the placement of these instruments around the baby's head, and we've already discussed the potential effects of this "little cut." But even without an episiotomy, the risk of injury during a forceps delivery, to the perineum and elsewhere, is high. One study concluded that of all women with tears into or through the anal sphincter following childbirth, up to 50 percent had either a forceps or vacuum-assisted birth. A landmark British study revealed that 80 percent of women who underwent forceps delivery experienced tearing of the anal sphincter that could be seen by ultrasound. Another report from Australia, involving more than three hundred women, concluded that women with prior forceps deliveries were up to ten times more likely to experience urinary incontinence after later deliveries. One recent study found that the odds of having stress incontinence seven years after a first childbirth was roughly ten times higher among women who had undergone a forceps delivery. And from Great Britain, it was reported that forceps delivery more than doubled the frequency and quantity of urinary leakage, compared with normal birth, at six months postpartum.

Finally, it's been shown that ten months after childbirth, women who had forceps delivery experienced a significantly weaker pelvic floor and decreased anal strength compared to those who had a spontaneous vaginal birth. That should come as no surprise. The average force of forceps against the pelvic tissues has been estimated at seventy-five pounds! Imagine a seventy-five-pound person standing on all of those nerves, muscles, and tissues and it's easy to understand how your brief sojourn inside the labor room might affect the function and control within this complex area of your body for many years afterward.

IF YOU HAVE TO CHOOSE: FORCEPS VERSUS VACUUM

An obstetrician's choice of either forceps or vacuum often depends upon the amount of room in your pelvis, the baby's position, and the degree of molding (cone head) visible. Your doctor's experience and professional judgment, in those instances, are invaluable. But perhaps you've been pushing for a couple of hours and just need a little help. In that case, either device will do. Faced with the two alternatives, what's the best choice for *your* body?

The short answer is that vacuum delivery appears to do less harm to your pelvic floor. A 1999 study randomly assigned women in need of an assisted delivery to one of these two instruments, and found that anal sphincter injury was significantly more common with forceps (79 percent versus 40 percent). Moreover, anal incontinence was also more common after forceps delivery (32 percent versus 16 percent). Another study using ultrasound found that up to 80 percent of women had anal sphincter injuries after forceps delivery, versus none after a vacuum procedure. And a report by the Cochrane Group—the British-led team of research analysts—concluded that vacuum delivery places you at a significantly lower risk of perineal injury than forceps. However, a recent review of more than ninety-one thousand births in Canada showed that both forceps and vacuum deliveries increased the risk of maternal pelvic injury. Vacuum delivery doubled the risk. Trying forceps after a failed vacuum proved to be the worst scenario, raising the risk of injury by almost sixfold.

In summary, while both methods increase the likelihood of perineal injury, vacuum devices tend to be less physically traumatic than forceps, from the maternal standpoint. Yet in a number of specific situations, vacuum-assisted delivery simply will not work as effectively as forceps—for instance, during the delivery of a fetus with thick hair or too much molding during labor. In these cases and others, forceps may remain the best choice. On this issue, your physician will need the flexibility to weigh a wide range of benefits and risks—including risks to the fetus—and to make an experienced professional decision.

Choice of Anesthesia

Whether or not they entered their labor suite planning or expecting to receive pain medication, a great number of women will eventually request it. The pros, cons, and controversies surrounding labor anesthesia have been widely discussed, but one aspect of the discussion is particularly relevant to us. Could your choice of anesthesia have an impact on your pelvic floor during childbirth and your function afterward?

INTRAVENOUS AND INTRAMUSCULAR PAIN RELIEF

Demerol, morphine, Nubain, and Fentanyl can provide partial comfort and improve your ability to relax but will not provide numbness equivalent to an epidural. Because lower-body sensation and muscle tone are generally unaffected, there is no reason to suspect that use of these painkillers will impact the course of your labor or the integrity of your pelvic floor.

EPIDURALS

The effect of this popular pain reliever on the overall course of labor has been a subject of debate. Some experts suggest that because epidurals help to relax the pelvic-floor muscles, they may facilitate a smoother and less traumatic delivery. Others have voiced concern that by leaving the delivering mother too numb and unaware of her labor, epidurals may increase her odds of needing assistance with forceps, vacuum, or even a cesarean delivery.

Is there evidence to support this concern? The potential effects of epidurals on perineal injury were assessed in a 1995 study from Brigham and Women's Hospital. Looking back at large numbers of women after delivery of their first baby, the investigators found that severe perineal lacerations occurred in 16 percent of women with epidurals, versus only 9.7 percent of those without. But further analysis showed that this difference most likely resulted from higher rates of episiotomy and forceps and vacuum delivery among women with epidurals. A more recent study, from Switzerland, evaluated eighty-two women during and after their first vaginal delivery. There were no differences in terms of bladder function, pelvic-floor strength, or sexual function when epidural and no-epidural groups were compared ten months after delivery.

In other words, rather than avoiding the epidural per se, avoiding forceps and episiotomy whenever possible appears to be the key to preventing injury in the delivery room. Could epidurals, though, somehow increase your risk of needing a forceps or vacuum delivery? This remains a subject for debate that future research hopefully will settle.

Selecting a Cesarean— *Should You Have the Right to Choose?*

Stop for a moment, refill your coffee cup (acid neutral and decaffeinated, of course), and give a few moments' thought to some eye-opening statistics. First, a 1996 survey of obstetricians published in

The Lancet (a British medical journal), revealed something remarkable about the way doctors view the effects of labor and delivery on the female body. Over 30 percent of female obstetricians in England reported that if faced with a normal full-term pregnancy, they would select cesarean over vaginal delivery. And 80 percent of these individuals cited concern over perineal injury as the main reason behind their choice. Another survey of female gynecologists found, somewhat more modestly, that 16 percent would personally choose cesarean delivery for delivering a full-term, normal-size infant. The reason, again, was pelvic-floor injury—specifically, the desire to prevent incontinence and pelvic prolapse.

The opinions of these female physicians are very telling, but they don't speak for all practitioners. A survey of 135 midwives found that only 6 percent of these practitioners would choose cesarean to protect their pelvic floor. Then again, midwives provide care to women only before and during childbirth—not years later, when the majority of the injuries we've discussed begin to occur.

THE GREAT DEBATE

It's truly a billion-dollar question, sitting right in the middle of a busy societal intersection where medicine, economics, politics, public health, and ethics all converge. Should women have the opportunity to accept the risks of cesarean—both maternal and possibly fetal, which we'll discuss in a moment—in order to possibly reduce their risk of developing incontinence, prolapse, and pelvic-floor dysfunction later on? The concept of routinely performing one major surgery to reduce the possibility of a future one is a big conceptual pill to swallow. Moreover, the notion of a woman choosing the route of childbirth, rather than her doctor, sounds equally foreign to our ears. But doctors, nurses, and others involved with childbirth are debating these ideas in many parts of the world. Their attitudes and conclusions are interesting, if often wildly divergent. Consider, for instance, Dr. W. Benson Harer, president of the American College of Obstetrics and Gynecology arguing on national television in June, 2000 that women should be given the option to choose a cesarean section to prevent injury to the pelvic floor. From a vastly different perspective, the former director of maternal and child health at the World Health

Organization—referring to the runaway cesarean rates in certain parts of South America—described that region's trend toward elective cesareans as an "expensive and dangerous luxury" in a June 2001 *Wall Street Journal* article. The debate has many sides, seasoned with not only medicine but also politics, economics, and ethics.

Let's boil a very complex set of issues down to one simple question: if 31 percent of British female obstetricians would choose a cesarean for themselves if given the option, should you have the right to choose? The views of nonmedical women, like yourself, appear to vary depending on how much information they receive. For instance, one survey found that women with no prior deliveries who were *not* informed of the link between childbirth and pelvic-floor injury would select cesarean only 5 percent of the time. Contrast this with another study, which presented young laywomen with the hypothetical scenario that vaginal delivery would carry a 15 percent risk of urinary incontinence later on. Roughly 50 percent of these women reported that they would choose the operative delivery over the incontinence. Obviously, women who are provided with accurate information tend to make different decisions.

Within our service-oriented society, it's unclear whether physicians should consider offering the "service" of cesarean delivery to patients who request it with the goal of protecting their pelvic floor. In a survey of Israeli physicians, 45 percent supported each woman's right to choose cesarean delivery, and half stated that obstetricians should inform their patients of this right. The bottom line is that in a medical world where other topics, such as hormones, herbs, and cholesterol, are discussed until we're all blue in the face, women deserve at least *some* open discussion of different childbirth strategies and their potential repercussions. Whatever her birthing philosophy or final decision, and whether or not she is permitted to choose cesarean, each woman should at least be provided with enough candid information to have her own educated voice in the debate.

HOW RISKY ARE CESAREANS?

Cesarean delivery under spinal or epidural anesthesia is safer today than at any time in the past, and that's a blessing for women with medical or obstetrical conditions that require one. But make no mistake, a cesarean section is still an operation and still carries risk. Even if the risk of later pelvic-floor or bladder dysfunction could be decreased, at what broad cost would this narrow gain be achieved?

For babies, temporary respiratory problems may be slightly more common when cesareans are performed before labor begins, since squeezing through the birth canal may help to expel amniotic fluid (water) from the baby's lungs. A small risk of a surface skin injury to the newborn during the incision into the uterus is another potential problem, though the great majority leave no lasting mark.

For Mom, cesareans entail higher amounts of blood loss, higher rates of infection and venous blood clots, temporary slowing of bowel function and anemia after delivery, and an overall longer recovery. The chance of needing a hysterectomy due to hemorrhage is increased up to ten times that of vaginal birth, though this complication is quite rare. In the long term, cesareans can cause adhesions (scarring inside the abdomen), which on rare occasion can lead to pain, bowel obstruction, or bladder injury during future operations. Because the degree of scarring may increase a bit after each successive surgery, it's often not the first cesarean that raises concern but rather the ones that follow. One cesarean will most often be followed by future elective cesareans. Future pregnancies may be complicated by abnormal growth of the placenta into the uterine scar (*placenta accreta*), placental separation (*placenta abruption*), growth of the placenta over the cervical opening (*placenta previa*), and rupture of the uterine scar—all of which can cause severe bleeding and serious risks to both baby and Mom. With multiple cesareans, the risks of these disorders can dramatically increase.

The risk of maternal death has fortunately become a rarity for any mode of delivery in the developed world—statistically less likely, in fact, than being struck by lightning. A 1998 study from the United Kingdom reported on more than a hundred and fifty thousand cesarean births performed before labor ever began, and concluded that although the risk of maternal death is extremely low for any delivery route, cesarean carried the greater risk of maternal death. In contrast, a more recent study of more than two hundred and sixty thousand women in Washington State concluded that cesareans were *not* directly responsible for a higher risk of death. Rather, it appeared that women who underwent cesarean were at slightly higher risk only because they entered childbirth with more complex underlying problems—in other words, medical baggage.

Finally, cesarean delivery carries psychological disadvantages for some women. Bypassing the natural birthing process may trigger feelings of failure or guilt, or a diminished sense of womanhood. Others fear that bonding with their newborn may be compromised if their baby enters the world suddenly, through an antiseptic abdominal incision, rather than slowly, through the natural birth canal. For countless others, greeting a newborn baby feels equally gratifying and miraculous, whether it occurs in the labor room or the operating suite. What should be common to all of these individuals, whatever their birthing philosophy, is that they're provided with all of the information necessary to make a truly informed choice.

The bottom line? Cesarean section is major surgery, carrying inherent physical risks from maternal, fetal, and even psychological perspectives. Although these risks are substantially lower than in years past, they remain significant. The debate over cesarean by choice is a perfectly legitimate one, so long as the potential hazards of this operation are never taken lightly.

HOW PROTECTIVE WOULD A CESAREAN REALLY BE?

Another billion-dollar question: do we have any proof that a cesarean would help prevent the postreproductive problems we've discussed? After all, there's reason to suspect that in a substantial number of cases, pregnancy itself may be enough to cause pelvic-floor injury, with the route of delivery playing only a minor role. Not enough research has been devoted to this challenging question in women's health; nevertheless, some basic patterns have become reasonably clear.

NERVE AND MUSCLE FUNCTION

A cesarean delivery can protect against nerve injury and spare muscle function, compared with a vaginal birth. But not all cesareans are equal in terms of their potential benefit. One study of ninety women in their first pregnancy found that when cesareans were performed before labor began, the women were completely protected against pudendal nerve injury; in contrast, cesareans performed after labor had begun resulted in a risk of nerve injury similar to vaginal birth. Other studies have confirmed that late cesareans don't fully eliminate the risk of injury to the pelvic nerves, or even the anal sphincter. The most protective cesareans of all—the ones that help to avoid injury to the key structures of the pelvic floor, and to prevent a number of postreproductive problems—appear to be those performed in the first pregnancy, before labor ever begins. In other words, *timing is key.*

URINARY INCONTINENCE

Though not totally eliminated, stress incontinence is far less common after cesarean, as compared with vaginal birth. One of the few studies examining this topic found that 24 percent of women were incontinent of urine three months after vaginal delivery, compared with only 5 percent after cesarean. A report from Britain tracked the symptoms of 1,169 women before and six months after their first childbirth. Impressively, cesareans performed before the onset of labor were associated with only 40 percent of the risk of stress incontinence seen after uneventful vaginal births, and lowered the frequency of accidental leakage by two thirds. A recent study of mothers of multiples found a 50 percent lower rate of urinary stress incontinence among those whose deliveries were all cesarean. A recent report from Washington State found that women undergoing cesarean reported a 60 percent decreased risk of urinary-voiding dysfunction (rather broadly defined as either urinary incontinence or difficulty emptying) during the postpartum period.

ANAL AND RECTAL INJURIES

Serious injuries to the anal sphincter are nearly nonexistent after elective cesareans that are performed before labor begins. But since "cesareans for all" could never be justified for this protective purpose alone, the challenge is to identify those women most at risk. For instance, it's been felt that for women carrying babies larger than four thousand grams, the benefits of cesarean may outweigh the risks. A 2003 decision analysis from the University of Louisville recently tested this assumption, concluding that a policy of elective cesarean delivery does appear to be a medically sound strategy for preventing anal incontinence among first-time mothers with babies larger than

4500 grams. Others argue against elective cesarean for this purpose, estimating that approximately twenty-three unnecessary cesarean deliveries would be performed to prevent a single woman from developing fecal incontinence.

THE MOST IMPORTANT DATA: YOUR FEELINGS!

Many women suffering prolapse or incontinence feel in retrospect that they would have strongly considered cesarean over vaginal delivery if they could have been assured of some protection against postreproductive problems. But for each of these individuals, a handful of others wouldn't change a thing about their vaginal birth experience. Childbirth will always be viewed through the lens of not only science and medicine but also politics, diehard opinions, and ultimately, very personal choices.

VAGINAL BIRTH AFTER CESAREAN: A PENDULUM OF POLICY STILL IN SWING

Vaginal birth after cesarean section (VBAC) has been an obstetrical topic mired in controversy. Up until the past few decades, VBAC was rarely attempted, due to the concern that the previous uterine incision might rupture under the forces of labor, risking a catastrophic situation for both mother and baby. As a result, few doctors deviated from the golden rule: once a cesarean, always a cesarean. But over the years, it became clear that VBAC could succeed for the majority of women who tried it—and although uterine rupture remained a potentially catastrophic event, the chances of it happening appeared small (0.5 percent if a standard low-horizontal uterine incision was made).

So the trends began to reverse. In 1987 the National Institutes of Health delivered a statement actively promoting VBAC as a safe and desirable alternative. The American College of Obstetricians and Gynecologists followed in 1998, with guidelines making VBAC a preferred rather than optional strategy for most women with a prior cesarean. A study of twenty-nine thousand Swedish women with prior cesareans seemed to bolster that shift in policy, since having a repeat cesarean was shown to triple the risk of needing an emergency hysterectomy due to unexpected hemorrhage, as compared with

VBAC. From 1989 to 1996, the rate of vaginal birth after cesarean rose by 50 percent. Insurance providers, managed-care organizations, and hospitals recognized VBAC as one of the ripest opportunities to lower the cesarean-delivery rate and rein in obstetrical costs. Patients and professionals were reeducated to expect an attempted vaginal delivery for women with a previous cesarean; not surprisingly, many women valuing the idea of natural birth met those trends with great enthusiasm. Entire books since then have been devoted to helping women achieve VBAC, and the range of situations considered suitable for attempting it has consistently widened. A recent Canadian study indicated that even women who underwent previous cesarean for a labor that failed to progress during the second stage—a group that earlier studies had identified as unlikely to succeed with VBAC— could achieve a vaginal birth up to 75 percent of the time in a modern obstetrical setting.

Yet with the latest swing of the pendulum, new concerns have been brought to the fore. Just because we can succeed with VBAC most of the time, should we? A 1996 study of more than six thousand women fueled the new debate, concluding that certain fetal complications (mainly fetal distress resulting from rupture of the uterine scar) were more common with VBAC than with a second elective cesarean. A 2001 study from *The New England Journal of Medicine*, the largest study to date, found that VBAC was riskier to both mother and child than a second surgical delivery in terms of uterine rupture, particularly if labor was induced with certain medications. Among the unfortunate women who had uterine rupture in this study, the rate of infant death increased tenfold. The risk of uterine rupture, though still small, has been on the rise as the practice of VBAC gained in popularity, even tripling in the state of Massachusetts between 1985 and 1995.

The ongoing push for VBAC has not been sufficiently scrutinized in one very important way: what are its effects on the overall risks for pelvic-floor injury and postreproductive problems? Not all cesareans are one and the same. Some may have been performed for reasons unrelated to the fit between mother and baby that aren't present the next time around, such as an abnormal fetal heart rhythm or breech presentation. Other cesareans are necessitated by bodily features and limitations of pelvic shape that don't change much from one pregnancy to the next, such as an android pelvis or a narrow pubic arch.

Could a cesarean for stalled labor during second stage sometimes indicate a pelvic shape that makes a smooth vaginal delivery no more likely with the next try? One Canadian study involving 214 such patients recently reported that VBAC can be achieved 75.2 percent of the time. But the question is, at what cost? In this study, the rate of forceps or vacuum delivery was fairly high, at 15 percent, and no mention was made of how long it took to achieve the vaginal birth or how these factors might affect pelvic-floor function. Many other questions remain unexplored. For instance, should an incontinent woman whose last labor arrested after many hours be automatically encouraged to try for vaginal birth again? A recent study from the University of North Carolina reported higher rates of stress incontinence, and worse quality-of-life scores, among women delivering by VBAC, compared to those having another cesarean. Sexual dysfunction was also more common after VBAC. More research is needed to clarify the relationship among VBAC, incontinence and prolapse, and other aspects of pelvic-floor function.

In 1999 the American College of Obstetricians and Gynecologists issued a statement rejecting an overall mandate for VBAC and stressing the importance of an individualized decision for each woman in each pregnancy. The National Center for Health Statistics has reported a small decline in the VBAC rate over the past few years—though whether this trend is significant is yet unknown. Wherever the pendulum may be when your due date arrives, individualize your decision making. Ask about the reasons for your last cesarean, the possible role of your pelvic shape, and any other reasons why your odds for a successful delivery might be different this time around.

CESAREANS A CURE-ALL? FORGET IT!

Incontinence, prolapse, and other pelvic-floor disorders are, as you've seen, very common among women who have had a vaginal childbirth. But are you aware that up to 5 percent of women who have never given birth by any route report incontinence? Or that a loss of bladder control may arise in up to 9 percent of women who have had a previous cesarean section alone? A number of experts have challenged the notion that labor and vaginal delivery are the most critical factors in the development of incontinence, and they propose that pregnancy and childbirth by either route may be enough to tip the tenuous balance of a healthy pelvic floor. Indeed, although birth mode is an important factor, certain women may be destined to develop incontinence regardless of their obstetrical road. As a result, cesareans are by no means a risk-free, clear-cut panacea for solving the problem of pelvic-floor injury. Determining the "best" obstetrical strategies will require ongoing debate and further research.

7

After Delivery

HOW TO MOST FULLY HEAL AND PREVENT PELVIC-FLOOR PROBLEMS DURING THE POSTPARTUM PERIOD AND BEYOND

I used to be able to do thirty-two changements (jumps) in ballet class; now, after the birth of my twins, I can't sneeze or cough without wetting my panties.

—Letter from Australia

After you strain a back muscle, common sense tells you to avoid heavy lifting for at least a week or two. After you finish the Boston Marathon, the days that follow should be filled with ice packs, rest, and massage. But despite the remarkable level of stress endured by your lower body during labor and delivery—leaving behind stitches and bruises, swollen muscles and battered nerves—most women devote little attention to recuperation. You can do better. Starting right after childbirth, be sure to consider some basic ways to care for yourself and help your pelvic floor get back to normal.

Starting With Postpartum Rehab

HEALING FOR YOUR PERINEUM

If you've had a laceration or an episiotomy, apply ice packs to the perineum for the first forty-eight hours to reduce swelling. Try ten minutes at a time followed by a twenty-minute rest. When you're lying in bed or on the couch, elevate your legs.

Hygiene is essential to proper healing. Keep the perineum clean and generally dry, with frequent pad changes to avoid infection and early breakdown of your stitches, which take several weeks to dissolve. Avoid the temptation to use lotions or ointments, and keep hemorrhoid creams away from the stitches. Don't directly scrub the healing area, and when drying your bottom, pat the area rather than wiping. Before you leave the hospital, the doctor or nurse will usually specify whether you should be cleaning with showers, sitz baths, or tub baths. Once again, simple is best. Lotions, soaps, and bath oils are unnecessary and may irritate your vulvar skin.

HEALING FOR THE PELVIC FLOOR

As you've already learned, the real action during childbirth takes place out of our view, closer to the bottom of the pelvic-floor "iceberg"—the levator muscles, fascia supports, and nerve supply. Well, your pelvic floor just finished the Boston Marathon, and it's time to give it the TLC it deserves.

RESUME KEGEL EXERCISES

Restoring the tone of your pelvic-floor muscles after each delivery will reacquaint you with the levator muscles and strengthen them at a time that they're most prone to neglect. One study discovered the rather discouraging fact that almost 79 percent of women were unable to properly contract their pelvic-floor muscles a year after childbirth.

With a bit of exercise during the postpartum months, the odds of your restoring this function before it's forever lost will increase dramatically. Strong levator muscles will help prevent vaginal laxity and give you the best resistance to postreproductive symptoms before they ever arise. Getting back to strong pelvic exercises will also restore your ability to brace the pelvic muscles and prevent urine leakage during sudden moments of stress or strain, a reflex that can be lost as the perineum and vagina heal.

Pelvic-floor education after vaginal delivery—in other words, having the doctor or nurse show you how to contract the correct muscles and get you started on a pelvic-floor exercise routine—has been shown to significantly reduce symptoms of stress urinary incontinence. One Swiss study demonstrated that this type of program, begun two months postpartum, reduced incontinence symptoms from 19 to 2 percent of women. A study from New Zealand indicated that an intensive pelvic-exercise program involving personal instruction and multiple daily workouts may be more effective than simple instruction. After one year, the intensive exercisers experienced less urinary incontinence, fecal incontinence, and lower levels of anxiety and depression. However, this study, like most others, showed that incontinence symptoms will improve only as long as you continue the exercise routine.

GOOD BOWEL HABITS

The way you empty is important after delivery. Avoid constipation to minimize the amount of straining against the levator muscles, pelvic nerves, and any perineal stitches. Some women may be instructed to support the perineum from the front side, with a flattened hand, during bowel movements. If you do so, just beware of soiling this area. Using plenty of dietary fiber and stool softeners, along with occasional laxatives or suppositories as needed, will hopefully make straining unnecessary and keep your perineal stitches safe. See chapter 10 for more tips on avoiding constipation.

DON'T DENY IT—YOU'RE HEALING!

We live in a society that places great value on a back-in-the-saddle spirit. Although that's a positive trend in many ways, the reality after childbirth is a bit more complex. It's wise to step back, consider the amount of healing taking place in your body, and do what you can to optimize your chances for full healing of your pelvic floor.

Work and Exercise Sensibly

After surgery in the pelvic area, women are usually instructed in great detail about what to do and what not to do to promote the strongest healing. Yet after delivering a newborn baby through the pelvis, you rarely hear about the rights and wrongs of physical activity in the same way. Although childbirth is a natural event if ever there was one, your physical recuperation is not unlike recovery after pelvic surgery—especially if you've had a long labor, a large laceration, or an episiotomy. In these cases, you're swollen and sore, and have stitches temporarily holding together parts of your lower body that you'd like to function as normally as possible for many years ahead. Leaping into a full and strenuous routine may stress these areas before they have a chance to properly heal.

Avoid Lifting

For new mothers, this may be the most practical and realistic single guideline: don't lift anything (or anyone) heavier than your baby. Don't make all of the countless new physical tasks—such as carrying the crib upstairs, baby-proofing the furniture, and hauling groceries—your sole responsibility during those first few weeks. That's what a partner, friends, and family are for.

Minimize Physical Stress

Position your baby's changing table and bathtub at waist level. Brace your pelvic floor if you happen to suddenly cough, sneeze, laugh, or lift (see Appendix A).

Exercise Right

The average woman gains twenty-five to thirty pounds during pregnancy; that weight (especially the last five to ten pounds) probably won't be shed immediately afterward. With a reasonable routine, you can bounce back while allowing these vulnerable areas of your body to properly heal.

- *After two weeks.* This is a great time to resume a walking routine: for example, thirty minutes each day with your baby. Your doctor may also approve pelvic tilts (see chapter 4) and mild abdominal exercises (like partial sit-ups) during this time. Twenty-minute light-duty workout sessions, three times a week, are a great start.

  If you had no exercise routine before or during pregnancy, start more slowly. Don't be hard on yourself or do too much too soon at this time, when your energies are needed for so much else. Also, if normal postpartum bleeding *(lochia)* becomes heavier, lighten up your exercise routine for a few more weeks.

- *After six weeks.* Check with your doctor or midwife about returning to more vigorous aerobic and muscle-strengthening routines, swimming, and bike riding, if you feel ready. Balance abdominal exercises (sit-ups and crunches) with lower-back strengthening. If you notice a wide space between your stomach muscles, have your doctor check it out at the next routine visit (separation of the abdominal muscles is fairly common).

  Fast-paced walking, weight training with light dumbbells, push-ups, postpartum yoga, and other resistance exercises are usually allowed. Exercise classes taught by postpartum specialists are increasingly popular. They focus on low-impact routines with nonstressful stretching and toning. At home, try an exercise video specifically geared to postpregnancy mothers. These group workouts can improve your technique and help make your transition back into shape feel less monotonous.

- *Listen to your body.* Just because the obstetrical textbook says the postpartum period lasts for six weeks does not mean that your healing process abruptly ends. In reality, it may take several months or longer for your energy level and muscle tone to return to their former state.

- *If problems persist, ask the urogynecologist.* If pelvic-floor symptoms become an issue, a number of high-tech treatments can be used even during the postpartum period. Generally speaking, urogynecologists will wait at least six to twelve weeks before recommending most of the therapies you'll read about in the chapters ahead. But it never hurts to ask.

Effects of Breast-feeding on Pelvic-Floor Symptoms

You probably anticipated the cracked skin, soreness, and engorgement that accompany nursing. But you might be surprised to learn that breast-feeding can also cause bladder, pelvic, or sexual symptoms. Lactation triggers a hormonal chain of events that leads the ovaries into a state of hibernation. That's why normal menstrual periods cease and the timing of ovulation becomes unpredictable.

Think of it as nature's own family-planning method, preventing Mom from getting pregnant while she's still caring for a very needy little newborn.

Unfortunately, this drop in estrogen may also cause a few less useful changes in some key pelvic areas. The vaginal skin, when lacking estrogen, becomes thinner, less lubricated, and often a bit irritated, making intercourse uncomfortable or even painful. Likewise, the urethra may become more weak, thin, and floppy. As a result, urinary stress incontinence and urge incontinence may both become more severe while you're nursing.

If you're breast-feeding and notice one such change, start a basic Kegel routine on your own, and use a water-soluble lubricant during intercourse—*then give it some time.* Symptoms that are truly estrogen-related will improve after you've stopped breast-feeding, as the normal function of your ovaries resumes. If your symptoms are mild, a full medical evaluation isn't necessary until a few months after you've finished breast-feeding. If changes down below remain a nuisance at that point, then it's time to see the doctor.

After a Rough Delivery: Managing Your Next Pregnancy

If a previous childbirth left you with postreproductive symptoms, approaching your next pregnancy and delivery can trigger a great deal of uncertainty and even fear. How should you approach the process this time to avoid making your problem worse? Should your next pregnancy be considered high-risk? Should you be thinking in terms of bed rest, extra time off work, or a planned cesarean birth?

FOR PERINEAL INJURIES

Although perineal injuries are most common during a first vaginal birth, as the tissues stretch out for the first time, repeat injuries are a possibility. One study, conducted at the University of Iowa in 1999, analyzed the first and second deliveries of more than four thousand women and discovered that those with a history of severe perineal laceration during their first delivery were 2.3 times more likely to suffer a repeat injury in their next delivery. Women at highest risk were those who underwent forceps, vacuum, or a repeat episiotomy in their second delivery—around one in five suffered a second severe perineal injury. Perineal massage during pregnancy and labor, attention to fetal size and position, and avoiding whenever possible the obstetrical interventions we know to be potentially traumatic, appear to be the most effective strategies.

FOR PROLAPSE

Mild prolapse—in other words, loss of uterine or vaginal supports to some degree—is an absolutely normal occurrence for most postreproductive women. But for women who already have more advanced pelvic prolapse causing problems, whether it's uterine prolapse, a cystocele, or a rectocele, the best strategy for future pregnancies remains a medical question mark. On one hand, studies have shown that pudendal nerve injury can accumulate with later deliveries. On the other hand, the majority of damage has already been done in most cases, and it's unclear which obstetrical interventions, if any, will counteract its progression. There is, at present, no evidence supporting an elective cesarean the next time around. Focusing on symptom relief and following a few simple tips is probably best.

- Understand that you absolutely *can* carry another pregnancy. Severe prolapse should be evaluated in order to determine whether any fertility or obstetrical issues need to be addressed. But prolapse itself should virtually never cause an inability to have another baby.
- To relieve vaginal bulging and prolapse discomfort during your next pregnancy, certain pessaries—for instance, a Smith-Hodge type—can be worn (see chapter 9).
- Limit your activity, especially until later in pregnancy. By eighteen to twenty weeks' gestation, you should feel less pressure as the enlarging uterus rises out of the pelvis and into the abdomen, usually staying up for the remainder of pregnancy. Prolapse symptoms usually improve after this transition.

- Strict bed rest may be recommended for very advanced cases, such as a prolapse bulge visible outside the vaginal opening. Absolutely avoid heavy lifting or straining.

- If your symptoms remain truly debilitating after delivery but you're still planning future pregnancies, then a pessary device (chapter 9) might become an appropriate option to discuss with your doctor. Having prolapse does not affect your ability to have another baby in the future.

FOR URINARY INCONTINENCE

As previously mentioned, one study looking at first pregnancies suggested that cesarean delivery could reduce the risk of incontinence from 25 percent to only 5. Another study showed that among mothers of twins or triplets, avoiding vaginal delivery reduced the risk of urinary stress incontinence from 60 percent to 39. But it's unclear whether postreproductive women who already have stress incontinence can prevent its progression by requesting a cesarean for the next birth.

FOR ANAL SYMPTOMS

Let's assume that an episiotomy or spontaneous perineal tear caused an injury to your anal sphincter. Will you be likely to experience the same injury during another vaginal birth, increasing your odds for anal incontinence or other pelvic-floor symptoms down the road? It has indeed been confirmed using ultrasound that a good number of hidden anal sphincter injuries occur during second deliveries, some of which may lead to anal-incontinence symptoms. As already mentioned, other studies have indicated that function of the pudendal nerve may diminish. At least to some degree, postobstetrical injury to this area of the body can accumulate from birth to birth. Your first trip to the labor room may be the most important, but a second or third delivery can cause new symptoms to arise, old ones to recur, or existing ones to worsen.

One 1999 study from Ireland published in *The Lancet* addressed this issue, tracking a group of women with some fecal incontinence after their first vaginal birth. For those who still had the problem at the time of their next pregnancy, almost all noticed that it became more severe afterward. For those women whose fecal incontinence had resolved by their second pregnancy, the second birth led to recurrence 40 percent of the time. The risk of having a cesarean was not studied, so it's uncertain how protective it would have been. On a slightly more hopeful note, another study estimated that only around 24 percent of women with anal incontinence after childbirth will find it aggravated after a subsequent delivery.

OPINIONS, OPINIONS

Some experts have suggested that every woman with postpartum anal incontinence should be offered cesarean delivery. After all, loss of bowel control is arguably the most distressing of all postreproductive pelvic-floor problems, and if we can help prevent its progression, then why not do so? According to physician surveys, the opinions you'll find on these subjects vary widely, depending on where you seek your advice. Surveys have revealed, for instance, that up to 71 percent of colorectal surgeons would advise women with previous anal injuries to deliver by cesarean, whereas only 22 percent of obstetricians would make the same recommendation. What about planning an episiotomy to protect a previously repaired anal sphincter? Only 1 percent of colorectal surgeons think it's a good idea, compared with 30 percent of obstetricians. Of course, there is a myriad of differences existing between these specialists, shaping their respective attitudes and opinions, and it's difficult to know whose advice is better. Hopefully, tomorrow's research will help doctors and their patients to reach a better scientific consensus on these and other questions of preventive obstetrics. In the meantime, find a provider who takes the time to discuss your situation, present the alternatives, and help shape a plan that feels most comfortable and rational to you.

Preventive Obstetrics of the Future: In Search of Red Flags

Each woman's body is different in shape, strength, and resiliency, and each new pregnancy and birth involves a completely unique fetal size, shape, and position. That's why we've put men on the moon but still are challenged by the task of predicting the precise physical impact of pregnancy, labor, and delivery on individual women. On the wonderful journey of childbirth—just like on that Hawaiian vacation—it's quite possible to still get burned, despite our best efforts.

You've learned, however, that there are prevention strategies that you can utilize during your reproductive years—perhaps not one simple cure-all like sunscreen, but a combination of diet, exercise, communication, and planning. A mind-set of prevention before, during, and after childbirth will make you more secure and more empowered, whether you're trying to prevent an initial injury or deal with symptoms.

TONE UP YOUR PELVIC FLOOR BEFORE, DURING, AND AFTER CHILDBIRTH

A regular pelvic-floor workout routine can prevent symptoms at each of these stages. In Appendix A, you'll learn step by step how to start your Kegel exercise program.

TRY PERINEAL MASSAGE

Start during pregnancy. It's right at your fingertips, costs nothing, and just might reduce your risk of perineal injury during childbirth.

AVOID EPISIOTOMIES

Over 50 percent of women in the United States have an episiotomy along with their first delivery, and that's unfortunate. As we discussed in chapter 3, there's a mountain of evidence indicating that this procedure is best to avoid whenever possible: for preserving pelvic-floor muscle strength, to prevent severe lacerations in the rectum, and to safeguard sexual function.

The American College of Obstetricians and Gynecologists formally stated in March 2000 that routine episiotomy should not be considered a part of current obstetrical practice. However, selective episiotomy remains an invaluable obstetrical tool, and in many cases, it represents the best care.

UNDERSTAND OTHER OBSTETRICAL FACTORS

We've explored the links between pelvic-floor function and forceps delivery, prolonged labor, macrosomia (very large fetal size), pelvic shape, and various styles for labor and delivery. As you plan for childbirth and its accompanying decisions, keep these factors in mind.

OPTIMIZE YOUR POSTPARTUM HEALING

Promoting an optimal recovery for the pelvic floor after childbirth has been a sorely neglected aspect of women's health care, but you can do better. If you're still having problems after utilizing the basic postpartum strategies discussed earlier in this chapter, then it's time to see the doctor.

COMMUNICATE

Your discussions surrounding forceps, laboring and pushing styles, perineal massage, episiotomies, cesareans, and other birthing practices do make a difference. Speak up, discuss the issues with your doctor or midwife, and make your feelings clear. Then—most importantly—understand that your provider may still need to rely on an unexpected strategy at the time of delivery. Although an intervention might not have been part of your best-laid childbirth plans, it will have been done to assure the safest birth for you and the baby.

Predicting and preventing pelvic-floor problems will, in the future, represent an increasingly principal task for the obstetrician and midwife. Perhaps through advances in prenatal pelvimetry and ultrasound, or through techniques that are yet to be discovered, the physical effects of childbirth and the likelihood of a postreproductive problem will be more accurately forecasted. With these advances, physicians and midwives will be better able to recommend vaginal delivery to some women and cesarean birth to others, and perhaps more effectively balance the pros and cons of forceps, episiotomy, and other obstetrical procedures. As our understanding continues to improve, the obstetrical red flags alerting mothers and their doctors to potential postobstetrical problems will become more comprehensible and reliable.

"I'm Way Past Prevention!": *Moving Ahead and Finding Relief*

In just a few short chapters, you've learned what's happened down there, and you have a good idea of how it all happened. You've bridged the gap between Ob and Gyn by understanding how physical changes that often occur during pregnancy and childbirth may connect with postreproductive symptoms. You've considered strategies for before, during, and after childbirth that might help prevent symptoms from arising. For those of you already having problems despite your best efforts at prevention, or those of you whose pregnancy and childbirth occurred years ago, let's explore the burning issue that brought you to the bookshelf in the first place: how to alleviate your symptoms and feel better—starting today!

PART 3

FINDING RELIEF FROM URINARY INCONTINENCE, PELVIC PROLAPSE, ANAL INCONTINENCE, AND SEXUAL DYSFUNCTION

THE WIDE WORLD OF SOLUTIONS, FROM
SIMPLE HOME REMEDIES TO THE
DOCTOR'S OFFICE AND OPERATING ROOM

ᔈ 8 ᔈ

Urinary Incontinence

UNDERSTANDING YOUR LEAKAGE AND RESTORING
CONTROL USING HEALTHY HABITS,
SIMPLE TIPS, AND HIGH-TECH THERAPY IN THE
DOCTOR'S OFFICE AND OPERATING ROOM

*How can you wear sexy underpanties when you're always wearing a pad?
I want to feel like a woman again.*

—Forty-one-year-old, before her operation
for urinary stress incontinence

*I gave up my walking routine . . . and keeping dry on business trips—
especially on airplanes—has become a major challenge. I've got to do
something!*

—Fifty-four-year-old, during her first office visit

Not long ago, a sixty-one-year-old woman came to the office, "at wit's end" over her long-standing pelvic prolapse and urinary incontinence. She'd "had it" with pads, and fear over accidents had taken the joy out of her regular walking routine. In the corner of the room sat her thirty-four-year-old daughter, herself a nurse at a nearby hospital, with, on her lap, her own four-month-old baby. I shared a simple anatomy sketch and explained the nature of the symptoms the older woman had experienced for the past thirty years. After we made a few arrangements for testing, our visit drew to a close. As I headed down the hallway, her chart in my hand, I felt a tap on my shoulder. It was the daughter. She'd been keeping her baby fully occupied with a rattle and a bottle of milk throughout the visit, as she closely followed my discussion with her mother.

Now she asked if she could have just another moment of my time: "By the way . . . since *my* daughter was born, *I've* been leaking sometimes when I cough or bend down to lift her up from the stroller. Is there anything I can do to avoid all this stuff my mom is going through?"

It was a question that most women with these early problems never find the opportunity to ask. I was glad this woman had—that along with caring for her daughter, she was also thinking about herself. After all, it had taken her mother a full three decades to seek help. Yes, I answered, there were things she could do to feel better, to avoid a bigger problem and "all this stuff" that her mother was facing. The way she worked and exercised, her choice of foods and beverages, her bathroom habits—all of these might have an impact. Whether you've recently noticed a loss of bladder control or have been struggling with symptoms for many years, familiarize yourself with all that can be done at home, in the office, and in the operating room to maximize your quality of life.

The Four Types of Urinary Incontinence: Understanding Your Problem and Finding Relief

TYPE #1: STRESS INCONTINENCE

As a young girl, I remember losing urine when jumping on a trampoline. But since childbirth, it's been a regular problem.
                    —Forty-one-year-old, during her first office visit

Although the symptom of stress incontinence (leakage at the moment of a cough, a sneeze, or other sudden physical stress) might not arise until years after pregnancy and childbirth, countless women can trace the physical changes setting the stage for incontinence back to their obstetrical past. According to a Danish study of more than three thousand women, two thirds of those with stress incontinence recalled that their condition began during pregnancy or just after childbirth. A study of nearly twenty-eight thousand women from Norway found that after just one childbirth, the risk of stress incontinence rose nearly threefold among those between the ages of twenty and thirty-four. According to a large study from the 1960s, 65 percent of women with stress incontinence first reported their symptoms during pregnancy, and 14 percent recalled that their leakage problems began during the postpartum period. Other studies have found that for women between the ages of thirty and forty-five, a history of vaginal childbirth carries a two-to-five-times higher risk of having stress incontinence.

Even if you've never had a child, you're not without risk for developing a loss of bladder control, particularly as you advance in age. Consider the survey of nuns that showed nearly half reporting some degree of urinary incontinence by the average age of sixty-eight. Although childbirth is the biggest factor leading to stress incontinence, it's not the only one. So don't swear celibacy or join the convent just yet.

TIPPING THE BALANCE OF CONTINENCE

To understand why stress incontinence becomes so common after childbirth, let's take a look at the basics of continence. What allows you to have normal control over your bladder in the first place? Whether you're coughing, lifting, or just trying to make it to the ladies' room during a powerful urge, your ability to hold it in boils down to a simple requirement: the urethra must stay closed and maintain a pressure between its closed walls that is stronger than the pressure building up in your bladder. It's similar to pinching the neck of a water balloon closed, to keep the water from leaking out. Simple, right?

Unfortunately, it's not so simple. Even before the physical stresses of childbirth, the maintenance of dryness is rather tenuous. Can you look back to childhood and recall a few times you laughed too hard at a slumber party and felt a dribble? Does the crossing-your-legs maneuver—womankind's most ancient method of incontinence prevention—ring a bell? Do you feel that you've often just gotten by on preventing an accident?

The illustration on page 123 shows the components necessary for good control at any age: a well-behaved bladder and a healthy urethra lying upon a strong vaginal wall. When these conditions exist, you'll have the best odds of creating enough pressure in the urethra to hold back the force of urine—even, for instance, when you're challenged with a full bladder during a tennis serve. These optimal conditions can be difficult to maintain. The anatomy of the female bladder and urethra places women at higher risk than men for developing stress incontinence. In fact, men are born with several innate advantages for maintaining dryness until their latter years—a longer urethra and a firm prostate rather than a flexible vagina lying beneath the urethral tube. But still, why such a steep rise in problems among women advancing in age?

Enter pregnancy, labor, and delivery—the likes of which men's bodies never have to withstand. As you'll come to appreciate, if you haven't already, the vagina, urethra, and bladder are among the areas of your body most exposed and susceptible to wear and tear through the process of childbirth. Like that last straw on the camel's back, the changes that occur during pregnancy and childbirth are often enough to tip the balance that had been keeping you dry.

STRESS INCONTINENCE: A MAJOR PROBLEM FOR YOUNG AND ACTIVE WOMEN

According to a 2001 nationwide survey conducted by the National Association for Continence, and sponsored by Eli Lilly & Company, 40 percent of women with the condition report that their problems started before age forty.

THE FLOPPY URETHRA

If you've developed stress incontinence during or after childbirth, one particular anatomical change is the most common culprit: weakening of the vaginal wall that lies beneath the urethra and provides its main support. Doctors refer to this problem as *urethral hypermobility*—meaning that the urethra is too mobile due to weakening of the vaginal wall beneath it. For the sake of simplicity, we'll call it the *floppy urethra*. It accounts for the largest number of stress incontinence cases in postreproductive women, and it's very much a product of pregnancy and childbirth.

To understand how and why this is the case, consider an analogy often described to patients in the doctor's office: the garden hose on the grass. Imagine you've returned from a weeklong vacation to find that your neighbor's six-year-old son, Kenny, whom you'd paid to water your flower and vegetable garden, has left a garden hose running in your backyard. After paying the taxi driver and setting down your suitcases, you raise your eyes to see water flooding your lawn and running like a suburban waterfall through your cellar window into your finished basement. You'd like very much, to say the least, to stop the flow of water in an expeditious manner. Rather than running around back to find the faucet valve, you hurry to the nearest loop of garden hose you can find on the ground, and step on it as hard as you can.

Now, if the garden hose was left lying on top of your driveway, your task is relatively easy—stepping down with minimal force, you compress the hose shut. Problem solved. On the other hand, imagine that Kenny left the hose lying on grass that hadn't been cut for weeks. In this case, you step on the hose, then a bit more firmly, and become quickly frustrated to see that the water has slowed but not yet stopped. You'll need to apply a much greater pressure—possibly even using the weight of your whole body upon your heel—to fully compress the hose as it sinks into the tall green grass. During the time it takes you to create this pressure, your basement continues to flood.

With that analogy in mind, take a look at the support of the urethra on the vaginal wall right beneath it. Like a garden hose, your urethra can lie across either a strong and intact upper vaginal wall, or a weakened vaginal surface. Childbirth causes this stretching and

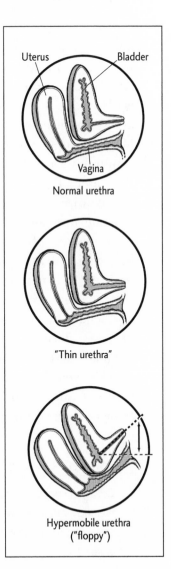

(Above) "Normal" urethra. (Center and Below) Changes leading to stress incontinence

weakening of the vaginal walls from their supports, thus reducing the firmness of the urethra's floor. When lying on a weakened vaginal wall, the floppy urethra sinks downward with the force of a cough, sneeze, or tennis serve, but is unable to compress itself shut. Luckily, the floppy urethra, while a very common cause of postreproductive incontinence, is also one of the most treatable.

THE THIN-WALLED URETHRA

The second major cause of stress urinary incontinence is thinning and weakening of the walls of the urethra. Imagine your garden hose again, but this time an older one with years of exposure to the elements, its rubber walls thin, dry, and brittle. The rigid, dry-walled hose is more open and less compressible. Even if it's lying across the firm pavement, without some rubbery thickness within to help compress the inner surfaces of the hose together, this hose would have a difficult time forming a watertight seal to hold back the water's flow.

Likewise, your urethra requires some thickness within its walls to function normally. If your urethral walls become too thin and lose their spongy softness, they won't effectively compress and seal to keep you dry. Stress incontinence due to a *thin-walled urethra* has been given a number of fancy names, including sphincteric deficiency, a low-pressure urethra, or drainpipe urethra. By any name, it's thought by many doctors to reflect a more severe type of incontinence—a gush rather than a squirt with a cough, or leakage with minimal exertion such as casual walking.

This type of incontinence usually calls for a different set of outpatient and surgical treatments, the objective of which is to re-create some thickness in the urethral walls.

YOU OUGHTA BE IN PICTURES

Collagen injections may look pretty good in Melanie Griffith's pillowy lips; but they can look even better in the urethra. Whether you're a Hollywood diva, a working woman, or a soccer mom, nothing is more beautiful than being dry!

If I Had Stress Incontinence During Pregnancy, Will It Become Permanent?

Experiencing stress incontinence for the first time during or right after your first pregnancy is by no means a guarantee that you're destined for leakage over the long run. But for large numbers of women, incontinence that arises in association with childbirth will eventually persist as a long-term problem, whether it's months, years, or even decades later.

When do you begin to worry? If you're still noticing leakage when you're lifting your baby at five months, eight months, or one year after delivery, you may have to concede that this problem is not going to disappear on its own. Actually, one study of more than three hundred women found that the presence of incontinence symptoms only three months after delivery meant a 94 percent chance that the problem would still exist five years later. That's quite a remarkable statistic.

But it doesn't have to remain that high. If you'd been noticing mild back pain and were informed that unless you began exercises, you had a 94 percent chance of long-term symptoms, wouldn't you pause to learn about proper lifting and physical therapy? Or if you were told about some early signs of bone loss, wouldn't you modify your diet and exercise routine to hopefully prevent osteoporosis and future fractures?

As with your bones and heart, prevention and planning deserve a place in the pelvis. If you're still bothered by incontinence after all of your postpartum visits, whether it's six months or six years later, optimism alone probably won't solve your problem. As with preventing osteoporosis, high cholesterol, or chronic back pain, you should take the time to evaluate your habits, assess your goals, and adopt a plan to preserve the long-term health and function of your pelvic floor. With the help of home exercises, office therapy, simple devices, and remarkable new procedures, *you can be dry.*

STRESS INCONTINENCE: IS IT VAGINAL CHILDBIRTH OR JUST PREGNANCY THAT INCREASES YOUR RISK?

Stress incontinence absolutely does occur among women who have delivered their children by cesarean—and even in some women who have no children. But labor and vaginal delivery *do* appear to increase your risk.

One survey of more than fifteen hundred women showed that twelve weeks after their first delivery, those who had a cesarean were less likely to be incontinent (5.2 percent) compared with those who had vaginal birth (24.5 percent). Other studies have arrived at similar conclusions, including one from Nova Scotia, which found that six months after a first childbirth, women who delivered vaginally had nearly three times the risk of incontinence compared to those who delivered by cesarean. Among women having twins or triplets, avoiding vaginal delivery reduces the risk by 50 percent. Despite these trends, as you've already learned, the issue of when to consider a cesarean to protect your body is far from simple, but it may be an important one to address.

MEDICATIONS FOR STRESS URINARY INCONTINENCE

Whether due to a urethra that's floppy or thin, stress incontinence is not often treatable with medication. Nevertheless, a few over-the-counter pills can improve mild stress incontinence.

- *Pseudoephedrine, ephedrine (Sudafed, Ephedrine).* This adrenergic medication, contained in a variety of over-the-counter cold, flu, and diet pills, has an effect similar to adrenaline. By improving muscle tone around the bladder neck and urethra, it can occasionally improve control over stress incontinence.

  These drugs can make you feel like you've just polished off a double café latte. The list of potential side effects includes agitation, insomnia, heart palpitations, elevated blood pressure, and confusion, among others. Even though these medications are available over the counter, they can be dangerous if you have high blood pressure or thyroid or heart problems. Be sure to read the package labeling and speak to your doctor before trying one on your own.

- *Phenylpropanolamine.* This caffeinelike medication was available until recently in many prescription and over-the-counter cold, cough, and allergy medications, and was shown to improve stress leakage for some women. However, FDA approval was recently withdrawn due to potentially serious side effects, including strokes. Phenylpropanolamine should no longer be used.

- *Imipramine (Tofranil).* This medication, which will be discussed mainly for its role in the treatment of urge incontinence, can also have occasional benefit for treating mild stress incontinence.

- *New possibilities.* Research trials are under way for medications that may provide more selective benefit to the bladder—in other words, targeting it with fewer side effects elsewhere in the body. One medication under investigation, Duloxitene, has shown a decreased frequency of incontinence episodes as compared with placebo. However, at the present time, the most effective treatments for stress incontinence are the wide variety of minimally invasive operations, office procedures, or simple devices, all of which physically support the urethra in some way.

IMPROVING STRESS INCONTINENCE THROUGH EXERCISE, PHYSICAL THERAPY, AND OTHER NONSURGICAL METHODS

Over half of women evaluated for incontinence will ultimately be nonsurgically treated. Beyond medications, the wide range of options available at the doctor's office—involving no scalpels, staples, or stitches—might help to put this postreproductive problem in its proper place and get you back to enjoying life again.

KEGEL EXERCISES

When it comes to treating stress urinary incontinence in the *least* invasive way—without the use of any devices, medications, or surgery—there is one time-tested technique that you need be an expert on, if you're not already: the Kegel exercise. Even if you ultimately select a more high-tech approach to your stress incontinence, pelvic-floor exercises can start you on the road to improving not only stress incontinence but also a number of other pelvic symptoms.

Kegel exercises are, in simplest terms, a physical workout for the pelvic floor. Their ability to improve mild urinary stress incontinence is clear. In order to maximize their impact, approach them with a structured exercise routine, just like signing up at the gym.

BEFORE GOING ANY FURTHER . . .

Turn to Appendix A, where you'll learn about Kegel exercises, how to get started, and all the dos and don'ts. Pelvic-floor exercises can be used alongside almost any other treatment for stress incontinence and won't cost you a dime.

Vaginal Cones and Biofeedback

For women who are motivated to give Kegel exercises a try but run into trouble finding and strengthening the right muscles, a few devices can help. *Vaginal cones* are small devices of varying weights that are inserted vaginally, improving your ability to work the correct pelvic-floor muscles. *Biofeedback* is a somewhat more high-tech office technique that provides a visual or audio signal when you're flexing the correct muscles of the pelvic floor, and another signal when you're flexing the wrong muscles. Biofeedback and vaginal cones are also covered in Appendix A.

Electrical and Magnetic Stimulation

Another physical therapy–type alternative for treating urinary stress incontinence involves stimulation of the pelvic-floor nerves and muscles. A number of devices using the controlled delivery of either mild electrical currents or magnetic fields can trigger a passive work-out for this area of the body. Rather than flexing your own pelvic-floor muscles, the device does the work for you by zapping your muscles and nerves into action. Because pelvic-floor stimulation can be used for both stress and urge urinary incontinence, it will be discussed in the section on mixed incontinence just ahead. However, this method has been shown to have only varying degrees of success, so it may not be right for you.

Vaginal Continence Devices
(Bladder-Neck Support Prostheses)

Specialized devices similar to a diaphragm have been designed to fit in the vagina and stabilize a floppy urethra and, in so doing, relieve urinary stress incontinence. Like any other indwelling vaginal device, they need to be regularly removed and cleansed, and can be worn only if enough vaginal and perineal support remains to hold them in place. They're inexpensive and worth a try if you're troubled by stress incontinence but don't want an operation. Remember, these devices are for stress incontinence only, and they will not relieve an overactive bladder or urge incontinence.

- *Continence ring, continence dish.* These devices are shaped like a dish or ring, with a knob on the outer ridge designed to compress the urethra between the vaginal wall and pubic bone during a cough, sneeze, or other moment of sudden stress.

- *Introl.* This flexible, ringlike device is inserted into the vagina like a diaphragm, with its two fingerlike prongs facing up toward the bladder. By stabilizing the upper vaginal wall and supporting a floppy urethra, 83 percent of stress-incontinent women may see improvement, according to one clinical trial.

- *Pessaries.* These vaginal devices, typically used for supporting prolapse bulges—which you'll learn about in chapter 9—can be used to manage urinary stress incontinence. A Smith-Hodge pessary, with a shape that gives more support to the bladder outlet than most other pessary types, is a common choice.

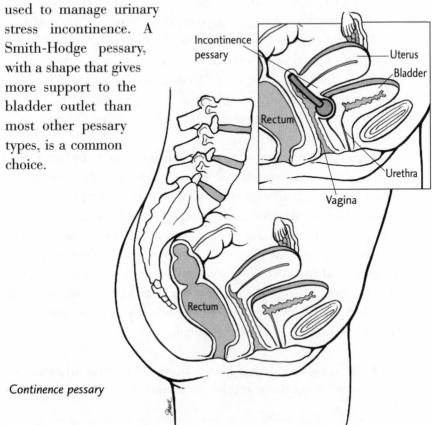

Continence pessary

- *Balloon-shaped tampons.* These have recently been developed for treating stress incontinence. One such product, the Conti-form device (not available in the United States at this time), can reportedly be left inserted for up to a month, with up to 75 percent of women reporting reduced overall leakage.

WHAT A LITTLE BIT OF PAVEMENT CAN DO

Remember the "garden hose on the grass" explanation for stress incontinence? Continence pessaries act like portable pavement that can be inserted beneath the urethra. By providing a firm surface for the urethra to compress against, one of these simple devices might help you to leave the doctor's office dry.

URETHRAL INJECTIONS

Collagen and "urethral injection" materials can plump up the urethra to treat urinary stress incontinence. This might provide a great option if you're looking to improve your control while avoiding surgery. These procedures are performed in the office, starting with an injection of local anesthesia around the urethra and placement of a catheter-sized telescope (see "Cystoscopy," chapter 13). Then the actual bulking material is injected into the wall of the urethra. By narrowing the garden hose, urethral injections help to create a better seal between its walls.

Urethral injections are generally safe and minimally invasive, allowing you to return home right afterward. If the injection is effective, you should notice the change right away. For doctors, it's truly gratifying when a successful injection allows a woman who walked into the office wet to walk out *dry,* amazed at such a sudden change. The greater challenge of urethral injections, however, is achieving long-term success. Several treatment sessions are usually required to reach dryness, and for most women, periodic booster injections will be necessary.

There are a few popular injection substances on the market, as well as several agents in development.

- *Collagen.* Collagen is a basic fibrous connective-tissue substance found throughout nature in various forms. It has become the most widely used product for urethral injection. Bovine collagen is relatively easy to inject and very well tolerated by the human body. The main disadvantage is its lack of permanence: the longevity of an injection is quite difficult to predict. For some women, the reduced leakage will last only a matter of weeks or months; for others, an injection may last for years. According to one study, improvement or cure was reported by 80 percent of women after one year; after two years, 50 to 69 percent were still improved. Estimates of long-term dryness vary widely, from 25 to 60 percent, depending on the severity of the stress incontinence and the type of injections used. Allergic reactions have been reported on rare occasion, so you will need a skin test several weeks before the first collagen injection.

- *Durasphere.* This newer substance, made of tiny carbon-coated beads suspended in a gel, is an alternative to collagen. Results for treating stress incontinence have been favorable. The major theoretical advantage is that unlike collagen, carbon beads do not dissolve or absorb. However, since the beads can lose their position over time, periodic reinjections may still be needed.

- *Macroplastique.* This product is composed of silicone rubber particles and has been a popular choice in Europe for years. FDA trials in the United States are currently under way, suggesting that Macroplastique might soon be available here.

Are injections for you? If you're in search of a hands-free, pill-free, and surgery-free treatment for simple urinary stress incontinence, then you might think about urethral injections. They can be especially useful for women who continue to have stress incontinence even after surgery, or those with a thin but not floppy urethra. Side effects—such as a thinner urinary stream or an inability to void right after

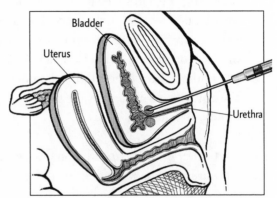

Periurethral injection

the procedure, usually requiring catheterization in the office—are infrequent and seldom serious. Infections or blood clots (hematomas) can occur on rare occasion. Several office visits will probably be necessary over time, since a truly permanent injectable substance does not yet exist.

WHAT *WILL* THEY THINK OF NEXT?

Can you guess what bone, ear cartilage, Teflon, carbon beads, and liposuctioned abdominal-fat globules might have in common? Each has been injected into the urethral wall in an effort to treat stress incontinence. Trials are under way for a number of other experimental substances, including pastes made of synthetic bone and even tiny inflatable balloons that are implanted into the tissues around the urethra; they can be adjusted after insertion depending on the amount of leakage. As researchers continue to develop urethral injections, and if longer-lasting effects can be achieved, you may see more and more women choosing this alternative as a first-choice therapy for incontinence.

BARRIER DEVICES: URETHRAL PATCHES, PADS, AND INSERTS

Patches, pads, and inserts that fit over the urethral opening provide another solution for simple stress incontinence. Though they've been made in various shapes and sizes, they share the goal of occluding the urethral opening, and are meant to be inserted depending on when simple stress leakage is most likely to occur. None of these urethral plugs or patches has ever attracted a large following, perhaps because they don't actually cure the underlying problem; they require more hands-on maintenance than most women are interested in; and they need to be removed if an active bladder or vaginal infection develops. Nevertheless, for those who are bothered by predictable moments of leakage—for instance, on the golf tee, tennis court, or ski slope—these devices may provide a handy alternative.

- *Patches and caps.* These devices, made of soft silicone or foam, are designed to stick over the urethra, creating a seal to block the flow of urine. They are removed before urination, then replaced. Most patches are recommended to be worn for five hours during the daytime and through the night.

- *Impress Softpatch.* A small disposable foam pad coated with a gentle adhesive.

- *FemAssist.* A nipple-shaped suction cup that affixes to the flat area around the urethral opening and sticks with the help of a bit of lubricating jelly.

- *CapSure.* Another suction-cup shield, which has demonstrated good success for reducing stress leakage.

- *Plugs and inserts.* These devices fit into rather than over the urethra, and need to be fitted by a physician. They're slightly more intrusive than a simple patch but may prove more stable during activity. They may provide a useful alternative to pads.

- *Reliance urinary control device.* A mini catheter that inserts into the urethra like a tampon and seals it shut like a cork. To urinate, a string is pulled to deflate the small balloon holding the device in place. The device is replaced around three times each day and removed before intercourse.

- *FemSoft.* A narrow silicone tube, surrounded by a soft sleeve containing mineral oil, which inserts into the urethra. Once inserted, the mineral oil pouches out the sleeve within the bladder, forming a tiny balloon that holds it in place. It's intended for onetime use.

COMMITTING TO SUCCESS

Success with a device or physical therapy won't come without a solid commitment. A 1999 study of more than a hundred stress-incontinent women compared pelvic-floor exercises (three daily sessions) with the use of electrical stimulation and vaginal cones. Surprisingly, pelvic muscle strength was most improved, and leakage most decreased, for the women doing regular Kegel exercises—but adherence to therapy was also greatest in this group. The lesson to be learned? *Those women least likely to abandon their routine were the most likely to succeed.* Whether you choose a low-tech or high-tech approach to finding relief, make it something you're prepared to keep up with. Dedication is the key to your success with nonsurgical therapy.

SURx: Radio-Frequency Shrink Therapy for the Bladder

This new, minimally invasive procedure for stress incontinence involves a handheld penlike device used to heat and shrink the previously stretched tissues around the urethra and bladder, using low-power radio-frequency (RF) energy. The procedure is performed in an outpatient setting and involves no artificial or implantable materials. Although some modest short-term success has been shown, long-term results are not yet available.

SURGERY FOR STRESS URINARY INCONTINENCE

SURGERY FOR STRESS INCONTINENCE: ON THE RISE

According to a recent report from Magee Womens Hospital at the University of Pittsburgh, the national rate of surgeries for stress urinary incontinence nearly doubled from 1979 to 1997. As stress incontinence procedures become less invasive, this rate continues to increase.

Over the past hundred years, more than a hundred different operations have been performed for the treatment of stress urinary incontinence. Although there's still no single best surgery, a few have risen to the top of the pack, with excellent odds of getting you dry.

Almost all of today's stress incontinence operations share a common goal: creating new support around the upper vaginal wall to stabilize and strengthen a floppy urethra. The operations fall into a few major categories designed to achieve this result.

Abdominal Operations
Burch and MMK Procedures

These two very similar operations, also known as retropubic bladder-neck suspensions, are the most common open abdominal operations for urinary stress incontinence. Through a small bikini incision, the upper wall of the vagina is strengthened and lifted in its most crucial area, beneath the neck of the bladder and urethra. Simple stitches (or, in some cases, surgical mesh or staples) are used to anchor the vaginal wall to specific ligaments or bones on the sides of the pelvis. The end result is to stabilize a floppy urethra.

- *Advantages.* The greatest advantage of these abdominal procedures is that they tend to work very well for long periods of time. Rates of cure at ten to twenty years have been estimated at around 70 percent; few other procedures have such a long track record and can claim such proven longevity. For some women, the operation's history offers a sense of confidence. Moreover, when compared with other stress incontinence operations, the Burch and MMK have usually fared well. One 1994 analysis showed that among the major stress incontinence techniques used at that time, these retropubic procedures resulted in the highest rate of cure: 86 percent at two years. Another study comparing outcomes after five years found that retropubic procedures had fared better than the vaginal alternatives available at that time: an 80 percent chance of dryness, as compared with only 50 to 60 percent. However, newer and more effective vaginal operations for stress incontinence have been introduced since this comparison was performed (see "Tension-Free Operations," below).

- *Disadvantages.* The most obvious disadvantage of open abdominal surgery is the need for a skin incision, general anesthesia, a hospital stay of one to two nights, and a longer convalescence. Cosmetically, there is a bikini scar, but in most cases, it becomes barely visible across the pubic hairline. Perhaps a more substantive limitation is that the procedures do not address all types of urinary stress incontinence. Specifically, if you have a thin-walled urethra, they may be more prone to failure over the long run, and a different operation (such as a sling procedure, described below) may be recommended.

Laparoscopic Burch

During laparoscopy, a small tube with a fiber-optic light and camera is inserted into the abdomen through a keyhole incision below the

belly button. This technology is also used for performing tubal liga-
tions or treating ovarian cysts. The laparoscopic Burch procedure
shares the same basic goal as the Burch procedure—suturing to stabilize the upper vaginal wall and support a floppy urethra—but it is
done through a laparoscope rather than an open abdominal incision.

- *Advantages.* Some surgeons feel that laparoscopy provides the
  clearest look at the sites of pelvic injury, and the closest restoration of this anatomy to its normal prechildbirth state. With the
  pelvis brightly lit, the defects in pelvic support leading to prolapse and incontinence can be directly seen and repaired.
  Laparoscopy involves relatively little postoperative pain, a
  quick return to activity, and is usually done as an outpatient
  procedure. Between three and four lower-abdominal keyhole
  incisions will be made and covered with Band-Aid dressings
  afterward.

- *Disadvantages.* Some early reports of the laparoscopic Burch
  raised concern over higher failure rates (up to 40 percent) and
  higher rates of complications, including injury to the urinary
  tract. But in the hands of surgeons performing these procedures
  regularly, very good results can be achieved.

VAGINAL OPERATIONS

Procedures performed through incisions in the vaginal skin, with
only tiny incisions on the abdomen or none at all, are a popular alternative for fixing stress incontinence. Not unlike vaginal childbirth,
operating through the vagina carries big advantages, including minimal pain, quick healing, and high patient satisfaction. The vagina
perceives relatively little in the way of pain and has an outstanding
ability to rapidly heal.

The Bladder Sling

Sling procedures place a band of tissue around the bladder's neck,
creating a floor for the urethra to compress against during a cough,
strain, or any other moment of stress. Like most stress incontinence
procedures, it transforms a floppy urethra into a stable one. If you
have urinary stress incontinence caused by a urethra that's both floppy

and thin-walled, a sling procedure may be recommended, since it has traditionally achieved the best results for this somewhat challenging type of incontinence. Dozens of sling procedures are performed today, using a number of materials and a variety of techniques.

Synthetic mesh, or strips of man-made material, comes in several types. Among the most common are Gore-Tex, Prolene, and Mersilene.

The natural-tissue grafts include *fascia* and *dermis.* Fascia, a naturally strong tissue layer, is found all over the body. Taken from beneath the skin of the patient's own leg or abdomen, it is particularly strong; during surgery, a small strip can be removed through a separate incision in one of these areas and inserted as a sling beneath the bladder and urethra. Prepared fascia can also be obtained from animal sources or human cadavers. *Dermis* is a skin graft, most often from a porcine (pig) source. As a natural substance, similar to fascia, it tends to be gentle on the body; the long-term durability remains to be seen.

The two techniques are *abdominal-anchored* or *pubovaginal,* and *transvaginal-anchored.* Abdominal-anchored is the original sling technique. It involves a regular bikini incision on the abdomen. The vaginal sling arms are passed around the bladder neck and up to the incision, where they are anchored around or into the abdominal muscles. The middle section of the sling lies beneath the urethra and lower part of the bladder.

In transvaginal-anchored, specialized devices enable the placement of slings through vaginal incisions, avoiding an abdominal incision altogether. Bone anchors (Vesica, In-Fast) are one such option, used to fix sling materials into the pubic bone with small metallic screws; however, concern has been raised over bone infections, which can occur in 1 to 2 percent of cases. Other devices (Capio CL) facilitate the anchoring of slings to ligaments, rather than bone.

- *Advantages.* In experienced hands, sling procedures can provide a cure for even severe types of stress incontinence. If you're entering surgery with stress incontinence accompanied by a large cystocele, a sling may decrease your risk of a cystocele recurrence later on, a nice secondary benefit to the surgery. Finally, compared to other operations for stress incontinence, slings are viewed by some surgeons as especially durable for overweight women, or for those who participate in regular heavy exertion.

- *Disadvantages.* Urinary retention and voiding difficulties are more common after traditional sling procedures, as compared with other Burch-type incontinence operations. Erosion of sling material into the adjacent vaginal tissues, bladder, or urethra can occur; this is more common when slings are made of certain synthetic materials. Infection can also occur, due to the presence of foreign material in the body, but is rare.

Tension-Free Operations

It was once generally assumed that a less invasive operation meant a slimmer chance of success, and that the most complete and successful operations required a traditional open surgical incision. But several revolutionary stress incontinence procedures have emerged as real phenomena over the past several years, successfully combining minimally invasive and relatively pain-free techniques with outstanding results. The *TVT*—tension-free vaginal tape—was the original procedure and has become enormously popular across the developed world. It involves placing synthetic mesh tape loosely beneath the urethra, using only one small incision in the vagina. The arms of the tape are passed through the small vaginal incision and up through two tiny incisions on the lower abdominal skin, using a stainless-steel surgical needle. During a cough, a sneeze, or any other moment of physical stress, the tape allows the urethra to compress itself shut and hold back urine. If performed on its own, the procedure can be done under local or spinal anesthesia with no overnight hospital stay.

The *SPARC* procedure entails placement of a similar synthetic mesh, using a slightly different technique but the same combination of small incisions. Even newer variations of this basic technique (for instance, the SABRE sling procedure) are now entering the medical marketplace. Based on the phenomenal success of this approach to date, the number of women choosing these operations will, by all predictions, continue to grow.

- *Advantages.* Despite the fact that the TVT doesn't tighten the urethra like a traditional sling procedure—instead resting rather loosely beneath it—rates of cure for stress incontinence have been excellent. At least 86 percent of women treated for stress incontinence (of the floppy-urethra type) report being cured after five years, and rates of patient satisfaction approach 95 percent. Because of these outcomes, along with its low rate of complications and voiding problems afterward, the TVT continues to generate great enthusiasm. SPARC is a newer procedure, with few reported outcomes. Will long-term results prove these to be the ideal operations for stress incontinence? Only time will tell. But even before the outcomes are known, it's safe to say that these procedures are revolutionizing the treatment of stress incontinence.

- *Disadvantages.* The most common complication during this type of surgery is that the operating needle may perforate the bladder, though this occurs in only 5 percent of cases. For most, it is simply pulled back out and replaced, with no long-term

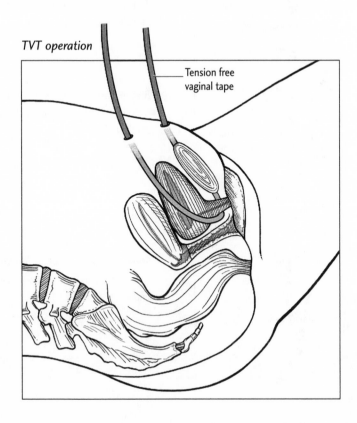

TVT operation

Tension free vaginal tape

consequence for the bladder. More serious concerns involve injury to blood vessels or bowel, but these complications are exceedingly rare.

Needle Suspensions

Needle procedures were once a very popular approach, performed through a few tiny incisions inside the vagina and a few more along the lower pubic area. Through these incisions, stitches are placed that stabilize the bladder neck and floppy urethra, but unlike the TVT or SPARC, without mesh material. Unfortunately, the success rates for most needle procedures have not justified their continued use.

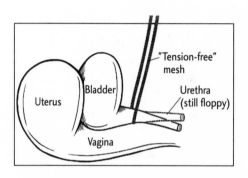

Surgery for stress incontinence: Three common options and the way they work:

• *TVT/SPARC: Narrow "tape" rests loosely beneath the urethra*

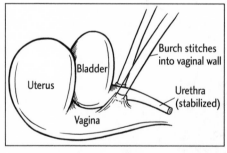

• *Burch/MMK: Stitches reinforce the vaginal "floor" supporting the urethra*

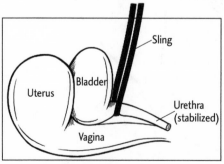

• *Sling: "Hammock" of supportive material placed around the urethra and lower bladder*

TYPE #2: URGE INCONTINENCE AND THE
OVERACTIVE BLADDER

My husband was a principal, and I was a teacher. When he retired, there
was a building and plaque dedicated to him. When I retired, my col-
leagues always joked that they would name the bathroom after me.
　　　　　　　　　　　—Janet, age sixty-two

As you might have gathered from the multimillion-dollar ad cam-
paigns for the latest overactive-bladder medications, urge incontinence (urine leakage when you feel a sudden urge to void) is an
extraordinarily common condition. The National Overactive Bladder
Evaluation (NOBLE) study, involving more than five thousand
adults, found that nearly 17 percent of all women suffer from an
overactive bladder—that's over 33 million individuals, far higher
than previous estimates. Among postreproductive women, the overactive bladder affects probably 30 percent. The NOBLE study found
that in comparison to women who have never given birth, those with
one to two previous births have 1.5 times the risk of an overactive
bladder, and those with three or more births had 2.1 times the risk.
Perhaps most surprising of all is the estimate that up to 80 percent of
affected individuals are not receiving treatment.

The same study confirmed a higher rate of depressive symptoms,
poorer quality of sleep, and overall reduced quality-of-life survey
scores among women with an overactive bladder. Moreover, a recent
report from the University of Washington found that urge incontinence, even more than stress incontinence, appears to be strongly
associated with depressive and panic disorders, perhaps a reflection
of just how distressing unpredictable accidents, as opposed to those
related to specific activities which can be avoided, can be.

MAPPING

Some women organize their lives around access to the bathroom. Those
with an overactive bladder or incontinence are the most likely to map the
nearest bathroom with each change of scenery. Every time they enter a
room, they seek out a position that assures easy access to the toilet; for
frequent flyers, these mental maps may eventually include toilets all over

the world. According to the National Overactive Bladder Screening Initiative in 1999, 46 percent of women with overactive bladder symptoms admit to the habit of toilet mapping. In Australia, a National Public Toilet Map on the Department of Health website even has a search engine for finding the location and hours of public toilets along your driving route in the land Down Under (www.toiletmap.gov.au). If you've become an amateur cartographer of this sort, consider it a sign—it's time to seek help.

Why should your bladder become overactive as you enter your postreproductive years? Aren't your muscles supposed to become *less* active with age? In many areas of the body, the answer is yes. But the bladder muscle behaves very differently from your biceps or triceps. The bladder is surrounded by a bundle of nerves called *autonomic* nerves. The bladder contracts in response to a surge in the activity of these nerves. All over your body, autonomic nerves control the behavior of organs such as your heartbeat, breathing, and other autopilot functions—those that you don't consciously control from minute to minute. But among all these organs, the bladder boasts a fairly unique distinction: it's an autonomic organ that you learn to voluntarily control.

As part of normal childhood development and toilet training, the bladder makes a transition from automatic emptying to controlled restraint. You learn to suppress the bladder's natural tendency to contract by reflex, emptying itself when it first senses fullness, and teach it to tolerate this feeling, emptying on command after you've reached the toilet seat. A normal bladder should tolerate at least a pint of fluid (eight to sixteen ounces) for long periods of time without contracting.

If you've developed an overactive bladder, it means your bladder has regressed to an untrained state and unshackled itself from your command. It no longer tolerates any sense of fullness at all and instead produces a strong urge from only small amounts of urine. Not only that, but like a distractible child at a carnival, it might begin to react whimsically to both physical and mental triggers. For instance, a mildly overactive bladder may associate the sound or feel of running water with the idea that a toilet is nearby, and hastily decide, "Hey . . . why not empty?" So it contracts, and you're forced to control the sudden urge wherever you happen to be. If an overactive bladder worsens, it begins to respond to even more far-fetched associations. You may notice that touching a doorknob triggers an overwhelming urge to urinate, as if your bladder were recalling times when you'd barely reached the bathroom following a long walk or car ride. The bladder's muscular walls contract, and again you find yourself fighting off waves of urge as you run to the toilet. For some women, an overwhelming urge to urinate is the extent of the problem; for others, it's actual leakage before reaching the toilet. Over time, the overactive bladder finds more and more excuses to contract on its own, and before you know it, your bladder is controlling you.

The good news? You *can* regain control. Let's take a look at the tools you can use to tame your overactive bladder and reduce urge incontinence, from simple tips to high-tech gadgetry.

IMPROVING URGE INCONTINENCE THROUGH LIFESTYLE AND HABITS

RETRAINING YOUR OVERACTIVE BLADDER FOR BETTER BEHAVIOR: "BORN AGAIN BATHROOM HABITS"

It's common for women with incontinence and other pelvic symptoms to adopt poor voiding habits. The strong urges of an overactive bladder, for instance, may lead to a habit of more and more frequent urination. Others begin to change their bathroom habits due to a sense of never feeling empty. Still others alter their toileting patterns out of fear over accidents: for example, staying as empty as possible to avoid potential embarrassment.

Some of these habits, as they become ingrained, can slowly but surely exacerbate certain postreproductive symptoms. Your bladder is a creature of habit—it craves routine, and it's largely up to you to decide whether these routines will be functional or dysfunctional, controlled or chaotic. The way you choose to empty can have a profound impact.

UNDERSTANDING THE WAYS YOU EMPTY

THE NURSE'S AND TEACHER'S BLADDER

Nurses and teachers display endless devotion to their patients and students, but they're notoriously unkind to their bladders and bowels. Shift by shift, class by class, their workdays seem to go by without a pause, and postponing bodily urges becomes a part of daily life. Unfortunately, too much postponement is *not* a good habit. Allowing your bladder to overfill can make it weaker and less able to fully empty, as the muscle is constantly stretched out.

EMPTYING JUST IN CASE

Some women make a habit of emptying more often than necessary. Do you urinate several times before leaving the house, just in case? Does the slightest urge send you for the bathroom even if you know there's not much inside? At night, after waking for reasons unrelated to your bladder, perhaps you empty because you happen to be awake. Women who work from home or are retired are often prone to these patterns. Emptying too often can have a very powerful effect on the way your bladder behaves, as it begins to expect a trip to the bathroom even at very low volumes.

VALSALVA

Although the name *valsalva* may at first conjure the romantic image of a wild-eyed fifteenth-century Italian sea explorer, its actual meaning is decidedly less glamorous. Valsalva refers to emptying your bladder by bearing down, in the same way you'd strain to push out a bowel movement or have a baby. Some women void in this way because they're simply not patient enough to let their bladder or bowels empty on their own; for others, it's the only way they can fully empty. Valsalva voiding is common among women, but over time, repetitive straining may erode the pelvic-floor support, and encourage prolapse or incontinence. Valsalva voiding is not the world's worst bathroom habit, but it's a good one to avoid.

DOUBLE VOIDING

Double voiding is a common habit among women who have a cystocele, an overactive bladder, or a weak bladder muscle. A short time after emptying what seem to be all the bladder's contents, the double voider senses a second urge and empties once again. For some women, this second urge will occur right away; for others, it doesn't occur until a minute or two later. In the vast majority of cases, double voiding is a harmless habit, but it's worth mentioning during your evaluation, in case you have a condition that may need further treatment.

CREDE

After you've urinated as much as possible, pressing on the lower abdomen and pelvis with a hand or closed fist can generate enough pressure against the bladder to force out any retained urine. This is the *Crede maneuver*, most often used when the bladder muscle has lost all its strength—for instance, by individuals with overflow incontinence caused by an injury or neurological disorder. If you rely upon Crede to empty your bladder, know that it is not a typical postreproductive habit. See a specialist for a full evaluation.

NO CAMELS

Camels are desert-dwelling beasts who very seldom urinate. Some humans—most notably teachers, nurses, and truck drivers who work long shifts without a trip to the toilet—challenge themselves over the years to become camels. *Don't become a camel!* Constantly stretching the bladder makes it weaker and less sensitive over the years. The way you choose to empty can impact your function and freedom in the years ahead.

ADOPTING NEW STRATEGIES

By now you should have identified the ways you most commonly void. Did you discover you have some bad habits? Not to worry. Just as bad bathroom habits were learned, they can be gradually unlearned. A few simple methods might help you to start regaining control.

THE BLADDER DRILL: TAMING AN OVERACTIVE BLADDER

My life has come to a screeching halt—I don't even bother with restaurants anymore.

—Forty-one-year-old with an overactive bladder

Bladder drills are the oldest trick in the book for improving your voiding pattern and controlling an overactive bladder. If you've developed frequent voiding, waking at night, urge incontinence, or silent leakage of urine, bladder drills may be the easiest first step toward fixing the problem on your own, and you can do them right at home.

Bladder drills are like enlisting for toilet training all over again. The overall aim is to gradually teach your bladder to tolerate more and more fullness, and to resist contracting until normal bladder fullness has been reached. In slightly more scientific terms, it's all about suppressing premature activation of the micturition reflex. Remember that bundle of autonomic nerves that can become unruly and lead to an overactive bladder or urge incontinence? You're about to send a clear message to that pesky bundle that *you're the boss.*

As with any behavioral approach, bladder drills will require you to be self-motivated and diligent, but they often work! One study showed improvement among 83 to 90 percent of women, versus only 23 percent in a placebo group. Especially if your major problem is an overactive bladder or urge incontinence, bladder drills can be a powerful tool when used on their own or alongside any other therapy you've chosen, with no added side effects. You might find they're more effective than even the latest medication or slickest device.

Voiding by the Clock

To begin bladder drills, you first need to decide on an initial voiding interval. From your voiding diary (see Appendix B), estimate how often you've been urinating during the daytime. Then choose a comfortable interval that you feel you'll be able to maintain throughout the day. Voiding every fifteen or thirty minutes is okay if that's been your recent pattern. The idea is to start comfortably and to avoid taking on too abrupt a challenge.

During your waking hours, you're now allowed to empty your bladder *only at your scheduled times.* For example, if you've started your bladder drills at a two-hour interval and wake at eight o'clock each morning with a trip to the toilet, then you should follow up with voids at ten A.M., noon, two P.M., and so on until bedtime. Your bladder drills apply only to the daytime; don't bother thinking about them after you've gone to bed. You should, however, always empty your bladder right before bedtime. With time, you might even find that the benefits of your daytime bladder drills eventually "spill over" into the night.

The Moment of Truth: Learning to Resist the Urge

When you feel an urge beginning to build before your scheduled time has arrived, don't run to the bathroom! Instead, hold your breath and run through the following simple steps.

Step #1: Avoid panic. Women with weak pelvic muscles usually respond to a sudden bladder urge by running to the bathroom, even when they know their bladder isn't very full. Unfortunately, this reflex of anticipating the toilet often fuels an even stronger bladder contraction that may be even harder to control. Although the trigger is largely psychological, the resulting bladder spasm is very physical and very real. Resisting the bolt to the bathroom and adopting a new reaction to the unexpected urge represent the essence of bladder drills. Remember the basic idea: *you're controlling your bladder now.* Breathe deeply and proceed to Step #2.

Step #2: Squeeze your strongest Kegel squeeze. Squeeze a Kegel (see Appendix A) like you really mean business, and hold it strongly. This immediate tightening of your pelvic-floor muscles will help to shut off the bladder's urge before it becomes stronger. The better shape your pelvic-floor muscles are in, the easier and more effective this squeeze will be.

Step #3: Distract yourself. Shifting focus away from the bladder is the next step. First distract your mind. Forgetting about your bladder may seem a laughable idea at first, but with time and improved pelvic-floor strength, you'll see it's possible. Try thinking about your child's next report card, or an upcoming business meeting—maddening or obsessive thoughts provide great distraction. Or try a mental puzzle, such as naming the planets of the solar system forward and then backward.

Next, distract your body. Try a change in position. If you're standing still, start walking, or try raising yourself up on your toes. If you're sitting, try pointing your toes down to the floor like a ballerina. By triggering nerve pathways that lead to your lower spine (the same area where nerves to the bladder cluster), these maneuvers can help to inhibit the bladder muscle and calm its urge.

Step #4: Cross your legs. All right, so it's not a very sophisticated tip, but clamping your thighs tightly together can be a last-ditch safeguard against leakage when you suddenly cough, sneeze, or feel an unexpected urge. Though it might be a bit conspicuous out in public, it's harmless and quite effective. Developing strong thigh (*adductor*) muscles with lower-body conditioning will allow you to reliably use this technique when you need it most.

DON'T BE A SOFTIE

Playing hardball with your bladder is the only way to achieve great results. That means *not* running to the bathroom out of fear; no exceptions, even when you're standing in the shower and that strong urge comes on. Once you've made the commitment to bladder drills, wear pads or other protection if you'd like, and don't fret over occasional leakage if you're truly playing by the rules.

Pushing Your Limits

Once you're feeling comfortable with your voiding interval, the next goal is to lengthen it, slowly but surely. Every ten to fourteen days, try increasing your interval by around thirty minutes. For example, if you've been comfortably voiding every sixty minutes for a few weeks, try increasing to seventy-five, and stay there for the next several weeks. Your ultimate goal should be a three-to-four-hour interval (no more than six to seven voids over twenty-four hours), assuming an average fluid intake. Just remember to approach that goal slowly, never extending your voiding interval by over thirty minutes every two weeks. Above all, remember to have patience while making progress. Working in small steps, you should take anywhere from three to twelve months to achieve your ultimate goal. If your symptoms remain a bother at that point, it's time to seek another strategy.

START YOUR MORNING WITH A SQUEEZE

As you improve with bladder drills, one part of the day often remains a big challenge: first thing in the morning. Many women notice that their over-active bladder is most difficult to control from the moment their feet hit the floor at the bedside, all the way to the toilet. That occurs not only because the bladder may be fairly full after a long night's sleep but also because the urine tends to become more chemically concentrated overnight, and irritates the bladder lining as a result.

Before getting out of bed, even if you don't feel an urge, make it your routine to stop for a moment. Now start with a strong Kegel squeeze, then another. Do a set of ten, and as with a bladder drill, try to distract yourself mentally. Think about the tasks waiting for you at work or at home. Then calmly, slowly, and confidently walk to the bathroom. No mad dash, no panic, and before long, perhaps to your surprise, a better start to your day.

MEDICATIONS FOR URGE INCONTINENCE AND OVERACTIVE BLADDER

Do you have an overactive bladder?
Is your life an accident waiting to happen?

If you've flipped through any of the most popular women's magazines, you might have come across one of these questions posed by the leading pharmaceutical companies, and caught wind of a whole new trend in women's health. Medications for the overactive bladder have emerged as a billion-dollar industry, and you're right at the epicenter of a modern marketing blitz. Colorful advertisements don't hesitate to remind you how disruptive constant bladder urges, urinary frequency, and incontinence can be for active women. Beyond the hype, do these medications work?

Actually, yes. Of all incontinence types, urge incontinence and the overactive bladder are the most likely to be fully relieved with medication. But finding the right medication for your symptoms, and arriving at the right dose, may require trial and error and a good deal of patience.

Anticholinergics and Antispasmodics

Remember the autonomic nerve supply to the bladder and how those nerves can act up to cause an overactive bladder and urge incontinence? Most available drugs are designed to diminish this nerve activity, relax the bladder, and prevent bladder spasms. *Anticholinergic* medications are the most common among them.

These pills don't truly cure the problem, and they're not magic bullets targeting the bladder. By entering the bloodstream, they eventually reach the salivary glands, decreasing their activity and causing dry mouth. They slow the activity of your esophagus and bowel, sometimes causing heartburn or constipation. Beyond those common side effects, a wide range of other, less common ones may also occur.

The generic medications include:

- *Oxybutynin (Ditropan).* This was the gold-standard overactive-bladder medication for several decades, and it remains an alternative today. It's been shown to reduce leakage episodes by 19 to 58 percent over placebo. Oxybutynin counteracts and even prevents bladder spasms by relaxing the smooth muscle of the bladder wall and calming the bundle of nerves surrounding it. It's available in generic form, so it costs less. Unfortunately, it needs to be taken three to four times daily, and side effects are very common. A newly developed skin patch was recently tested and found to be effective for urge incontinence; it remains to be proven whether certain women will experience fewer side effects with this approach, as compared with oral therapy. But by far, the most widely used novel nongeneric form of oxybutynin, already on the market, is Ditropan XL (see below). Side effects may include: dry mouth, dry eyes (especially if you wear contacts), constipation, drowsiness, blurred vision, and a host of other, less likely side effects.

Several other anticholinergic medications are available, with a chance of success comparable to oxybutynin and a similar probability of side effects. They can occasionally provide effective and inexpensive relief.

- *Hyoscyamine (Levbid, Levsin, Cystospaz, Urised).* Tablets are usually taken twice daily. Levbid is also available in sublingual form (placed beneath the tongue rather than swallowed).
- *Propantheline (Pro-Banthine), flavoxate (Urispas), dicyclomine (Bentyl).* Tablets are taken several times daily, with side effects similar to oxybutynin's.

The name-brand medications include:

- *Ditropan XL.* Ditropan XL looks like a pill but actually is a capsule-size delivery system with a microscopic hole drilled into its center and filled with regular oxybutynin. Over a twenty-four-hour period, it releases medication through the tiny opening at a slow and regular rate. It avoids the sharp peaks and valleys in medication levels, so side effects are considerably fewer. Only around 7 percent of women need to discontinue due to side effects, and many are able to reach dose levels they would never have been able to tolerate with the generic pills. Ditropan XL also offers the convenience of taking only one pill daily.

   Side effects are the same as generic oxybutynin's but less common.

- *Tolterodine (Detrol in the U.S., Detrusitol in Europe).* Detrol entered the market in 1998 and has become widely popular across the United States and Europe. According to animal studies, it may target the bladder wall more selectively than standard anticholinergic medications, avoiding the salivary glands and thus raising hope that dry mouth might occur less frequently. Indeed, huge numbers of women have found relief with this medication, with very manageable side effects. It is taken twice daily. Detrol LA is becoming a popular first-line option and offers once-daily dosing.

   Side effects are the same as oxybutynin's but less common.

TRICYCLIC ANTIDEPRESSANTS
If your doctor prescribed an antidepressant for your bladder or pelvic symptoms, don't be too surprised. It's not a thinly veiled message that this bladder problem is all in your head. Certain antide-

pressants have been used for decades to treat overactive bladder symptoms.

- *Imipramine (Tofranil).* This drug boasts the unique ability to not only alleviate urge incontinence but also to occasionally improve mild forms of stress incontinence. Because of this dual action, and because it's available in relatively inexpensive generic form, imipramine has remained a popular choice even in our "designer-drug" era. Because of its tendency to cause sedation, it's best taken after dinner, so you'll sleep off the peak medication levels during the night. Small doses can also be taken during the day.

  Side effects may include: sleepiness, dry mouth, constipation, confusion, altered blood pressure, and a long list of less likely symptoms.

- *Doxepin (Sinequan), amitriptyline (Elavil).* Similar to imipramine and often chosen for patients with conditions causing a very sensitive or painful bladder.

- *Desmopressin (DDAVP).* This is a different type of medication altogether, not specifically targeting the bladder but useful for treating nighttime urinary frequency *(nocturia)* or leakage resulting from an abnormally high nighttime production of urine. It's an antidiuretic that signals the kidneys to slow their output—causing you to temporarily retain fluids in the rest of your body. When starting DDAVP, you need to work closely with your doctor to avoid risks relating to fluid overload and altered body salts. If you can avoid these side effects, DDAVP is effective for some types of nighttime urgency and incontinence. A recent multinational trial of DDAVP indicated that it may also be useful for treating daytime urinary incontinence.

COPING WITH SIDE EFFECTS

The latest generation of anticholinergic medications, such as Detrol and Ditropan XL, maintains the beneficial effects of older overactive-bladder medications with fewer side effects. Still, side effects occur. Some doctors will begin with a mild dose, slowly increasing it as necessary over a period of weeks. If you've noticed no relief of your bladder symptoms once you've reached your maximum tolerable dose, or the side effects become too much to bear, you may need to switch to another medication. But if you're generally happy with your medication and are facing side effects that you'd like to minimize, here are a few ways to cope.

- *Dry mouth.* This common anticholinergic side effect can be quite a nuisance, and can even pose a risk to dental health over time. Carry a water bottle and stay well hydrated, swishing sips of water to keep your mouth moist throughout the day. To stimulate the production of saliva, try chewing gum or sucking on hard candies, especially those with bitter flavor, such as lemon drops or peppermints. Artificial-saliva products are available in sprays, gels, or lozenges, but they offer little advantage over less expensive options.

- *Dry eyes.* Artificial tears, available over the counter, are especially useful if you wear contact lenses. Contact your doctor for any blurred vision or eye discomfort.

- *Constipation.* Counteract the bowel-slowing effects of these medications with plenty of dietary fiber, adequate fluids, regular exercise, and a daily stool softener.

- *Retention of urine.* Your stream may feel slower and less forceful; this is a normal side effect. Double voiding (see chapter 8)— waiting an extra minute or two after you've urinated for the arrival of a second bladder contraction—is a harmless way to be sure you're emptying completely. Avoid the temptation to strain, since this can damage your pelvic-floor supports and their nerve supply. If you feel you're not emptying as fully as before, mention this to your doctor.

- *Less common.* Confusion, drowsiness, headache, and rapid heart rate. Report these side effects to your doctor.

"WILL I NEED TO TAKE THIS STUFF FOREVER?"

Overactive-bladder medications can be used indefinitely, for years and years, but that's often not necessary. For many women, medication provides just a first step toward regaining confidence and control—a sort of temporary crutch allowing them to begin a more long-term process of behavioral retraining (see "The Bladder Drill," page 145). Over time, as these improved voiding habits influence bladder control, you'll depend less and less on the medication.

SURGERY FOR URGE INCONTINENCE

NEUROMODULATION: THE PELVIC PACEMAKER

Now for one of the most fascinating advances in overactive-bladder treatment: the Interstim device, or the pacemaker for the pelvis. The procedure involves placement of a tiny permanent electrode beside the key sacral nerves that exit the spine and head toward the pelvic floor. The device has received FDA approval for urge incontinence and overactive-bladder symptoms, and it is being investigated for a handful of other problems, including fecal incontinence (see chapter 10).

The first step involves an office procedure called the *test stimulation*. The doctor inserts a small, thin wire beneath the skin of the back, using just a bit of local anesthesia. When the tip of this wire is positioned correctly, it's securely taped to your back. Over the next three to five days, a small battery-powered device stimulates the pelvic nerves and muscles, producing a mild pulling or tightening sensation in the pelvic and vaginal area. If the test stimulation is a success—meaning that your symptoms improve with the temporary wire in place—you can proceed with the second phase: *implantation*. This involves surgical placement of the actual pacemaker—around the size of a

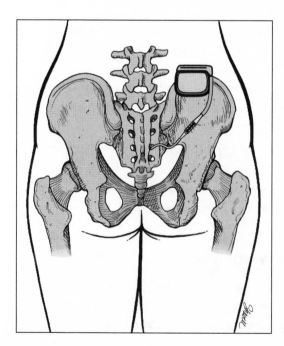

The Interstim "pacemaker"

large stopwatch—beneath the skin, during a relatively short operation requiring general anesthesia. It provides constant stimulation to the pelvic nerves.

Assessing the long-term results for this treatment will require several more years of follow-up. But to date, the response of many different pelvic and urinary symptoms has been remarkable. Urge incontinence and the overactive bladder, urinary retention, bladder pain, and even constipation can improve dramatically. One large report on the Interstim device reported 61 percent excellent response, and 22 percent good response for the overactive bladder. According to another series testing seventeen women, 94 percent considered it a success and would do it again. Impressively, success can be achieved for some of the most challenging patients, those who failed to improve with all other treatments.

As with any operation, complications can occur, including infection, low-back pain, or shifting of the pacemaker from its proper position, which sometimes requires another operation. According to initial reports, around a third of recipients needed additional surgery to either alleviate pain or replace the device; however, this appears to be less common as techniques improve. In the near future, modifications of this amazing technology are anticipated to make the implantation procedure even less invasive. In the meantime, its early success has already raised enormous excitement.

"A TREATMENT IN MY BACK SIDE FOR A PROBLEM IN MY FRONT?"

Neuromodulation, the pelvic pacemaker, may change the way we view many common female symptoms. A number of disorders once thought to arise in the bladder and pelvis may really begin higher up in the nervous system, closer to the spine.

OTHER OPERATIONS FOR URGE INCONTINENCE

Major surgical procedures aren't generally considered for urge incontinence except in very unusual cases, which usually involve severe underlying neurological problems. In these circumstances, bladder augmentation (which surgically enlarges the bladder) may be considered.

TYPE #3: OVERFLOW INCONTINENCE

This type of leakage occurs when the bladder is unable to empty fully and remains in a constantly overfilled state. Unlike the overactive bladder, with overflow incontinence, the bladder muscle is usually underactive. From time to time, the bladder reaches its absolute capacity and excess urine simply spills, overflowing like an overfilled pail of water, often without urge or warning. The bladder never fully empties with overflow incontinence; it just remains a bit less full for a while. Overflow incontinence is uncommon. Nevertheless, you should understand it, because it can indicate an elevated risk of an underlying neurological condition, spinal injury, diabetes, or a blockage problem such as narrowing of the urethra. Also, if left untreated, it can increase your risk for kidney infections and damage to the kidneys resulting from slowing of their drainage.

How would you know if you have overflow incontinence? Most commonly, you would notice small, frequent leaks of urine with a weak stream, and you probably wouldn't feel truly empty even after urinating. One tricky aspect of overflow incontinence is that it might also cause leakage with coughing or straining, mimicking the more commonplace stress incontinence. The critical difference is that with overflow incontinence, the bladder never fully empties; the problem is caused by bladder weakness rather than urethral weakness.

During your first office visit, the doctor will test you on postvoid residual (see chapter 13): after you urinate, the amount of urine left inside your bladder is measured with either a small catheter or an ultrasound machine. If this test shows you're retaining urine, your doctor may recommend more complex office testing to better understand whether you have overflow incontinence, and to rule out an underlying neurological or medical cause.

TYPE #4: MIXED INCONTINENCE

Mixed incontinence signifies two or more of these incontinence problems (stress, urge, overflow) occurring together. By far, the most common pairing is stress incontinence alongside urge incontinence. The symptoms caused by this dynamic duo can be truly incapacitating. Between all of the uncontrollable urges—and the anxiety that begins to accompany coughing, exercising, or even changing positions— mixed incontinence can leave you with very little worry-free time to enjoy your life.

While there's no need to make yourself an overnight expert in each of the several varieties, you should understand a few take-home points. First of all, mixed incontinence makes guesswork more difficult from your doctor's point of view. While somebody with simple overactive-bladder symptoms may be offered a trial of medication before any testing is done, the presence of mixed symptoms makes early testing more important. These tests will help your doctor to decipher exactly what is happening beneath a frequently nebulous mix of bladder symptoms, and to decide what needs treatment most (see "Urodynamics," chapter 13). The second key aspect of mixed incontinence relates to how quickly and easily you can expect to achieve total relief. You may start a trial of medication for urge incontinence but still leak; and that's probably because your stress incontinence has yet to be addressed. Likewise, surgery for stress incontinence may be performed perfectly but fail to leave you completely happy and dry. In most cases, this is because the urge incontinence has persisted even after the stress incontinence has resolved. If you're diagnosed with mixed incontinence, you may ultimately need a mix of at least two different treatments in order to fix your leakage. Finding the right combinations of therapy will often require trial and error and a good deal of patience on your part.

Since mixed incontinence usually includes overactive-bladder symptoms, all of the previously discussed tips for better bladder behavior still apply. Kegel exercises, cones, and biofeedback (discussed in Appendix A) are also useful tools.

MEDICATIONS FOR MIXED INCONTINENCE

The same basic medications for urge incontinence and stress incontinence are also used to treat mixed incontinence.

ELECTRICAL AND MAGNETIC STIMULATION THERAPY: A NONINVASIVE OPTION FOR STRESS, URGE, AND MIXED INCONTINENCE

PELVIC-FLOOR ELECTRICAL STIMULATION

Electrical shock therapy for your pelvis? Sounds like a bad scene from a B horror film—but actually, it's a real-life medical alternative used to treat certain types of urinary incontinence, fecal incontinence, even sexual dysfunction and pelvic pain. Have you known someone suffering from back pain or muscle spasms who uses electrical stimulation? *Pelvic-floor stimulation* (PFS) is similar, using a mild electrical current to recondition the muscles and nerves of the pelvic floor.

Electrical stimulation devices consist of a probe around the size of a tampon, inserted vaginally or rectally, attached to a small portable device that delivers a mild electrical current to the pelvic-floor muscles and nerves. If you can insert a tampon, you should be able to insert a probe. Daily treatments are self-administered, beginning frequently—sessions of fifteen to thirty minutes, twice daily, in most cases. Ideally, different current strengths and frequencies are used, depending on the condition. As you gain awareness of the muscles and supports being stimulated, you can join in with your own Kegel squeeze. After symptoms have begun to improve, often over a period of several weeks to months, the number of sessions can be tapered off.

- *For urge incontinence.* Overactive-bladder symptoms, such as urge incontinence, urinary frequency, and bladder irritation or pain, can respond favorably to pelvic-floor stimulation. The odds of success appear to be greater (50 to 70 percent) for treating these symptoms than for treating stress incontinence.

- *For stress incontinence.* Pelvic-floor stimulation has been reported to help up to 48 percent of women, though surprisingly, roughly 13 to 28 percent of women treated with a placebo in published series have also reported improvement.

THE MAGNETIC STIMULATION CHAIR

Electromagnetic fields exist all over our world—in outdoor power lines, cellular phones, airplanes, computers, and televisions. The same basic type of energy is used in medicine to treat a number of common pelvic and urinary symptoms, ranging from an overactive bladder to an underactive one. Magnetic stimulation chairs deliver twenty-minute treatment sessions, involving no discomfort, while you remain fully clothed. The rather magical scientific feature is that magnetic stimulation can be targeted to areas deep in the body, passing through skin and other tissues without irritating them at all.

Although the device has not been tested in a placebo-controlled study (the only true way to prove its effectiveness), improvement has been reported for up to 69 percent of women with urinary incontinence in one clinical trial of biweekly treatments for six consecutive weeks. Improvements have also been seen in overactive-bladder patients for reducing the frequency of urination, nighttime voiding, daytime leaking, and overall quality-of-life survey scores. Trials are under way to test the magnetic chair right after childbirth for preventing urinary incontinence, and also for treating fecal incontinence. In its present form, magnetic stimulation can be performed only in the doctor's office, requiring multiple visits. Regardless, it remains yet another nonsurgical treatment option worth considering if low-tech alternatives have failed and you're intent on avoiding more invasive therapy.

WHAT TO EXPECT FROM SURGERY IF YOU HAVE MIXED INCONTINENCE

If you're heading into surgery, mixed incontinence means mixed news. The bad news is that surgery for stress incontinence may have an unpredictable effect on overactive-bladder symptoms: they can get worse, stay the same, or improve. So even if your operation keeps you from leaking with coughing, sneezing, or lifting, don't be shocked if you're still bothered by urinary frequency, nighttime voiding, and/or urge incontinence. The good news is that both components of your problem can still be effectively treated. A combination of medications, behavioral tips, gadgets, and procedures can eliminate both culprits causing your mixed incontinence. Just don't expect an operation for stress incontinence to cure your overactive bladder—after all, that's not what it was designed to do!

General Treatments and Tips
for All Incontinence Types

DIET AND SELF-HELP REMEDIES

Everything you eat and drink affects the way your body feels. Cajun spice can burn your stomach; grapefruit juice can make your whole chest feel sour. Too much caffeine can leave a throbbing headache in its path, and a bag of salty chips may leave your mouth feeling parched and dry. But how often are you aware of the connection between what you eat or drink and how your body feels down below? When substances in your diet reach their final destination in your bladder and bowels, they can profoundly affect postreproductive symptoms. If you're looking for quick and easy relief at home, take a careful look at your diet.

Take Stephanie, an avid diet-cola drinker who came to the office complaining of urinary frequency, urge incontinence, and waking several times each night with a strong need to void. At work, it had been her routine to drink three cans of pop, one before lunch and two afterward. At night, she kept a caffeine-free standby on her nightstand for after-hours thirst quenching. Though her bladder irritation and incontinence had been an increasing bother for several years, she had never associated her pesky symptoms with her love for soda. At our first visit, I shared with her a list of foods and drinks to consider avoiding, and she was surprised to see diet cola near the top. Not a medical miracle performed on my part, but Stephanie accepted my simple advice and kicked the habit, and her problem gradually improved.

Even if you're not a card-carrying member of the Pepsi generation, read on—you might not be off the hook. Less obvious foods and drinks may be contributing to your bladder symptoms. An innocent cup of decaffeinated tea, perhaps a weakness for pasta with red sauce and a glass of wine on the side, or a cappuccino after dinner. Your postreproductive body might feel a great deal better with the help of a few culinary tips.

HYDRATING RIGHT
- *Not too wet.* For better or worse, we're living in a water-bottle culture, where sleek marketing has transformed our least expen-

sive resource into a costly craze. Thousands of years from now, the relics of our era will be excavated not as mosaic-tiled floors and Doric columns but in the form of countless sixteen-ounce plastic sport bottles. For some women, life in the water-bottle culture translates into excessive water intake; those on weight-loss diets, in particular, are likely to overhydrate. Drowning it with fluid will challenge even a very strong bladder and should be avoided if you have incontinence or other urinary symptoms.

• *Not too dry.* Dehydration, on the other hand, is also a problem. Women who are concerned over a loss of bladder control often develop a habit of drinking less to reduce their odds of an accidental leak. Intentional dehydration is not a healthful habit. Chemicals in the urine can become highly concentrated and irritating, leading to spasms of an overactive bladder and sometimes even worse incontinence.

• *Just right.* Good hydration usually means a basic goal of six to eight glasses each day, and more in hot weather or during exercise. Prefer a more mathematical guideline? If so, aim for a half ounce of water per pound of body weight each day. If your symptoms tend to flare at night, try restricting your fluid intake starting around two to four hours before bedtime. Urine color is a very reliable indicator of whether you're ahead or behind with your daily fluids. A pale straw appearance usually indicates that you're in a healthy balance.

THE BLADDER DIET

If you have bladder symptoms, take a close look at the foods and drinks you choose each day. Irritants in the diet can lead to symptoms that feel just like cystitis, cause patterns that mimic an overactive bladder, or even make incontinence suddenly worse. A bladder diet can have the opposite effect, helping to prevent infections, relax an overactive bladder, and reduce incontinence. For starters, take a look at Table 1 (see page 165), which lists most of the foods and drinks that could irritate the bladder. Foods that acidify the urine are often the biggest offenders, but as you can see, a number of other substances may also spell trouble. You'll notice that the table lists most of the world's healthiest foods and beverages. Don't worry—you won't be asked to avoid them all. Though some of these items might be contributing to your symptoms, the vast majority are not.

Step #1: Scan the list. First, take a look at the foods on the list, then write down any of the items that have been a regular part of your diet. You're creating a suspect list. Next take a look at the drinks. Again, list any that have been a regular part of your diet.

Step #2: Make a change. Once you've scanned the bladder diet, it's time to look back at your suspect list and start your investigation. Try eliminating one possible offender at a time for a week, keeping track of your symptoms during that time, and reassess for any changes. If things felt better—for instance, less urinary frequency and urgency, better control, more restful nights—then keep this food or drink out of your routine. If the dietary change made no difference, then add the item right back.

Tweaking your bladder diet may take several weeks or months, but if you're lucky enough to find a genuine trigger, you'll have made a small investment of time for a rich payoff. Just don't abandon a fully balanced diet for daily meals of Pop-Tarts and water with the hope of doing some good for your body. Your task is to seek out one or two bad apples, not to throw out the whole bushel.

The Bad: Dietary Suspects

- *Spicy and sweet.* Chilies, chocolates, corn sweetener, honey.
- *Fruits and veggies.* Apples, cantaloupes, citrus, cranberries, grapes, lemons and limes, guava, peaches, pineapple, plums, strawberries, tomatoes.
- *Juices.* These acidic drinks may help to decrease your risk of bladder infection, but what's not often realized is that they can also act as bladder irritants, causing urinary frequency, the urge to urinate, and discomfort or pain within a sensitive bladder.

    Cranberry, orange, and tomato juices are acidic and may spell trouble. In addition to being acidic, grapefruit juice is a mild diuretic—in other words, a substance that causes the body to excrete water. That is one reason why the grapefruit diet became so popular several years ago, and also why it can overwhelm an overactive or irritated bladder. As a rule of thumb, opaque juices (tomato, grapefruit) are generally more irritating than clear ones (apple).

- *Miscellaneous and hidden triggers.* Carbonation, artificial sweeteners (Nutrasweet and saccharine), vinegar, mayonnaise, and soy sauce. Watch out for salad dressings, marinates, ketchup, and tomato-based sauces.

The Really Bad: Prime Suspects

- *Coffee and tea.* You're probably well aware from personal experience that coffee and tea can rev up a bladder like almost nothing else. For postreproductive women already struggling with control, the hours after the morning brew might present a clear and present danger. Why? For one, caffeine is a strong diuretic. Even without the caffeine, the chemical texture and acidity of coffee and tea can be highly irritating to the bladder's inner lining, making it less likely to behave.

  Because coffee and tea can undermine your control over both bladder and bowels, women with certain postreproductive symptoms are often advised to quit the habit cold turkey. For many a soul, that's easier said than done. If you're like me and find it hard to start your day without the company of Earl Grey or Juan Valdez, here are a few tips that may help you maintain better control while satisfying your craving:

  - *Decaffeinated coffee or tea.* The chemical texture of decaf can be almost as irritating to some bladders as the regular stuff, but at least caffeine's diuretic effect won't be a problem. It's worth a try.
  - *Low-acidity coffee beans.* In general, for any coffee, a darker roast means lower acidity. Specially marketed low-acid coffee beans may be better tolerated by sensitive bladders. Freshness of the beans also matters—try to avoid that wicked truck-stop blend in your office percolator, especially after it's been sitting for a while.
  - *Coffee substitutes and grain or malt-based drinks.* Kava (instant, low-acidity), Postum, Pero, Roma, Cafix, Breakfast Cup.

- *Non-citrus herbal teas.*
- *Hot water.* Try it with a lemon.
- *Cranberry juice.* The juice from those little red berries just might be the most underused and overused home remedy for the female bladder. As you've undoubtedly heard, cranberry juice is a great means for prevention of some postreproductive conditions; for other conditions, as you might not know, it's the pits. When it comes to its effect on your bladder, cranberry can play both Jekyll and Hyde.

  Countless women over the years have sworn by cranberry for preventing cystitis. It does appear to reduce the amount of bacteria in the bladder by keeping the urine more acidic and preventing bacteria from sticking to the bladder's inner surface. One study of postmenopausal women in *The Journal of the American Medical Association* concluded that a ten-ounce daily dose of cranberry-juice cocktail reduced the amount of bacteria in the urine by up to 40 percent. Another, smaller study, this one of sexually active younger women, showed a reduced risk of infections over a six-month period. So remember—ten ounces each day just may keep the bugs away. If juice therapy entails more fluid and calories than you can afford, consider these alternatives:

  - *Unsweetened cranberry juice.* Available at some natural-food stores.
  - *Artificially sweetened juice.* Keep in mind that synthetic sweeteners can act as bladder irritants themselves.
  - *Dried cranberries, or fresh cranberries ground with honey.* Another option for those of you who have a little extra time and a bit of Martha Stewart in your blood.
  - *Cranberry extract or capsules.* Can help you achieve the same effect as juice, minus the fluid load.

  Don't assume that cranberry is a panacea. Acidifying the urine—with the help of juice, tablets, or extract—is great for *preventing* bladder infections and stopping symptoms in their tracks (see chapter 12). But if you're dealing with an existing infection, an active inflammation, or an overactive bladder, acidifying might make your bladder feel much worse.

• *Your bladder on booze.* You know all about the dizzying effects of alcohol up above, but what about its effects down below? For at least a few reasons, liquor can present a real challenge to your postreproductive body. Alcohol in any form causes the kidneys to draw water out of your body and flush it into the bladder. If a brisk diuresis leaves you suddenly more full than usual, it may create a recipe for leakage. Also, the chemical texture of alcohol can directly irritate the bladder lining. This can trigger an over-active bladder, urge incontinence, even stress incontinence—and require some quick thinking! So before you pop that cork or cap, be prepared for the consequences.

TABLE 1
DIETARY TRIGGERS

FOODS	**Fruits and veggies:** Apples, cantaloupes, citrus, cranberries, grapes, lemons and limes, guava, peaches, pineapple, plums, strawberries, tomatoes
	Sweets: Chocolate, artificial sweeteners, honey, corn sweetener
	Spicy: Chilies, peppers
BEVERAGES	**Coffee and tea:** Even decaffeinated
	Acidic juices: Cranberry, orange, tomato, grapefruit
	Carbonated Beverages
MISCELLANEOUS	Vinegar, soy sauce, marinates, salad dressings, ketchup and tomato-based sauces

The Good: Dietary Substitutes

Try olive oil and garlic on your pasta instead of red sauce. Pears, apricots, and watermelon are a good alternative to other, more acidic fruits. Papaya is low in acidity but may have a diuretic effect.

THE LOW-OXALATE DIET

Oxalate is a chemical found in plant products, including green vegetables, wheat bran, coffee, tea, and chocolate. It's been proposed that dietary oxalate can trigger bladder irritation and vulvar symptoms. As a result, a low-oxalate diet is sometimes recommended to women with unexplained complaints in those areas.

- *Avoid:* Coffee, tea, beets, beans, peppers, celery, berries, grapes, nuts, tofu, peanuts and peanut butter, chocolate, spinach, orange and lemon peel, celery
- *No Problem:* Bananas, cherries, grapefruit, peaches, melon, plums, onions, peas, avocado, bread, pasta, white potatoes, rice, beef, fish, pork, poultry, cauliflower, mushrooms
- *Consider:* Calcium citrate (Citracal), a chemical that neutralizes oxalate in the bladder; may be taken after meals in the case of diet-sensitive bladder symtpoms

---

THE NOT-SO-WONDERFUL DEVICES: PADS AND ABSORBENT PRODUCTS

Despite the number of fancy, flashy, and high-tech treatments and cures available, there will still be times when women need temporary protection. For some, stress leakage might occur only at specific times, such as during pregnancy or on the tennis court. Others may have more regular incontinence but simply haven't addressed the issue with a physician. As we've seen, these symptoms can be effectively treated or cured in a number of elegant ways. But if protection rather than cure is your present strategy, then understand a few aspects of this multimillion-dollar absorbent-product industry to help minimize your fear of embarrassment and maximize your quality of life.

Pads, Shields, and Liners

Far too often, postreproductive women make a transition from menstrual pad to incontinence pad, considering it a normal aspect of life during their postchildbearing and perimenopausal years. Postreproductive women who worry about daily control over their bladder or bowels can easily spend hundreds of dollars each month on pads, shields, and liners. Here are a few guidelines that may keep things more effective and affordable:

- *Don't economize by using homemade substitutes.* Some women use folded paper towels or tissue paper in their underwear; others use newspaper, once they discover that it can reduce the odor of urine. These solutions may be cheap, but they're not very effective. Their absorbency is limited, compared with specialized pads and liners. Occasionally, chemicals and dyes in these materials may irritate the vulvar skin.

- *Choose the right product.* Incontinence liners and full-size pads (Serenity, Dignity, Depends, Poise) have a plastic backing, with absorbency capacities varying by pad thickness and design. Very light leakage may require a simple thin liner, which is barely visible even through sport clothing. Moderate leakage may require a thicker pad, with layers designed to pull moisture away from the surface and toward the core. Heavier-duty pads are lined with chemical additives that absorb urine and react with it to form a gel. This process stores urine in a drier form and prevents moisture from accumulating. The absorbent gel also allows pads to remain relatively thin, easily concealed beneath regular underpants yet able to absorb many times their weight in water. Their typical absorbent capacity ranges from 100 to 350 milliliters.

  Adult diapers and briefs (Depends, Attends, Surecare, Promise) may be a bit more challenging to conceal underneath clothing, but they can absorb the equivalent of several pads (1,000 to 2,000 milliliters). Recent improvements have made them far less bulky and conspicuous; some are nearly identical in appearance to regular underpants. Products designed for the most severe leakage combine undergarment briefs with gel-containing pads capable of absorbing large amounts of urine, in both daytime and overnight forms.

  Boutique incontinence garments are available from specialty vendors, combining washable briefs with built-in pads holding up to 200 milliliters of urine. Specialty swim suits, fitted with similar systems, can also be found.

  About one of every three menstrual pads is used for urinary incontinence rather than menstruation. But often they are not the optimal product. First, they have much lower absorbent capacities than gel-containing incontinence pads. Second, the chemical additives in menstrual pads, when mixed with urine, can cause skin irritation around the vulva and vagina. Switching to incontinence pads may prove to be not only more economical but also more comfortable.

Disposable and washable bed pads can be used for nighttime leakage. If the vulvar skin is irritated, sleeping underwear-free is often recommended. A bed pad can allow your skin to better breathe and heal.

- *Obey the laws of good skin care.* The wetness and rough chemical texture of urine can spell hard times for skin, which can become irritated if you're not careful. The use of poorly absorbent pads and shields can worsen matters by trapping moisture against the skin. Whatever product you choose, remember to change pads as often as necessary to keep the skin dry. Try going pad-free at night, using a bed liner if necessary, to allow your skin some time to breathe.

  Shower with nonperfumed hypoallergenic soaps, avoid overly aggressive scrubbing of the area, and steer clear of perfumed or medicated creams. Barrier creams can help protect raw areas from the chemical irritation of urine, providing a second skin. Try cocoa butter, zinc oxide, lanolin, parafin, Balmex, Carlesta, or A&D emollient cream.

- *Consider cost.* Absorbent products aren't usually covered by insurance. Be sure to weigh their cost and inconvenience against that of medications, devices, physical therapy, and operative treatments. A curative approach may cost far less than pads and diapers over the long run. Consider, for instance, a woman using just two pads each day—that's fourteen per week, 730 per year, and thousands of dollars over each decade devoted to pads rather than movies, books, restaurants, and vacations. Finding a long-term solution for your problem may prove to be a wise financial investment.

- *Kick the habit once you can.* Though it may seem odd, many women who use pads for years have a very difficult time breaking free of these security blankets, even after their incontinence has been cured. Doctors will sometimes beg and plead with patients to give up their pads long after they've made it to dry.

HIDDEN TRIGGERS: EFFECTS OF OTHER MEDICATIONS ON BLADDER CONTROL

A wide range of postreproductive symptoms may be affected and even caused by medications you're taking for totally unrelated medical conditions—and the connection might not be obvious at first. Take a close look at your medicine chest, both prescription and over-the-counter products. Just remember, don't start or stop any medications without first checking with your doctor.

ANTIHISTAMINES, COLD MEDICATIONS, DIET PILLS, DECONGESTANTS

As already mentioned, several over-the-counter pills (such as Sudafed, Alka-Seltzer Plus Cold, Dristan, Sinarest, TheraFlu, NyQuil, Afrin). can occasionally improve mild stress incontinence. But since part of their effect is to promote retention of urine, they can occasionally cause the bladder to overfill, leading to overflow incontinence. Difficulty passing urine or frequent urges may be the first indications of this problem and should be mentioned to your doctor.

BLOOD-PRESSURE MEDICATIONS

- *Beta blockers (Propranolol, Inderal).* These are very common medications used for treating high blood pressure, which can occasionally make urinary incontinence worse. They can also diminish sex drive.

- *Alpha blockers (Prazosin, Minipress, Hytrin, Cardura, Aldomet).* Another family of blood-pressure medications that can aggravate incontinence by overrelaxing the urethra and its surrounding muscles. Women who become incontinent after starting one of these medications may sometimes be switched to another.

- *Ace inhibitors (Vasotec, Zestril, Monopril, Lotensin).* These blood-pressure medications have no expected effects on urinary control. Just one potential concern regarding your pelvic-floor symptoms: on rare occasion, ace inhibitors can cause a chronic cough. If this side effect happens to arise, the physical stress associated with coughing may place you at greater risk for incontinence and even progression of prolapse over time.

DIURETICS

Diuretics such as Lasix, Maxzide, and Diuril cause the transfer of water from around your body into your kidneys and bladder. These "water pills" are prescribed by doctors for the treatment of high blood pressure and heart disease, and also to relieve swelling from fluid retention (edema). By causing a rapid excretion of bodily fluids, diuretics can flood your bladder with urine; certain types can also irritate the bladder lining. If you're coping with incontinence, some diuretics may be better for you than others—an issue worth discussing with your doctor. Never stop or start one on your own.

ASTHMA MEDICATIONS

Asthma puffers (Albuterol, Ventolin) often consist of adrenaline-like chemicals capable of causing urinary retention, overflow incontinence, and urinary frequency. Oral steroids—used for asthma and a wide range of inflammatory conditions, including skin rashes—can occasionally tip a weak bladder over the edge.

PAIN RELIEVERS

Certain pain or headache medications (Excedrin, Anacin) contain caffeine, which, as you've already learned, is not only a diuretic but also a bladder stimulant. Narcotic pain medications may cause constipation.

SEDATIVES AND SLEEPING PILLS

Certain antianxiety medications (Valium, Ativan, Xanax, Serax). relax the urethral sphincter muscles, in some cases enough to cause leakage.

PSYCHIATRIC AND ANTISEIZURE MEDICATIONS

Side effects of these drugs (Thorazine, Haldol, Clozaril) can include incontinence, urinary frequency, urgency, and nighttime urinary loss.

SOME ANTIDEPRESSANTS

Drugs such as Elavil and Prolixin might occasionally affect urinary symptoms or control.

CONSTIPATING DRUGS

Watch out for iron tablets, pain pills, or cough medicine containing codeine or another narcotic, and antacids containing calcium or aluminum.

GOUT MEDICATION

Colchicine, a common antigout medication, may aggravate urge incontinence.

JUDY AND HER MEDICINE CHEST

Judy was forty-two years old when she was evaluated for mixed stress and urge incontinence, as well as a small cystocele that hadn't changed for years. It seemed, she said, that her bladder symptoms were almost intolerable in the spring and late summer, with greater frequency of urination and uncontrollable urges; yet during the rest of the year, they were manageable.

So we talked and charted her observations. What was making her so uncomfortable during those seasons? Her daily routine and diet seemed very consistent from month to month. She exercised regularly year-round. But medically, every month was not so equal. Judy was a mild asthmatic, bothered only during cold winter days and the dry weeks of the ragweed season. Ever since she could remember, she'd carried a small puffer in her purse, along with an antihistamine for her allergies. She showed them to me, and it became quickly clear that we'd found the culprits. These medications were each capable of tipping the balance of her bladder control; when she took them together, she didn't stand a chance. In the end, finding relief for Judy was as simple as looking into the medications she'd been taking for years.

If you notice a change in your pelvic symptoms after taking medication for an unrelated problem, it's probably not your imagination. More likely, it's the effect of drugs on the nerves and muscles of the bladder, bowels, and pelvic floor.

QUICK AND EASY MEDICATION CHECKLIST

If You've Noticed One of These . . .	Check if You're Taking One of These
Difficulty starting your urine stream Weakening of stream Incomplete emptying Frequent urges	Antihistamines Antidepressants Blood-pressure medications Cold medications (containing pseudoephedrine) Steroids or antiinflammatory pills Irritable-bowel medications
Worse stress leakage (with sneezing, coughing, lifting, exercise)	Certain blood-pressure medications Sleeping pills and muscle relaxants Psychiatric medications
Frequent need to urinate Incontinence Large amount of urine	Diuretics/water pills
Constipation Rectocele pressure or discomfort	Pain medications (containing narcotic) Iron supplements

WHAT ABOUT HERBS?

Just reading the labels of some herb supplements can inspire hope for curing your most persistent maladies. Their extensive claims of bodily benefits often stop just short of promising world peace. One herbal site that I stumbled across on the Internet even said, for instance, that oatmeal can rejuvenate your sex life (would you have guessed it, given the look of that Quaker Oats man?). Enticing as these claims may be, they're rarely backed by science and shouldn't be taken at face value without some medical advice.

So, what about herbs for the bladder?

- *Buchu tea (Agathosma betulina).* Tea from the leaves of this South African shrub have been used by some for its diuretic and anti-inflammatory action in the urinary tract, and reportedly even as an antibacterial for treating cystitis.

- *Bearberry (Uva-ursi).* Leaves from this plant have been used in diuretic and laxative preparations and as a popular urinary disinfectant in Europe. It's sometimes recommended as a urinary aseptic for bladder and urethral inflammation. Bearberry is available in concentrated drops or tea to mix with water, or as a capsule or tablet.

- *Alfalfa.* Taken as a pill, alfalfa is reported to reduce the odor of urine, like a deodorizing tablet for women prone to leakage. Vitamin C, according to some, may serve the same purpose and may also have an antibladder-infection effect.

- *Cornsilk.* A few cups of cornsilk tea each day has been touted traditionally as bladder-soothing and a means for preventing cystitis.

- *Horsetail (Equisetum arvense).* Horsetail is an herb that's rich in silicon, cited as a urinary diuretic. It's prepared as tea and also available in tablets and capsules.

- *Catnip tea (Nepeta cataria).* Catnip has been touted as an antispasmodic. The Native Americans used it for colicky babies and gastrointestinal disorders.

Herbal remedies can be interesting to investigate, but an herbal panacea for bladder problems simply does not exist. The touted effects are rarely proven with medical research and should be discussed with your doctor.

DRUGS OF THE FUTURE: MAGIC PELLETS AND RED-HOT CHILI PEPPERS

In years to come, your medical options for treating incontinence and bladder dysfunction will look completely different from those of today. Trials are under way, for instance, to test a specially engineered capsule that inserts like a magic bullet into the bladder, slowly releasing medication for several months. Too tame for your imagination? How about capsaicin, an extract of red-hot chili peppers from the genus *capsicum*, instilled directly into the bladder? Not hot enough? Then imagine resiniferatoxin, another essence of peppers that's a thousand times more potent. Even Botox has been used experimentally for treating the overactive bladder, with some encouraging early results. Only time will tell which innovations will fall by the wayside and which will become the next cutting edge. The field of urogynecology is moving fast—and the landscape up ahead looks promising.

QUICK AND EASY TIPS: KEEPING DRY AT THE GYM

One in every three women report leakage that occurs only during strenuous exercise. Are you one of them? Sure, you could decide to eliminate bouncing and straining activities from your routine, which would probably improve your symptoms. But who really wants to give up Tae-Bo for a stationary bike, or a brisk jogging routine for lazy walks on the treadmill? If you're anxious to get a head start before even seeing the doctor, try these low-tech tips:

- **Use tampons.** A regular tampon may sometimes provide just enough support beneath a weak vaginal wall to stabilize a floppy urethra and keep you dry during exercise. Especially if you experience only mild incontinence symptoms triggered by a high-stress workout, a tampon might prove helpful. After a shower or bath, the tampon can be more comfortably removed than when it is dry; or try lubricating it with a bit of K-Y jelly. Occasionally, a large diaphragm can serve the same purpose. Whenever using a tampon for a reason other than your period, discuss the idea with your doctor first, and remember to *never* leave a tampon inside beyond its recommended time.

- **Try over-the-counter medications.** A few common decongestants may alleviate mild stress incontinence if taken an hour before exercise. Because they can increase your heart rate and blood pressure, they're not recommended for everybody. Check with your doctor first.

- **Cool it with that water bottle.** Proper hydration is important, especially when you're exercising in dry or hot conditions. But some individuals (you know who you are) take it to the extreme. Overhydrating will challenge even the strongest bladder. Drinking only when you're thirsty, and chugging just a bit less from that ever-present water bottle, may be the simplest way to make it through your workout without a dribble.

- **Tread lightly.** Harsh landings may increase leakage. If you jump, try landing on the balls of your feet with some bend in your knees, rather than on a flat heel.

～ 9 ～

Pelvic Prolapse

BULGING, DROPPING, AND FALLING OUT:
CAUSES, SYMPTOMS, AND TREATMENTS

I had only one itty-bitty baby, thirty years ago. Why did this happen?
—Sixty-one-year-old, during a preoperative
visit for uterine prolapse

*P*elvic prolapse has complicated women's lives from time immemorial—in fact, probably ever since women started having
babies. So, how come you'd never heard of it before you started feeling symptoms? How come it hasn't been mentioned in history books?
Well, it has—as far back as the writings of Hypocrites. And it's been
treated in countless ways, many of them unfortunate. Women have
been suspended from their feet upside down, or cauterized with hot
iron and acids. In nomadic desert tribes, some women were known to
place salt in their vagina after delivery to help shrink the vaginal
walls and prevent prolapse.

Not until the nineteenth century were safe and effective treatments developed. Only then did most women with prolapse feel
empowered to confess this problem to their doctors. Yet even today,
the social embarrassment associated with these highly personal problems causes many women to underreport symptoms relating to prolapse, and as a result, it remains among the most challenging surgical
conditions to diagnose, let alone treat. What we do know is that by
age eighty, the estimated likelihood of undergoing an operation for
prolapse or incontinence is 11.1 percent. Give that statistic a
moment's thought—you're about as likely to have a major surgery for

weakening of the pelvic floor as you are to experience breast cancer during your lifetime.

Only a Problem . . . If It's Causing Problems

Almost all women enter their childbearing years with normal, strong pelvic supports. Depending upon childbirth, exercise habits, and work routines over the years, almost all women will eventually develop some degree of weakening down below, at least enough to be visible to a doctor during a pelvic exam. Fortunately, only a fraction of women with mild changes to their pelvic supports will be bothered by symptoms. For the rest, prolapse remains a physical feature that just happens to be there—the pelvic equivalent of wrinkling, of no consequence to daily function. Unlike high blood pressure or diabetes, which must be treated even during their silent early stages, asymptomic pelvic prolapse is rarely of medical importance. Prolapse is a problem only if it's causing problems and diminishing your quality of life.

So . . . You've Noticed a Bulge

Did you first notice the problem while cleaning yourself on the toilet? Did you feel it during intercourse or actually see it in the mirror? However you discovered your prolapse, no doubt you wondered what it could possibly be. What *could* it be? A bulge at the vaginal opening almost always means you've lost some pelvic support. The more challenging question is where?

Figure 9–1 shows perfectly normal pelvic supports. The vagina is like a horizontal tube with strong upper and lower walls. As you've seen, the vagina's upper vaginal wall provides the major support underneath the urethra and bladder, like a hose lying on the pavement. Beneath a sturdy lower vaginal wall, the rectum is kept down in its proper place. Finally, several ligaments that attach to the bones of the pelvis support the uterus, cervix, and upper apex of the vagina. So under normal conditions, as we've discussed in previous chapters, the strength within the vaginal walls, and their attachments to the pelvis, play essential roles in keeping the nearby organs—including bladder, rectum, and bowel—where they're supposed to be.

When a bulge has developed, support might have been lost around one or all of these individual areas, including the vagina, cervix, or uterus. Even within the vagina, the bulge could be arising from the upper wall, lower wall, entrance, or apex. Not all bulges are alike. Different types of prolapse often cause their own distinct symptoms and call for different treatments.

"MY MOTHER NEVER HAD THIS PROBLEM . . . WHY ME?"

Prolapse is common among postreproductive women, even those whose mothers and sisters were never affected, though family history may play a role, according to one recent study from the Netherlands. The odds of vaginal prolapse appeared to be five times higher for those individuals who could recall that their mother had prolapse, in comparison to those who could not.

Normal pelvic anatomy (without prolapse)

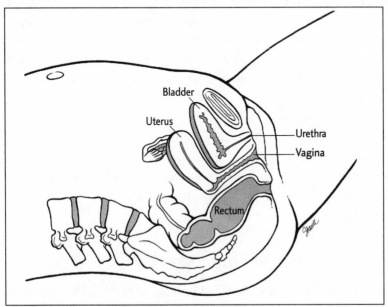

Types of Prolapse

CYSTOCELE: THE DROPPED BLADDER

A *cystocele* is what women have long referred to as a dropped bladder and it is one of the most common prolapse bulges in postreproductive women. A cystocele forms when your normally flat upper vaginal wall loses its support and drops downward. Because the bladder is located right above the upper vaginal wall, when that wall starts to drop, the bladder will drop right along with it (see Figure 9–2A). In advanced cases, the bulge may become visible outside the vaginal opening.

Cystoceles can cause a number of symptoms, ranging from vague to quite specific. Vaginal pressure is common, especially when the full bladder bulges down from its normal pelvic location and is felt in the vagina. During intercourse, pressure may be even more pronounced against the vaginal bulge.

Slowing of the urinary stream may occur when the urethra and bladder sink lower, as the normally straight urethral tube develops a slight bend or kink. Postvoid fullness—the sensation of bladder fullness even after you've tried to empty—may be caused by retention of urine inside a cystocele bulge that fails to fully empty while you're on the toilet. To compensate for this difficulty in emptying, many women with cystoceles begin a habit of double voiding, as discussed in chapter 8—several moments after they urinate, the urine retained inside the cystocele triggers a second urge, and they void a second time.

Finally, a cystocele bulge can also cause bladder infections. Like still water in a pond without a running river, cystoceles contain a pool of retained urine that doesn't flush out of the bladder normally. As a result, any bacteria finding its way into the bladder will have the opportunity to linger, multiply, and eventually cause a full-blown bladder infection.

RECTOCELE: THE BULGING RECTUM

Just as a cystocele is a downward bulging of the bladder into a weakened upper vaginal wall, a *rectocele* results from upward bulging of the rectum into a weakened lower vaginal wall. Figure 9–2B shows a weak lower vaginal wall allowing the rectum to bulge upward, forming a rectocele. This abnormally wide area in the rectal tube can, in turn, lead to a number of troubling symptoms.

First, if you've developed a rectocele, it's quite possible that your rectum never fully empties itself of stool, in contrast to a normal rectum, which fully empties after each bowel movement. As a result, rectocele-related symptoms include the sensation of rectal fullness and pressure, and difficulty pushing out stool even when it feels like it's right there. These symptoms can become aggravated by constipation, as hard stools are more likely to become stuck in the rectocele. Some women with rectoceles rely on *splinting* to empty their rectum, placing a finger in the vagina and pressing down on its lower wall during bowel movements. Splinting straightens out the weak and bulging lower vaginal wall, flattens the rectocele bulge, and allows stool to pass through.

With a rectocele, you're also prone to experience some loss of bowel control. Soiling of your underwear becomes more common, since stool left behind within the rectocele bulge is located just a short distance from the anal opening. Even more distressing is fecal incontinence. This can become a problem, as the stool within the rectocele can accidentally slip by the anal sphincter while you're exercising, lifting, or changing position.

If you have a cystocele, or a dropped bladder, your bladder itself is actually normal. It's just sinking down into a weakening in your upper vaginal wall. By the same token, if you have a rectocele, there's nothing wrong with your rectum—it's just bulging up into a weakened lower vaginal wall. Cystoceles and rectoceles are not diseases of the bladder or rectum—they're just mirror-image changes to the vaginal supports that allow those other organs to wander from their normal locations. Later in this chapter, you'll learn about simple devices and surgical procedures that relieve cystoceles and rectoceles by restoring vaginal supports closer to their prechildbirth state.

UTERINE PROLAPSE

Uterine prolapse, or a dropped womb, occurs when the uterus and cervix drop down toward the opening of the vagina after the pelvic ligaments supporting them have weakened. Sometimes diagnosing uterine prolapse is easy—you see the cervix (an irregular bulge with a small, slitlike opening at its center) protruding outside the vagina, or feel it while inserting a tampon. But most of the time, your doctor will make the diagnosis during the office exam. Uterine prolapse is one reason for needing a hysterectomy, usually performed through a vaginal incision. The symptoms caused by uterine prolapse can vary widely. A dropped uterus may cause pressure sensations in the vagina or rectum, or even lower back pain. Or sexual discomfort can develop from the penis striking the cervix, which has dropped from its location high up in the vagina, to somewhere in the middle or lower portion. Finally, if the uterus drops a lot, you may actually see the cervix outside the vaginal opening. If the cervix hangs low for prolonged periods, it can become irritated and significantly enlarged, even causing a heavy vaginal discharge.

VAGINAL VAULT PROLAPSE

If you've had a hysterectomy, part of your surgery involved securing the top of the vaginal tube (also called its apex) to nearby pelvic ligaments. When these new attachments are strong, the posthysterectomy vagina will have a length and depth that allows normal sexual function; the absence of a uterus and cervix will, of course, mean no more periods. However, if these attachments weaken, the upper vagina can begin to bulge downward, causing *vaginal vault prolapse.* By definition, this prolapse type can occur only in women who have had a hysterectomy. To the untrained eye, prolapse of the vault can appear quite similar to prolapse of the vagina's upper wall or lower wall—all three look like a bulge of tissue at the vaginal opening. In fact, all three can be similarly managed with pessaries, diaphragmlike devices that you'll learn about later. But repairing vaginal vault prolapse requires its own specific surgery, called a *vault suspension.*

ENTEROCELE

An *enterocele* is a bulging of the small intestine into the top of the vagina: in medical terms, an actual hernia into this especially vulnerable area of the female body. In terms of their general appearance, enteroceles look much like any other vaginal prolapse bulge. The difference is that lying behind an enterocele bulge are the intestines, rather than the bladder or rectum.

Because virtually any physical exertion tends to cause pressures to rise in the intestinal cavity, an enterocele bulge can expand like a balloon during activity and will often progress rapidly once it reaches a certain size. During periods of reduced physical activity, an enterocele may bulge much less, or even fully reduce. Just like a hernia, an enterocele will progress more rapidly if a woman performs heavy lifting, strains on the toilet, or fails to treat a chronic cough.

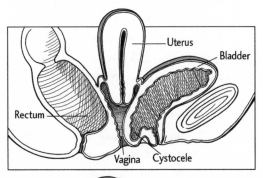

Although large enteroceles are usually easy to identify, determining whether or not you have a small enterocele can be somewhat difficult. Sometimes they're found only during surgery. On rare occasions, high-tech radiology tests are used to help make the diagnosis. Finding and repairing enteroceles is one of

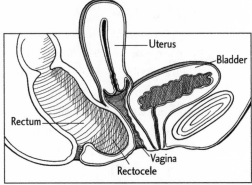

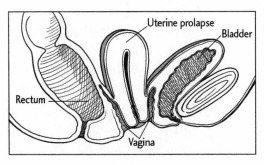

Common prolapse "bulges":
(A)cystocele, (B) rectocele,
(C) uterine prolapse

your doctor's important tasks, to reduce your chances of a recurrent prolapse. If a small enterocele is not recognized, it may grow in size, begin to protrude, and weaken the nearby areas of surgical repair.

IS THAT PROLAPSE I'M FEELING?

If you've been aware of pelvic symptoms and feeling that something's not quite right down there, it's not always easy to decipher which of them are being caused by prolapse. Early prolapse symptoms tend to be vague and can be easy to confuse with other common symptoms arising in the pelvis, bladder, vagina, and even lower back. But determining the cause of your symptoms is important, not only so you'll know what might improve with treatment, but also to avoid unnecessary procedures. After all, you wouldn't want to go through a major operation for what seems to be worsening prolapse symptoms when all you need is a stool softener for chronic constipation or a lower-back massage for muscle strain. Here are some useful clues to keep in mind.

- *Do you have bulging, pelvic or vaginal discomfort, or a dragging sensation in the lower abdomen or back that becomes worse when you're standing and improves when you lie down?* This is how prolapse symptoms often behave. If the reverse is true, and your symptoms worsen while you're at rest or sleeping, consider other causes. Try keeping a diary of your symptoms and activities for two to three days. This diary may be your first step toward finding relief (see "Voiding and Symptom Diary" Appendix B).

- *Are your symptoms worse at the end of the day?* That's pelvic prolapse's typical pattern. Pressure symptoms tend to become more severe after a long day of activity, exercise, and the simple downward force of gravity. The morning hours, after a good night's sleep, are usually the most symptom-free.

- *Do your symptoms improve when you're wearing a tampon or diaphragm?* For mild cases of prolapse, inserting a tampon or diaphragm can provide enough support to the vagina, rectum, and bladder that you'll notice an improvement in symptoms of either prolapse or incontinence. If you're familiar with the use of these devices, it's safe to try them before seeing your doctor, as long as you follow the usual instructions for use and *never* leave them inserted for longer than the recommended time. If they make you feel better, speak with your doctor about a longer-term support device (see "Vaginal Continence Devices," chapter 8).

• *Do your symptoms improve with the pessary test?* Pessaries are diaphragm-like devices inserted vaginally for the nonsurgical relief of prolapse, which you'll learn about in the next section. Trying one, even if only for a few days, might help you to better understand vague symptoms. For instance, is your lower-back discomfort arising from the prolapse of an enterocele or vaginal vault, or just a simple muscle strain? If pelvic symptoms disappear with the pessary in place, that's pretty good evidence that they're related to the loss of vaginal supports. The pessary test can help you to predict how you might feel after your prolapse is surgically repaired.

• *Has your urinary stream become weaker?* As prolapse bulges enlarge around the bladder and urethra, it's common to notice a weaker urinary stream.

• *Did your long-standing stress incontinence start to improve on its own?* Ironically, as prolapse becomes more advanced, you may notice an improvement in stress incontinence. That's because a large prolapse bulge will actually cause a bend or kink to form in the urethral tube (like putting a bend in that leaky garden hose we discussed), reducing the odds of accidental leakage during physical stress (see "Increased Incontinence," page 188).

• *Do you double-void, dribble, or feel full right after urinating?* Signs of urinary retention or incomplete voiding become common as certain prolapse bulges enlarge.

• *Does urinating become much easier after you've emptied your bowels?* Sometimes the stool filling a rectocele can actually push the bulging lower vaginal wall up against the urethra or bladder. After the rectocele is emptied with a bowel movement, the urinary stream will usually flow more easily.

Nonsurgical Remedies for Prolapse

MEDICATIONS FOR PROLAPSE-RELATED SYMPTOMS

There is no medication to fix pelvic prolapse, no wonder drug to address this challenging area of gynecology. There are, however, a handful of medications that can help you to deal with the symptoms that pelvic relaxation might cause. Anal incontinence (loss of stools), fecal soiling (staining of the underwear), and fecal urgency (sudden strong desires to have a bowel movement) can each result from the presence of a rectocele bulge. A high-fiber bowel diet and the bowel drill for behavioral therapy (see chapter 10) may be enough to relieve symptoms. If not, they can be alleviated with the help of a few simple products that maintain the right consistency of your stool. You should know the differences between the various common stool softeners, laxatives, and cathartics discussed in chapter 10, so you'll be able to improve your symptoms while doing no harm.

WHY ALL THE FUSS OVER CONSTIPATION?

We've said it before, but just in case you haven't heard: constipation is an archenemy of the pelvic floor. If you have a rectocele, constipation and hard stools can make the symptoms associated with this type of prolapse feel much worse. Occasionally, a rectocele filled with hard stool may even partially obstruct the urethra, making urination slow and difficult until the bulge finally empties along with a bowel movement. Good hydration and lots of fiber will minimize your troubles; if not, be sure to discuss other strategies with your doctor.

PESSARIES

The *pessary*—a device that fits into the vagina to support a bulging prolapse—may be the most enduring tool in the history of medicine. For millennia, in various forms, it has provided the major nonsurgical approach to supporting prolapse and relieving symptoms of pressure and discomfort. As early as 1500 B.C., pessaries were made of vine and natural extracts in Egypt. Three thousand years later, in eighteenth-century Paris, mothers were fitted with pessaries made of cork surrounded by layers of wax, "to hold her womb where it belongs . . . its ligaments . . . loosened by the strains of childbirth." Repeatedly dipping the device into wax would make it larger and more likely to stay in place, and a hole was left in the center to allow for conception.

Pessaries have, of course, changed in appearance over the years— thank goodness, we've come a long way since the 1700s—but they're still very much a part of gynecologic practice today. Modern pessaries are made of silicone and latex, in various shapes and sizes—such as rings, donuts, cubes, and bridges. When fitted properly, they can hold back bulging pelvic tissues and provide an invisible, effective, low-tech treatment alternative for prolapse.

Which women usually choose pessaries? In general, pessaries tend to be less popular among young and sexually active women, who are often more attracted to the quick fix of surgery. Women who are uncomfortable with the idea of wearing a device inside their body, don't like inserting or removing a pessary on their own, or cannot make fairly regular visits to the doctor's office also tend to choose another option. But for women of any age who wish to avoid surgery and are willing to accept these management issues, pessaries can be a real help.

HAVING A PESSARY FITTED

The right pessary is different for each woman, varying with her individual body shape and size. The only rule is a simple one: whichever pessary works for you is the right one. Pessaries are fitted in the doctor's office, where the doctor or nurse will most likely try a few different shapes and sizes, fitted according to the type and severity of your prolapse. In general, the largest pessary that fits comfortably is the most effective. Each will be checked for stability and comfort while you're lying down, standing, straining, and walking around. Fitting a pessary is a process of trial and error, and for better or worse, it has become something of a lost art as the popularity of surgery for prolapse has increased. Not every gynecologist will stock every type of pessary. So if your prolapse is advanced, you may be referred to a specialist.

When a pessary fits just right, you shouldn't be able to feel it

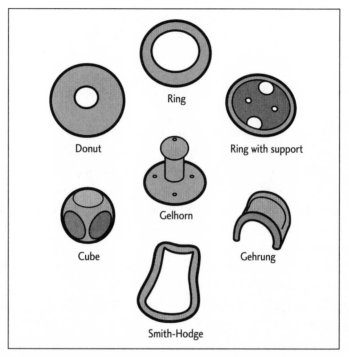

Common pessary types

inside, and it shouldn't block your flow of urine. An occasional awareness of something inside isn't unusual, but any pain or strong pressure will indicate it's not a good fit. Before leaving the office, you may be asked to empty your bladder to assure that the pessary isn't causing any sort of obstruction. Some pessaries need to be changed at the doctor's office, and others can be easily inserted and removed at home. Here are some of the most common:

- *Ring.* The simplest pessary type, for supporting mild prolapse bulges. Easy to remove and insert on your own.
- *Ring with support.* A simple variation of the ring pessary; looks just like a diaphragm.
- *Shotz.* A pessary shaped like a flying saucer, able to stay inside more firmly than a ring in situations where vaginal and perineal supports are very weak.
- *Smith-Hodge.* Specifically designed to support prolapse of the uterus and cervix.

- *Gelhorn.* Can provide very strong support but is rather difficult for women to insert and remove on their own. Inserted with the stem pointing out.

- *Gehrung.* An arch-shaped pessary, good for large cystoceles and/or rectoceles. Its awkward shape can make it difficult to insert and remove on your own.

- *Cube.* This type of pessary is designed to support very advanced prolapse bulges. Because the cube relies on suction against the vaginal walls rather than muscle support to stay inside, it may be effective even after almost all vaginal and perineal tone has been lost or as a last-ditch option when simpler pessaries have failed. However, because of its odd shape, it's difficult for most women to remove on their own and will often predispose to a buildup of (usually noninfectious) vaginal discharge, due to irritation of the vaginal walls, and partial blockage of the normal outflow of vaginal moisture.

- *Donut.* Another last-ditch pessary; bulky and difficult for most women to manage without frequent office visits.

CARING FOR YOUR PESSARY, AND POTENTIAL PROBLEMS

Some women can comfortably manage a pessary for years, with nothing more involved than regular removal and cleansing. But certain issues and problems can arise.

- *Vaginal discharge and irritation.* These can sometimes result simply from contact of the device against the vaginal skin and blocking of its normal drainage. Removing your pessary at bedtime, thoroughly rinsing it with warm water, and leaving it out for the night to rest the vaginal skin will reduce the odds of this problem. Most pessaries can be removed once or twice a week, or even much less often, but larger pessaries sometimes require nightly removal. The doctor or nurse will instruct you on the most appropriate routine. If you're not comfortable managing your pessary at home, then you'll need to make more frequent visits to the doctor's office.

  Applying a dollop of lubricant on the pessary surface can help to prevent irritation during insertion and removal. Remember to always use a water-soluble type (*Trimo-San, K-Y jelly, Astroglide*).

For some women, an occasional dilute vinegar douche may help counteract odor or discharge resulting from a pessary. This is by no means necessary for all pessary users, and douching should never be done regularly (otherwise, the vagina will have trouble restoring its normal balance of bacteria).

Atrophic vaginal skin is far likelier to become irritated and occasionally eroded by the friction of a pessary. Treatment with estrogen vaginal creams will make the vaginal skin less prone to irritation or erosion. Alternatively, an estrogen ring can be inserted right along with some pessaries, then exchanged for a new estrogen ring every three months.

- *Pressure sores.* If a pessary fits too tightly or sits inside for too long, or the vaginal skin is abnormally thin or dry, a pressure sore, or ulcer, may develop. In this case, the device must be removed and left out for a period of time specified by your doctor or nurse, to allow for proper wound healing. Again, the best way to prevent this problem is regular nightly removal of the pessary to rest the vaginal skin, along with maintaining proper lubrication and a healthy estrogen supply to the vagina.

- *Infections.* While wearing a pessary, some women may notice more frequent bladder infections, due to the sometimes heavy vaginal discharge that might allow bacteria easier access to the urethra. You can minimize this problem with regular removal and a healthy estrogen supply to the vaginal skin. Likewise, occasional yeast infections or other forms of vaginitis may occur. The risk of a more serious infection is extremely low.

- *Increased incontinence.* Urogynecologists constantly face this rather tricky paradox: when a large prolapse bulge is supported, stress incontinence may appear for the first time, or already existing stress incontinence may worsen. The reason for this is actually quite simple: when prolapse is unsupported and bulging out, a slight bend will often form in the urethral tube and serve to hold back leakage of urine, like an artificial valve. Compare it to bending the garden hose, which produces a kink that stops the flow of water. Conversely, supporting or reducing the prolapse bulge may increase the tendency to leak urine as the urethra is unbent. This is called *potential stress incontinence.* With surgery, prolapse and incontinence can be simultaneously fixed with good success. But with a pessary, addressing both problems in tandem poses a much greater challenge.

• *Still bulging.* If prolapse becomes more advanced, a pessary may need to be upsized. Even women who have been satisfied with their pessary for a long time may eventually find their prolapse has progressed, and surgery becomes the only effective option.

• *Urinary obstruction.* As already mentioned, during your pessary fitting, the doctor or nurse will usually check to be sure your pessary isn't blocking the urethra. Nevertheless, if you're ever unable to void when your bladder feels distended, call your doctor.

CAN PESSARIES CURE PROLAPSE?

Pessaries can definitely make a case of prolapse *feel* better. But can wearing one actually halt its progression? Common sense would suggest that a well-fitting pessary might reduce the burden on weakened pelvic supports bearing the weight of a prolapse bulge—and perhaps, as a result, slow its progress. On the other hand, the pessary itself can further stretch the surrounding tissues and may not hold back the entire bulge when prolapse becomes advanced. The bottom line? Wearing a pessary successfully for years does not eliminate the possibility that your prolapse will continue to progress, ultimately requiring an operation.

WHEN A PESSARY MIGHT NOT BE THE RIGHT CHOICE

Sometimes very advanced prolapse simply can't be propped up by an odd-shaped piece of plastic. For most pessaries to stay inside and work effectively, some degree of pelvic support is required within either the levator muscles or the perineum. By strengthening these areas, Kegel exercises may help to improve the support around a pessary. If all pelvic supports are gone, then there's little hope that the pessary will be the answer for you.

Surgery for Prolapse

Surgery for pelvic prolapse has always been one of the gynecologist's most difficult tasks. After all, prolapse often means the coexistence of several bulges, such as a cystocele, rectocele, uterine prolapse, vault prolapse, or enterocele; and the problem isn't fixed until every bulge is gone. Surgeons usually need to draw from a number of techniques to address every unique case, and they tailor them a bit differently each time. Permanently curing prolapse remains a challenge for even the most skilled and innovative reconstructive surgeons.

Fortunately, the number of techniques known for reconstructing the pelvic supports continues to expand. Prolapse bulges can be pushed up from below during vaginal surgery, or pulled up from above by abdominal or laparoscopic techniques. They can be folded up with stitches, covered with a graft or mesh, or sometimes stretched back and attached to their original supports along the pelvic bones or ligaments. In most cases, a combination of procedures will be used to repair the various components of prolapse that usually coexist.

REPAIRING CYSTOCELES

Cystoceles—the bladder dropping or bulging into a weak upper vaginal wall—come in two types. Your pelvic exam in the office will determine which type you have and what kind of repair would be most appropriate.

THE CENTRAL CYSTOCELE

A central cystocele occurs when the vaginal wall stretches and weakens, allowing the bladder to sag into the middle or central part of the upper vaginal wall. Imagine the Golden Gate Bridge stretching out at its center, allowing the road to droop in the middle under the weight of too many trucks.

Anterior colporrhaphy is the basic repair for a central cystocele. It involves tucking up the upper vaginal wall by bunching together the connective tissues beneath the vaginal skin, restoring a stronger floor for the bladder. It's one of the oldest reconstructive procedures in gynecology and is still commonly used. Following an anterior colpor-

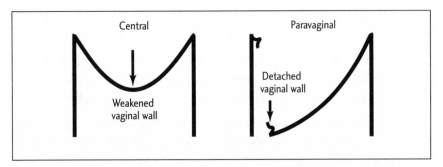

Two types of cystocele: "central" and "paravaginal"

rhaphy, the upper vaginal wall is flat and strong; over the long run, however, recurrent cystocele bulges can develop in somewhere between 3 and 30 percent of women.

THE PARAVAGINAL DEFECT

This type of cystocele develops during childbirth, when the vaginal walls tear away from their attachments along the sidewalls of the pelvis. In this case, it's not the middle of the Golden Gate Bridge that's sagging, it's the ends of the road detaching from their vertical supports and falling inwards after a San Francisco earthquake.

Paravaginal repair involves reattaching the sides of the vagina to the pelvic walls. It's a newer approach than the anterior colporrhaphy and is favored by some experts who consider paravaginal defects the most common and critical injuries occurring to the upper vagina during childbirth. Paravaginal repairs can be performed through an abdominal incision, by laparoscopy, or sometimes even through the vagina.

REPAIRING RECTOCELES

You've learned about the symptoms that can be caused by a rectocele, often the most bothersome of all prolapse types. Surgically repairing a rectocele can relieve or at least improve many of these complaints.

- *Bulging.* With repair, bulging of the lower vaginal wall and rectum will be improved, with at least 90 percent success. Among all the operations for prolapse, rectocele repairs tend to be among the most durable and effective over the long run.

- *Constipation and splinting.* The majority of women with difficult bowel movements will experience relief after this surgery and will be able to stop relying on the splinting technique.

- *Fecal incontinence and soiling.* Bowel control may improve after a rectocele repair, as the rectum is more likely to be completely empty of stool between bowel movements.

Rectoceles are typically repaired with a vaginal operation. *Posterior colporrhaphy* is a mirror image of the anterior colporrhaphy. This traditional rectocele repair involves finding the connective tissues between the vagina and rectum and bunching this layer together more strongly.

The newest surgical approach, *site-specific rectocele repair,* involves finding discrete areas of injury (or defects) in the connective tissues between the vagina and rectum—ones that were caused, in most cases, by childbirth. After the defects are identified, they are repaired, just like stitching closed a cut in the skin. It's not yet clear whether the site-specific rectocele repair is more or less successful than the standard posterior colporrhaphy technique, but its potential for success has raised interest in learning more about how childbirth injury affects each woman's pelvic function during her postreproductive lifetime.

WHEN YOU NEED A GRAFT OR MESH

Whenever possible, most surgeons prefer to use each woman's own pelvic connective tissues and ligaments to repair prolapse. But if your natural supports have become too weak, synthetic materials or grafts may sometimes be utilized for reinforcement. These foreign substances can be anchored to nearby muscles or ligaments, or placed loosely over the cystocele or rectocele bulge.

- Synthetic mesh (Gore-Tex, Prolene, Vicryl, Mersilene) is an entirely man-made woven material. Both absorbable and permanent materials may be used.

- Fascia is a layer of connective tissue that exists throughout the body. When implanted as a graft during pelvic surgery, a strip of fascia will stick around for a period of months or years before it is slowly absorbed. During this process, the fascia is replaced by a new layer of scar. A strip of the patient's own fascia can be taken from beneath the skin of the leg or abdominal wall, through a separate incision. Sterilized and processed strips, originating from cadavers, are also commercially available.

- Dermis is a strip of skin, obtained from either animals (pigs, for instance) or human cadavers. Like fascia, dermis does not last forever; over time, it is absorbed and replaced by scar.

- Skin and fascia grafts reprocessed for extra strength have been recently developed, possibly adding more durability.

REPAIRING VAGINAL VAULT PROLAPSE

These procedures are used when the vaginal vault, or the top of the vagina, has come loose from its attachments deep in the pelvis. Three operations are most common, each using a different anchoring point for reattaching the vagina.

UTEROSACRAL LIGAMENT SUSPENSION

This procedure, which can be performed through abdominal, laparoscopic, or vaginal incisions, attaches the upper vagina to the *uterosacral ligaments.* These strong tissue bands run along the sides of your pelvis, back toward the upper vagina. When reasonably strong uterosacral ligaments exist, this operation can provide excellent long-term support while keeping the vagina straight and wide at the top; in other cases, however, the uterosacral ligaments are simply too weak and stretched, so another technique must be used. When performed vaginally, the procedure is referred to as the McCall culdoplasty, named after a famous surgeon.

SACROSPINOUS LIGAMENT SUSPENSION

This operation is performed only through a vaginal incision; it fixes the top of the vagina to a very strong ligament along the floor of the pelvis called the *sacrospinous ligament.* It is a particularly useful approach for advanced cases of vaginal vault prolapse, and also for women with very weak uterosacral ligaments, since the sacrospinous ligament is a consistently strong anchoring point even in these situations. Although the top of the vagina angles slightly to the side after sacrospinous suspension, this rarely poses a problem during intercourse or otherwise.

Sacral Colpopexy

This operation uses an open abdominal technique for repairing vaginal vault prolapse. It utilizes a graft of material, either synthetic mesh or a natural-tissue graft, to fasten the upper vagina back to the sacrum at the rear of the pelvis. It is a sturdy repair (over 90 percent successful, comparable to sacrospinous ligament suspension) that keeps the vagina straight. The major disadvantage is the abdominal incision, resulting in a longer average hospital stay and recovery time. Also, the mesh or graft introduces other risks, including infection or erosion through the vaginal skin, requiring partial or full removal.

Laparoscopic Sacral Colpopexy

The sacral colpopexy can also be done through a laparoscopic camera and keyhole incisions, rather than a bikini cut, by experienced laparoscopic surgeons.

REPAIRING ENTEROCELES

Enteroceles are most often repaired vaginally, through the same type of incision used to repair a cystocele, rectocele, or uterine or vaginal vault prolapse. This type of prolapse bulge actually contains loops of intestine, just like a hernia. During the operation, the enterocele bulge is carefully entered; then the intestinal loops are replaced back up into the pelvis, and the area where the enterocele originated is closed off and strongly reinforced with stitches.

Enteroceles can also be repaired during abdominal surgery for prolapse. Special support sutures are used to reinforce the very bottom ligaments and connective-tissue supports of the pelvis, so that the bowel contents are supported more strongly above the vagina. Laparoscopic repair is similar to the other two methods but uses laparoscopy.

Hysterectomy and Other
Surgical Options for Prolapse

Surgical removal of the uterus, or *hysterectomy*, has historically been one of the most overused operations in gynecology, at least in the United States, where rates have been up to twice those among British women and four times those in France. In years past, up to a third of women over the age of sixty-five had one. The landscape of gynecology has changed dramatically, and the recent declining rate of hysterectomy in the United States is encouraging. A number of less invasive treatment alternatives are available for a wide range of problems, including fibroids, abnormal bleeding, and pain—and for prolapse, as we've discussed.

On the other hand, if you have pelvic prolapse or incontinence, hysterectomy can be a necessary part of surgical treatment. When properly used, it can have definite benefits. So, under what circumstances is a hysterectomy the right choice for you?

- *Bulging of a prolapsed uterus.* For advanced prolapse of the uterus, hysterectomy is often the best treatment; around 15 percent of all hysterectomies are performed for prolapse. Despite the understandable impulse to avoid hysterectomy whenever possible, a bulging uterus will usually result in persistent symptoms and may, over time, seriously jeopardize any repair done to the nearby vaginal anatomy. The weight of a prolapsed uterus may simply pull down the vaginal stitches and supports until a new cystocele, rectocele, or other prolapse bulge appears. On the other hand, if the uterus isn't part of your prolapse bulge, cystoceles and rectoceles can be repaired just as effectively without a hysterectomy. Performing an unnecessary hysterectomy, in these cases, may even raise the risk of recurrent prolapse by weakening the natural supports that surround the upper vagina, and by removing the blocking effect that an enlarged uterus sometimes has at the bottom of the pelvis.

- *Sexual pain.* A prolapsed cervix that has dropped closer to the vaginal opening can become a source of discomfort when it's bumped during intercourse.

- *Big fibroids, bleeding, and other problems.* Factors that are not directly related to your prolapse might also steer your decisions about hysterectomy. Have you been dealing with heavy or irregular bleeding, fibroid tumors (benign growths on the uterus), or abnormal Pap smears? Peripheral conditions such as these sometimes make it advisable to treat definitively with hysterectomy during incontinence or prolapse surgery.

When is hysterectomy not right?

- *For urinary incontinence alone.* If you have incontinence without prolapse, hysterectomy is rarely necessary. A recent systematic review showed that hysterectomy might even be associated with higher rates of urinary incontinence later on. All of the operations for stress incontinence can be done just as easily in the presence of a normal, well-supported uterus.
- *You're just not ready.* Hysterectomy for many women is not simply another surgery—it's a symbolic life event that should never be taken lightly. The operation shouldn't be performed for these benign postreproductive problems until you're finished with childbearing, informed of your alternatives, and feel that you're emotionally ready.

TYPES OF HYSTERECTOMY

VAGINAL HYSTERECTOMY

This technique to treat a prolapsed uterus has been around for a hundred years; it remains a standard approach for most cases. Through an incision at the top of the vagina, the uterus and even the ovaries can be removed. In most cases, you can expect relatively mild postoperative pain, a short hospital stay, and quick recovery. At times a vaginal hysterectomy might not be feasible—for instance, if your uterus is too large, your pelvic bones are too narrow, or if prior surgery left you with scarring around the pelvic organs.

ABDOMINAL HYSTERECTOMY

Abdominal hysterectomy involves a skin incision, usually a bikini cut just above your pubic hairline. Surgeons who favor an overall abdominal approach to prolapse or incontinence surgery may perform abdominal hysterectomy because it can be naturally combined with other abdominal-route prolapse techniques. The abdominal hysterectomy may also sometimes represent the only option for removing a uterus that is very enlarged or stuck with scar tissue to surrounding structures due to a previous pelvic surgery or infection.

LAPAROSCOPIC HYSTERECTOMY

Beyond vaginal and abdominal hysterectomies lies the more high-tech alternative of laparoscopy, taking place through tiny incisions and projected onto a video screen. Laparoscopy can be used to partially detach the uterus in order to make a vaginal hysterectomy easier (*laparoscopic-assisted vaginal hysterectomy*). In some cases, it can be used to perform the entire hysterectomy (*laparoscopic hysterectomy*), using special devices that detach the uterus and then remove it in small pieces. Recovery after these procedures is generally rapid, similar to a vaginal hysterectomy—with the added possibility of some upper abdominal or shoulder pain for a few days after surgery, resulting from residual gas bubbles in the abdomen irritating the nerves running to those areas. Critics of laparoscopic hysterectomy argue that it necessitates a longer operating time, can incur greater financial costs, and may increase the risk of certain injuries. Nevertheless, if used in the right instances for the right women, laparoscopic hysterectomy can be a useful and well-tolerated option.

SUPRACERVICAL HYSTERECTOMY

This variation involves removal of the uterine body while leaving the cervix attached to its pelvic supports and in its usual position above the upper vagina. It can be performed through either a standard abdominal incision or laparoscopic keyholes, but not as a vaginal surgery. Supracervical hysterectomy involves a few pros and cons.

- *Pro.* It's been claimed (more often in checkout-aisle magazines than in scientific journals) that leaving the cervix may help to maintain sexual pleasure and orgasmic function by preserving a bumping sensation against the cervix during intercourse.

- *Con.* Even if that claim holds true for some, it's probably least likely to apply to those women with uterine prolapse, whose bulging cervix contributes more often to sexual discomfort than pleasure. Studies have confirmed that among women with prolapse, a substantial percentage of those with deep sexual pain will find improvement in their sexual function after hysterectomy involving removal of the cervix.

- *Pro.* Could a supracervical hysterectomy help to better preserve your pelvic supports? It's been proposed in years past that fewer nerves and connective tissues may be injured with supracervical as compared with complete hysterectomy, helping to preserve bladder, bowel, and sexual function.

- *Con.* A group of British investigators appear to have debunked this claim. Their study involved 279 women scheduled for hysterectomy who received either the total or supracervical operation by random choice. The authors found that contrary to popular belief, supracervical hysterectomy did not result in better bladder, bowel, or sexual functioning one year after surgery. Particularly if you're having the hysterectomy for prolapsed pelvic supports that have already proven themselves weak, then removing the entire uterus and suspending the upper vagina to more solid structures is probably the best plan.

Finally, after supracervical hysterectomy, your risk for cervical cancer will remain the same as before, so you'll still need regular Pap smears.

OTHER SURGICAL METHODS FOR UTERINE PROLAPSE

Several operations can lift a partially prolapsed uterus back into the pelvis by securing it to pelvic ligaments or other supports. If you're still considering future childbearing and simply can't succeed with a pessary, then these alternatives may be worth looking into. These uterine sparing alternatives are appropriate only in very specific circumstances, however, and may offer limited long-term success compared with hysterectomy.

SACROSPINOUS OR UTEROSACRAL FIXATION

These are the most common vaginal operations for suspending the uterus, using no abdominal incision in most cases. A 1993 report of nineteen women included five who later had a successful vaginal birth. Through a vaginal incision, the ligaments connected to the uterus are secured to the sacrospinous or uterosacral ligaments, located deep in the pelvis.

LAPAROSCOPIC UTERINE SUSPENSION

This method involves shortening the ligaments between the uterus and pelvic walls, or fixing the uterus to the tailbone with a graft or strip of mesh through a small laparoscopic Band-Aid incision.

WHAT ABOUT THE OVARIES?

If a hysterectomy will accompany your prolapse or incontinence repair, you'll need to decide whether to have your ovaries removed (*oophorectomy*) or to have them left behind. You're probably well aware that up until menopause, the ovaries are your main source of estrogen; as for afterward, the debate surrounding estrogen replacement has become enormously complex.

If you're postmenopausal, many gynecologists will favor oophorectomy. Ovarian cancer will develop in approximately 1 percent of women during their lifetime, and it remains one of the most difficult to detect of the female cancers; surgically removing the ovaries nearly eliminates this risk. Others disagree, arguing that the ovaries continue to play a valuable role in producing male hormones in small quantities, even after menopause, and that these substances may influence libido, sexual function, mood, and mental acuity. This data is interesting but by no means conclusive. Also, hormone replacement containing both male and female hormones is now commercially available.

If you're premenopausal, the issues can be even more perplexing, since removal of the ovaries will induce the onset of menopause in women who haven't yet naturally passed through "the change." The presence of functional ovaries, as we've already discussed, is an important protector of so many aspects of your health, including a healthy heart and strong bones. As a result, removing the ovaries would typically be recommended only for women at an elevated risk for ovarian cancer, or those approaching natural menopause. Your age, family history, and personal feelings regarding hormone replacement after surgery all need to be carefully weighed.

A full exploration of the issues of oophorectomy before menopause, risk assessment, and hormone replacement are beyond the scope of this book. Work with your doctor to choose the approach that feels right for you.

⚘ 10 ⚘

Bowel Problems
and Anal Incontinence

EXPLANATION AND REMEDIES
FOR A NEGLECTED FEMALE PROBLEM

I thought that these problems were the price that all women pay for having children.

—Jennifer, thirty-nine, teacher and
mother of two

Diminished control over the bowels, whether it's stool or gas, is one of the most distressing and embarrassing problems faced by postreproductive women. Unfortunately, it's far more common than once believed. By age forty-five, it is eight times more prevalent in women than men, occurring in around 25 percent of women who have had a previous vaginal delivery. Awareness and recognition of this problem have lagged far behind other problems of women's health, but can you imagine one that is more elemental? If you've noticed symptoms in this department, or are concerned about your risk, it's time to educate yourself.

Fecal Incontinence

To keep you continent of stool, the anal sphincter muscles normally encircle the anal opening like a donut. When functioning properly, these muscles provide constant involuntary pressure at the anal sphincter, even while you're sleeping. Beyond that, we depend on the ability of these muscles to voluntarily contract. If you're faced with a sudden urge while window-shopping after lunch, these muscles should be able to flex even more strongly, at least long enough to get you back to the office.

During childbirth, the anal sphincter muscles can be torn partially or completely, leading to a loss of bowel control. Vaginal delivery is the main cause of fecal incontinence in women. Among three million vaginal deliveries each year in the United States, it's been estimated that nearly 5 percent (one hundred and fifty thousand) are complicated by a torn anal sphincter, and 25 percent of these injuries (forty thousand) will lead to anal incontinence later in life. A study from Sweden found that among those with a recognized anal sphincter tear at their first delivery, 32 percent had some form of both anal and urinary incontinence five years later. Another British study of 286 women during their first pregnancy found that anal incontinence increased from 1.4 percent, before pregnancy to 8.7 percent afterward. Some women will have trouble controlling only soft stool or diarrhea; others will become incontinent of solid stools also.

Even more surprising, a 1993 lead article in *The New England Journal of Medicine* showed with anal ultrasound that hidden injury to the anal sphincter occurs in up to 34 percent of seemingly uneventful first deliveries, and in up to 44 percent of women after two or more vaginal births. That's a remarkable reflection on the physical stress of childbirth; only a fraction of these hidden injuries will cause a problem later on, depending on how a "problem" is defined.

Beyond that, a great number of women develop *fecal urgency*, meaning the presence of very strong urges to defecate. Reports of fecal urgency, an often overlooked bowel symptom, increased from 1 to over 10 percent after childbirth.

Flatal Incontinence

Flatal incontinence is the inability to avoid passing gas even in social situations. It's as common among women in their postreproductive years as it is embarrassing, found in up to 26 percent of women after delivery. Many postreproductive women find that no matter how much they change their diet or bowel habits, this problem won't go away. Why should this become a problem after childbirth?

Even if your external anal sphincter survives childbirth intact and keeps you continent of stools, damage to the less visible internal anal sphincter may have occurred, leading to flatal incontinence. Unlike the external anal sphincter, which resembles a donut, the internal sphincter muscle is a thin, sheetlike layer surrounding the rectal tube. An intact internal sphincter makes the rectum a high-pressure area, giving you the ability to sense the presence of gas and appropriately deal with it. If your internal sphincter is no longer functional after childbirth, you'll often be completely unaware of gas until it's too late.

Repairing or even looking for injury to the internal anal sphincter is uncommon in routine obstetrical care. Probably because women rarely mention flatal incontinence, doctors are unlikely to give its obstetrical causes a great deal of thought. Amid all of the drama on childbirth's stage, this issue simply hasn't drawn the attention it deserves, during birth or afterward.

Other Bowel Problems After Childbirth

If your pelvic floor weakens after childbirth, the overall function of your bowels can also become slower and weaker. Due to a diminished functioning of nerves and muscles, a shift in anatomy, or both, some women will notice a change in their bathroom habits, requiring more proactive strategies for keeping the bowels moving, which we'll discuss soon.

Of all bowel problems, it's fairly common to notice *hemorrhoids* for the first time during or after pregnancy. If you already had them before childbirth, chances are they got worse. Whether they're old or new, for a good number of postreproductive women, hemorrhoids become a steady companion and a source of burning, itching, bleeding, and pain.

There are specific reasons why hemorrhoids grow during and after childbirth. As the pregnant uterus expands, its size and weight become large enough to compress the hemorrhoidal veins that run through your pelvis and carry blood back to the heart from your lower body. Compression of these veins leads to sluggish blood flow and pooling into varicose veins. Imagine a tourniquet tied tightly around your upper arm, causing the downstream veins in your hand and wrist to bulge. That's very similar to what occurs in the pregnant pelvis. As the growing uterus begins to compress the nearby blood vessels, varicose veins in the lower legs often flare. They flare around the anal area as well. The only difference is that the anal variety is given a special name and a shelf in the pharmacy aisle.

If all of this sounds alarmingly familiar, don't despair. Did you know that up to 80 percent of anal incontinence can be alleviated without procedure or surgery?

LIFESTYLE AND HABIT CHANGES FOR COPING WITH ANAL INCONTINENCE

THE BOWEL DRILL

Your bowels are yet another creature of habit, and somewhere along the line, after childbirth, you might have noticed that habits in this area began to change. Anal incontinence, frequent sudden urges to move your bowels, trouble urinating unless your bowels have emptied, never feeling finished after trying to empty, or soiling your underwear: all of these are potential signs of a postreproductive change, and many can be improved with behavior alone. For instance, using only dietary changes and pelvic exercise, fecal incontinence can be improved or eliminated at least 50 percent of the time. As with the bladder, the bowels can be retrained to some degree. The following three steps should help to keep your bowels well behaved.

Step #1: Prevent Constipation. Chronic constipation occurs in up to 25 percent of the population, and it's more than just an inconvenience: it's one of the genuine archenemies of your pelvic floor. Hard stools and constipation encourage heavy valsalva straining on the toilet, a habit that can further stretch and weaken the pelvic nerves and muscles. Over time, this may lead to increased floppiness, causing incontinence, and the bulges of pelvic prolapse. Less commonly, *impaction* can occur, meaning that the colon is temporarily blocked by hard stool resulting from severe constipation. If the rectum is filled with impacted stool, it can form a bulge that presses against the urethra or bladder outlet, making urination more difficult and causing the bladder to over-fill. For that reason, women with rectoceles, especially, may notice that their urine flows easier after their bowels have been emptied. For these reasons, although maintaining regular bowel movements is a healthy habit at any stage of life, it's particularly important for your postreproductive body.

- *Fiber and hydration.* These are the key ingredients to keeping your stools bulky yet not too hard. Just ahead, you'll learn the basic ingredients for a healthy bowel diet. Good hydration is another component, although the mantra of eight glasses a day is not necessary for most women.
- *Exercise.* This may be the most overlooked aspect of bowel control. A regular exercise routine is critical for keeping the bowels moving, and it may also keep your pelvic floor healthier over the long run. Even a brisk twenty-minute walk each day will greatly improve your function.

Step #2: Time your movements. Preventing constipation is sometimes as simple as making the effort to move your bowels regularly. Amid a hectic daily schedule, it's common to postpone trips to the bathroom; this can lead to constipation, as the stool loses its water content and the bowel muscles pass up their best shot at fully emptying. Unlike bladder drills—where resisting the urge to urinate can be therapeutic—with the bowels, it's almost always best to go to the toilet as soon as you notice an urge. Empty your bowels, or at least try to do so, after breakfast and other meals. At those times, your colon and rectum will tend to most fully evacuate due to the natural stimulation of the bowels that occurs after eating. As a result, rectoceles will be less likely to retain stool contents, leaving you less prone to soiling and accidents. Take your time on the toilet, and *avoid straining.* Between one and three movements each day is considered normal.

Step #3: Learn your patterns. You may need to tailor your habits for different times of the day or even month. For instance, some women notice variation in their bowel habits during different phases of the menstrual cycle. In the week before your period, high levels of progesterone tend to encourage constipation by relaxing the smooth muscle of the bowels, causing them to fail to move stools along as efficiently. As a result, you may need to add stool softeners during these times. Your Voiding and Symptom Diary (see Appendix B) may help you to identify these patterns.

SPLINTING

This term refers to using a finger, or several fingers, to push down on the lower vaginal wall in order to defecate. Though it's rarely discussed outside of the doctor's office, this is a common habit among women with rectoceles, due to stool becoming stuck in the bulge. It's a habit that's unnecessary, as the problems causing it are treatable. If splinting has become a necessity for you even after following these simple tips, be sure to discuss the problem with your doctor.

DIET AND SELF-HELP REMEDIES

THE BOWEL DIET

If you're dealing with postreproductive bowel symptoms, such as a loss of control over stool or gas, fecal urgency, or soiling, simple changes to your diet may help.

Fiber, or roughage, is the part of plant food that passes through the bowels without being absorbed or digested. Fiber promotes larger, bulkier stools, making them easier to control—either holding back or letting go, depending on the situation. A bulky stool will be far less likely to accidentally slip past a weak anal sphincter or rectocele bulge to cause incontinence or soiling. Most Americans consume less than half of the recommended daily fiber intake.

You'll find both major types of fiber, water-soluble and insoluble, in a number of basic food products. Aim for 28 to 30 grams of daily fiber, along with plenty of water. Introduce fiber into your diet gradually, to allow your bowels to adjust.

- *Bran: wheat or oat.* Bran is the outer capsule of grain and a great source of fiber. Try bran cereal and muffins, oatmeal or high-fiber wafers, along with fruit or applesauce.
- *Wheat germ.* Try one to six tablespoons in your daily diet, along with your favorite cereal, fruit, or cottage cheese.
- *Seeds, brown rice, fiber breads, fiber cookies.*
- *Popcorn.* An inexpensive, low-calorie source of pure roughage.
- *Psyllium.* When soaked with water, psyllium husks become gelatinous, and when eaten, make the stool soft, bulky, and hydrated. Seeds and husks from the psyllium plant, or psyllium bran, are the raw product for several popular stool-softener supplements (Metamucil, Per Diem fiber, and generic equivalents).
- *Prune juice.* Six ounces each morning to start the day.
- *Cooked or stewed fruits.* Prunes are fat-free and even available in different flavors. Applesauce or cooked fruits can provide a tastier substitute.
- *Leafy vegetables and fresh fruits.* Just like Mom always said, make lettuce, spinach, celery, or broccoli a regular part of your lunch and dinner.
- *Avoid fast food.* Don't just "hold the pickles, hold the mayo"; go one step further and hold the whole darn order. Fast foods are mostly fatty, low in soluble fiber, and likely to leave your bowel movements soft, fatty, and slow.

Watch for what stimulates, and know what slows:

- *Stimulates.* Caffeine, spicy foods, and lactose can stimulate the bowel, loosen the stools, and make control a much bigger challenge.
- *Slows.* Cheese and yogurt may have a binding effect on the bowels. On the other hand, for women with an irritable or lactose-intolerant bowel, they can sometimes act as stimulants. Bananas and rice are sometimes helpful for binding the stools and harnessing a runaway bowel.

TAKE THE PLEDGE: BECOME AN LOL

Little old ladies (LOLs) are known for eating fiber and stewed fruit and drinking prune juice by the six-pack. Why do you think, good reader, that might be? It's not because these ladies' taste buds are any different from yours, or that they've somehow lost their marbles. Quite to the contrary. The reason is that little old ladies know what works. Through daily fruit and fiber, they stay regular with the time-tested tricks that work the best. When it comes to a good bowel diet, remember that you're never too young to become an LOL.

MEDICATION AND HORMONAL REMEDIES FOR ANAL INCONTINENCE

If you have anal incontinence—whether it's the actual loss of stool or just fecal urgency or soiling—*don't skip this section.* The majority of bowel problems such as these can be fixed with a combination of diet, behavior, and one or more basic remedies found in just about any pharmacy. Understanding the different products that can help to regulate your bowels is the first step.

BULK-FORMING STOOL SOFTENERS

Bulky stools will naturally stimulate the bowel, encouraging better peristalsis (intestinal activity) and more efficient emptying. If you have a rectocele, well-formed stools will make you less prone to fecal soiling and incontinence.

- *Psyllium (Metamucil), calcium polycarbophil (FiberCon), ducosate sodium (Colace, Surfak), and generic equivalents*
- *Husk supplements, malt extract*

Add these agents slowly to your routine, and drink at least eight ounces of water with each dose. Using fiber supplements without adequate fluid intake can actually worsen constipation. Because they're nonaddictive, you can use them daily without concern.

LAXATIVES

If your bowel movements remain infrequent (fewer than three or four per week) despite high fiber and good hydration, an occasional laxative may stimulate some action. But avoid regular use. Because certain laxatives fail to soften the stools, you may be better off with a more aggressive regimen of stool softeners. Also, the intestines can become dependent upon laxatives if they're used too regularly, causing a lazy bowel. When you see the word *laxative* on the package, remember to use sparingly, and don't hesitate to consult with your doctor. If your doctor okays their use, laxatives come in a few forms:

- *Water magnets.* These agents, also known as osmotic laxatives, stimulate bowel activity by pulling water into the intestines. They are made of specific salts or sugars that are not absorbed by the bowels. Use these substances with care. If used excessively, they can cause abdominal cramping or an upset stomach.

- *Magnesium citrate, magnesium hydroxide (milk of magnesia).* A relatively mild and fast-acting laxative.

- *Lactulose (Chronulac), lactitol, sorbitol.* Stronger osmotic laxatives; less common for at-home use.

BOWEL LUBRICANTS

These products, also called *emollients,* are inserted from below to promote emptying of hard, constipated stool.

- *Mineral oil (Fleet).* Can be used orally or as an enema, but unpleasant side effects are common.

- *Glycerine suppository.* Occasional use may help a rectocele bulge to empty its stool contents.

CHEMICAL STIMULANTS

These substances act to stimulate the smooth muscle of the intestinal wall, with an effect that may last up to several days. They should be started only with your physician's guidance and *not* used on a regular basis.

- *Bisacodyl (Correctol, Dulcolax).* Oral and suppository forms are available.

- *Senna, Cascara.* Natural substances available in pills (Senokot) or herbal forms ranging from tinctures to seedpods or tea.

- *Per Diem.* Fiber supplement available in a few forms, one including a stimulant laxative.

Remember to consult with your doctor before starting a bowel regimen that includes laxatives. Some of these medications contain salts or sugars that should be avoided by women with certain medical conditions. Overstimulation of the bowel with chemical laxatives can lead to dependence and even more severe constipation. Constipation and other changes in your bowel patterns may sometimes signal a more serious underlying problem. Speak with your doctor before treating yourself to be sure that an examination or testing isn't necessary.

BOWEL SLOWERS

For women dealing with even a subtle loss of control over the bowels, routine situations can quickly become a nightmare when diarrhea strikes. For some individuals, a waxing and waning pattern of diarrhea and constipation called *irritable bowel* is a chronic state. In this case, you should be evaluated by a gastroenterologist, who can confirm the diagnosis and recommend dietary and medical strategies. But for others, sporadic and unexpected attacks occur infrequently and unpredictably. A few key medications may provide short-term relief by slowing the bowels. These pills should always be used very sparingly so that constipation doesn't result. But when you just can't risk an accident—for instance, during your well-deserved winter trip to Mexico, or your daughter's graduation ceremony—they can be a cherished companion.

Some options are loperamide, Lomotil, cholestyramine resin, and diphenoxylate.

PELVIC STIMULATION, IMPLANTS, AND PACEMAKERS: NEW NONSURGICAL OPTIONS FOR ANAL INCONTINENCE.

As you learned in chapter 8, a number of stimulation devices and relatively easy office procedures can be used to help restore bladder control. If you're coping with a major loss of bowel control and dietary and behavioral changes have failed to solve the problem, these alternatives may be worth checking into. In general, their use for anal incontinence is relatively new, even experimental in some cases. But a number of specialists are looking into the use of these options before recommending surgery.

- *Biofeedback.* Just as with urinary incontinence, learning to identify and strengthen your pelvic muscles could help to improve anal incontinence in up to 72 percent of cases.
- *Interstim.* The pelvic pacemaker, an amazing new therapy for urge incontinence and other bladder problems, may have a future use for anal incontinence. A clinical study is ongoing—stay tuned for results.
- *Neotonus.* In general, responses to magnetic therapy are difficult to predict, even for its main indication of urinary incontinence. But its effectiveness for fecal incontinence is being tested, and since from the patient's perspective, it's as easy as sitting in a chair fully clothed, it might be worth asking about.

SURGERY FOR ANAL INCONTINENCE

Surgery to repair an anal sphincter injured during childbirth is best performed right after delivery, during the episiotomy repair; years later, the healing is far more complicated and the outcomes are far from guaranteed success. Only a very select group of women troubled by poor bowel control should consider the option of surgery later in life.

REASONS FOR SURGERY
- Your doctor has identified an anal sphincter defect by physical examination and/or ultrasound tests.
- You have fecal incontinence with solid and well-formed stools.
- You've been unable to control the problem using dietary and behavioral strategies, such as the bowel drill and the bowel diet.

- You've tried physical therapy: for instance, biofeedback, pelvic-floor stimulation, or the Interstim pelvic pacemaker.
- You're willing to accept the possibility that even after a challenging recovery, the operation may fail to improve your fecal incontinence.

TYPES OF SURGERY

Anal sphincteroplasty is by far the most common surgical approach for anal incontinence. Through an incision in the perineum extending to the anal opening, the torn edges of the anal sphincter muscle are stitched back together, re-creating its circular donut shape. Often the edges of the circle are overlapped during surgery, forming a double-layer of muscle where the "defect" previously existed—this is called the "overlapping sphincteroplasty."

The *postanal repair, levatorplasty,* and other procedures utilizing nearby muscles to wrap around and strengthen the anal sphincter are performed only on rare occasion, usually by colorectal surgeons. The *artificial anal sphincter* is an even more uncommon procedure and is considered an option only for highly symptomatic patients who have failed other repairs.

YOU'RE IN GOOD COMPANY, AND YOU *CAN* RESTORE CONTROL

Problems with bowel control are common and can be devastating to an individual's self-confidence and quality of life. A number of childbirth-related changes—to nearby nerves, muscles, and connective tissues—help to explain why women are more often left to cope with these problems than men. Between 10 and 25 percent of all postreproductive women report symptoms to some degree; fortunately, their taboo status is quickly changing.

Whatever your age and whatever the nature of your problem, start with the simple tips we've discussed and mention the problem to your doctor. Most importantly, don't stop pursuing help until you've found relief.

⛬ 11 ⛬

Sex After Childbirth and Beyond

RESTORING SATISFACTION, SENSATION, AND SELF-CONFIDENCE

I feel almost nothing during intercourse anymore.
                              —LeAnne, age thirty-six

I had a wonderful, fantastic, empowering home birth . . . but I went to feeling basically sexless for months and actually years.
                              —Demi, age forty-eight

*I*t's been estimated that sexual dysfunction affects anywhere from 19 to 50 percent of women. In the United States National Health and Social Life Survey of more than 1,700 women, sexual dysfunction was reported by 43 percent. Sexual disorders have been reported in approximately 14 percent of women following routine vaginal delivery; the risk is thought to be even higher after a forceps or vacuum delivery. If things haven't been the same between the sheets ever since you had your baby, rest assured that you're *not* alone.

Why, then, amid all the hype over hormones, osteoporosis, and heart disease, haven't you heard much about this aspect of your postreproductive health? The answer is simpler than you might think—physicians haven't asked. Medical office records show that questions relating to sexual function are asked of women at their routine doctor visits only 2 percent of the time. Another study has shown that adding just a few brief sex-related questions can trigger up to a sixfold increase in reported complaints. So it's not that sexual dysfunction never existed in years past; rather, it's that most women quietly accepted it as an inevitable change and weren't told otherwise.

The time is long past due that you're not only asked about these legitimate problems but informed of their causes and provided with the best preventive strategies.

Sex is like a physiological play that takes place in several acts; not surprisingly, postreproductive sexual problems may take a number of different forms. A simple change in sexual energy or desire (*libido*), a diminished physical response (*arousal*), an inability to reach orgasm (*anorgasmia*), or perhaps even physical pain during intercourse (*dyspareunia*): all of these may be grouped under the broad umbrella of sexual dysfunction. By menopause, decreased libido can affect up to 40 percent of women; vaginal dryness affects a similar number; and over 20 percent of women report pain with intercourse. Overall, up to 59 percent of menopausal or postmenopausal women report some negative association.

For some women, sex starts to feel different long before "the change" ever arrives. For the vast majority of individuals, postreproductive sexual problems are short-lived and resolve on their own—but sometimes they don't. Whatever your age, diminished sexual satisfaction should never be shrugged off as insignificant, if it's enough to bother you. If you've felt a change in this department, it's worthwhile to pause, consider the potential underlying causes, and take steps to restore this important bond between you and your partner.

Right After Childbirth: Maximizing Healing and Rekindling Intimacy

Although most doctors give the green light to resume sexual activity at around six weeks after delivery, the reality of resuming intercourse is not necessarily that simple. During the first three months after delivery, up to 50 percent of women report diminished sexual desire, and 21 percent report a complete loss of desire or aversion to sexual activity. After all, life changes in wholesale ways from the moment you leave the hospital with your new bundle—physically, emotionally, hormonally, and logistically. Right from the start, these changes can take a toll in the bedroom. Because parenting books, support groups, and postnatal classes place little or no emphasis on a woman's sex life after childbirth, keeping the flame of your relationship glowing bright is usually left up to the two of you, with little guidance at all.

THE MIND

Although we'll see that physical anatomy and hormones are prerequisites for normal female sexual function, a woman's sense of intimacy and sexuality, at any age, is at least as strongly shaped by psychological and emotional factors. An active sex life is more likely to be experienced by happy women: and that activity contributes, in turn, to happiness. Being stressed or depressed is a reliable predictor of trouble in the bedroom. It would be an understatement to say that in the aftermath of childbirth, many psychological and emotional transitions arise. It's a time of unparalleled joy accompanied by inevitable doses of stress, anxiety, and fatigue; your perspective on the world has radically shifted, and your whole self feels different. Though the bond with your partner may stay strong or even grow stronger, your shared life begins to center around new and less sensual topics. Getting in the mood quickly gives way to getting the kids washed and ready for bed. Countless diaper changes and feedings sap your emotional and physical energy, making sexiness seem obsolete. Sheer fatigue can make sleep a higher priority than romance.

- *Find time for yourself.* Make a conscious, planned effort to recharge your own energies from time to time. Let the kids spend some time with their father, aunt, or baby-sitter while you escape the house for a movie, an afternoon with a tall stack of magazines at a café, or a long walk with a friend. During those precious hours, try to reconnect with the activities and roles that gave you a sense of pleasure and independence during your pre-mommy adult life.

- *Make time as a couple.* Resuming sex after childbirth means two partners getting reacquainted with each other in some basic ways. Simply finding time alone for adult interaction, of any kind, becomes a major challenge. Schedule a date for just you and your partner. Even if it's only once or twice each month, a date night will allow at least a partial escape from the roles of Mom and Dad for a short time, and hopefully an opportunity to resexualize your relationship. You may worry about still being attractive, which is natural considering the physical experience you've had. While your mutual physical attraction may never be exactly the same, with the right nourishment and a bit of patience, it can be even stronger. Parenting, though exhausting, can awaken attributes and passions that partners never appreciated in each other before building a family. Like taking a few steps back from an impressionist painting, you may discover entirely new and attractive dimensions in your partner and yourself that you'd never noticed before.

• *Rebalance work and play.* Sex works better when you're content with yourself. For some women, that means keeping a professional identity at work; for others, it's freedom from the job and undertaking the new challenge of raising children. Striking the balance that's fulfilling to you, whether that means being a working mom or a soccer mom, will always be best for your love life.

   According to one study from the University of Wisconsin, working moms place their sex life no more at risk than those who stay home. Among five hundred couples, the frequency of intercourse did not differ between individuals who worked full-time or part-time and those who did not work at all; only women who overworked, more than forty-five hours per week, were more likely to report a lack of sexual satisfaction.

THE BODY

However important are the countless psychological and emotional factors contributing to sexual function, our focus in this book is on a different set of postreproductive factors, often overlooked: the purely physical ones. Some of these you probably anticipated—physical symbols of femininity feeling different, your stomach stretch-marked and no longer washboard-flat, your lower body a bit wider. You feel physically more like a mom, perhaps, than a romantic partner. But apart from the superficial transitions, less visible changes to your lower body and pelvic floor can set the stage for other problems in the bedroom—

sometimes right away but often not until years later. Facing them squarely, and learning how to optimize your postdelivery healing process, will be your best insurance policy for a healthy love life.

Keep in mind that only a decade ago, male impotence was labeled as psychological in all but a few cases; the physical causes of female symptoms, likewise, are only now starting to receive the attention they deserve. If physical changes have taken a toll on your sexual function, rest assured, it's not all in your head.

PERINEUM AND VAGINA

The perineum is a highly sensitive area that is crucial for sexual function, and one, as we've discussed, that's prone to injury. Poor healing or scarring can lead to painful intercourse during the postpartum period; even up to three months after delivery, perineal tenderness and pain will often persist. One Australian study found that one in five women took longer than six months to resume comfortable intercourse. A recent study from Harvard Medical School and the University of Nebraska found that women who had a perineal injury, or underwent forceps or vacuum delivery with their first vaginal birth, were at significantly higher risk of painful intercourse six months later.

Perineal laxity can occur if the perineum and vagina are put back together too loosely, or if stitches break down before they fully heal. This anatomic change can have a major impact on sexual pleasure, including a loss of sensation or lack of fullness during sex, or difficulty reaching orgasm during intercourse.

Anal sphincter injuries during vaginal delivery have been associated with painful intercourse in up to 48 percent of women afterward. Whether you had an episiotomy or a spontaneous tear of your perineum during childbirth, you should give this area all the attention that it deserves, and maximize its odds for a full recovery.

- *Avoid swelling and infection.* During the first forty-eight hours after delivery, ice packs may help to reduce swelling around your sutures; switching to warm compresses may then be recommended in certain situations. Check with your doctor before using ice packs, especially if you've had an anal sphincter or rectal injury, since coldness can sometimes cause the muscular sphincter to spasm and feel worse.

Cleanliness is central to avoiding infection and breakdown of a perineal and vaginal repair. Shower regularly, or spray the perineum with a peri-bottle or handheld shower attachment. Let the water gently wash over your bottom; don't scrub or use a high-pressure stream directly on the area of healing. Sitz baths, which are small plastic basins that fit onto a regular toilet seat, can be used to bathe your bottom without maneuvering into the tub. Finally, avoid tampons and douching during the healing process.

- *Avoid dryness.* Vaginal dryness is common during breast-feeding, due to a drop in hormones, and may lead to sexual discomfort and even pain. Try a generous amount of water-soluble lubricant (Astroglide, Replens, K-Y jelly, Liquid Silk) when your doctor says it's okay to do so. Avoid petroleum jelly and other nonwater-soluble lubricants.

- *Positions and perineal massage.* The woman-on-top and side-by-side positions may give you the most control over the angle and depth of penetration, and allow you to reduce friction against the tender areas. You may notice that the perineum feels less flexible as the tissues heal; this does not necessarily indicate a problem. After six weeks, try massaging and gently stretching the perineum and vaginal opening with lubricant or a dab of olive oil, to familiarize yourself with the anatomic change, and get this area accustomed to pressure and touch. Estrogen-containing vaginal creams are also sometimes recommended. If tenderness is occurring deeper in the vagina during penetration, it might indicate a tender cervix or a repaired vaginal laceration that needs more time to heal. Finally, if you've had a cesarean, you'll need to find positions that minimize pressure against your abdominal scar, which will probably remain sensitive for several months.

- *Timing.* Returning to sex may sometimes prove a slower process than you or your partner had expected; healing, after all, is a dynamic process that occurs over a span of months, with many stages of wound remodeling. Some women feel ready and able soon after delivery; others have zero interest or too much discomfort for quite some time. The Harvard/Nebraska study found that six months after their first vaginal childbirth, around a quarter of women still reported decreased sensation, worsened sexual satisfaction, and a reduced ability to achieve orgasm. When the time feels right for you and your partner, choose a part of the day or night when the baby sleeps deeply, if such a time exists. Start by relaxing with a bath and massage, and take it slow. If you notice bleeding or feel a strong pulling or tearing sensation, listen to your body and stop. A bit more time for healing is usually all you'll need.

- *If all else fails.* If tenderness persists along the perineum or inside the vagina after the full healing process is complete, on rare occasion, other treatments may be warranted. For instance, antiinflammatory injections, referred to as *trigger-point injections,* can be used to treat certain tender areas. In other cases, removal or revision of scarred or stretched tissue, with a minor surgical procedure, may ultimately provide the best relief.

DON'T RUSH IT

There's a long-standing belief out on the street that returning to sex is a breeze after childbirth. Doctors typically give couples the green light somewhere around four to six weeks. But how often are couples able to return to having sex at this point? One study in *The Journal of Family Practice* reported that less than 20 percent of couples had resumed intercourse by four weeks, and not until four months had 90 percent of them resumed. The average time to resume activity was seven weeks. A report from the University of North Carolina found that 17 percent of women still reported pain with intercourse at six months after delivery. Similarly, in Australia, it was found that one in five mothers needed up to six months to feel fully comfortable during sex. Resuming relations after childbirth needs to occur at your own personal pace.

- *Pelvic floor.* A strong and careful repair of your perineum after childbirth—whether it follows an episiotomy or a spontaneous laceration during delivery—will often restore a normal anatomy and tone to the vaginal opening. But it can't restore the function of the deeper muscles, nerves, and connective tissues of the pelvic floor. Weak and deconditioned levator muscles may decrease sexual satisfaction by making you feel too loose. In other cases, tenderness or spasm of the levator muscles may lead to pain and hesitation during penetration. As mentioned earlier, starting a Kegel routine (see Appendix A) can improve your vaginal tone and ability to find pelvic muscles that are overly tense and tender during penetration. In doing this you may improve your ability to relax the muscles during intercourse.

  Pelvic-floor physiotherapy may also help to reacquaint you with the pelvic-floor muscles after childbirth, even if Kegel exercises fail. Biofeedback sensors signal when you're contracting the correct pelvic-floor muscles, and will improve your workouts. Pelvic-floor stimulation, with electrical or magnetic energy, is a means to rehabilitate the pelvic nerves and muscles when exercises have failed.

- *Hormones.* It's impossible to discuss the postpartum transition without some mention of hormones and the roller-coaster swings they can undergo after childbirth. Bodily chemicals that were surging during pregnancy are suddenly in free fall until the return of menstrual cycles, when a natural nonpregnancy hormone mix resumes.

  The hormonal changes accompanying lactation can have a negative impact on sexual function, lasting until breast-feeding ends. Reduced estrogen levels account for the majority of problems by causing severe vaginal dryness and temporary atrophy. It's also been proposed that breast-feeding temporarily decreases male-type androgen hormones responsible for libido. The short-term use of vaginal estrogen cream or tablets can improve vaginal blood flow and sexual lubrication, if approved by your doctor. Urinary incontinence during intercourse (coital incontinence) can result from estrogen-deprived bladder, urethra, and vaginal supports. Extra Kegel exercises, and low-dose estrogen cream if approved by your doctor, may help.

- *Postpartum depression and the blues.* Whether these postpartum mood disorders are of hormonal origin remains a subject of debate. Whatever their biological or psychological cause, sexual interest can be among the first bodily functions to fall by the wayside.

AND NOW FOR SOME GOOD NEWS

Lest you begin to feel that statistics are all gloom and doom, here's one to cheer you up. Around 25 percent of women will enjoy sex *more* after their first childbirth than before they conceived. This was reported in *The British Journal of Obstetrics and Gynaecology* in the early 1980s and confirmed by a more recent study; this study also found, though, that women with perineal injury during childbirth were only about half as likely to enjoy this unexpected natural boost.

The Postreproductive Years Before and After Menopause

LIBIDO, AROUSAL, ORGASM: POTENTIAL PROBLEMS IN EACH "ACT"—AND THEIR TREATMENTS

ACT 1: LIBIDO

For the average woman (not that *average* applies to you!), sex drive does decline to some degree as years go by. On the other hand, many individuals notice no change for the worse during their postreproductive years, continuing to enjoy an active sex life just as before, and sometimes even more so. What's the secret? Is it their hormones, the quality of their relationships, or their physical health? Actually, a combination of several factors is at work.

- *General health.* Anemia, diabetes, and thyroid disease are among the more common specific medical conditions that can affect libido. But even without a specific medical problem, your general physical shape and well-being can strongly influence sexual function. Feeling well tuned and well toned—close to your optimal weight, body shape, and cardiovascular conditioning—is one of nature's most potent aphrodisiacs.

- *Depression, stress, and substance abuse.* Sex drive is often the first bodily function to fail when you're coping with emotional baggage, or battling an addiction with alcohol or drugs. Women who are happy outside of the bedsheets are far more likely to feel contentment between them.

- *Medications.* Antidepressants, blood-pressure medication, and sedatives are among the drug types that should be reviewed by a physician to be sure they're not contributing to a flagging sex drive, slowed arousal, or difficulty with orgasm. In some cases, substitutes can be found. Never discontinue a medication without your doctor's approval.

- *Hormones.* During your postreproductive years right on through menopause, sexual interest and function can mirror your hormonal swings. A lack of androgens (the male hormones that are also present in women) occurs naturally after menopause, and a more dramatic drop occurs after surgical removal of the ovaries. Abnormally low testosterone levels may sometimes lead to diminished libido. *Testosterone-replacement therapy* can be used to improve sex drive, which you'll learn all about in the section ahead.

  Levels of estrogen, the staple female hormone, may fluctuate more widely as your postreproductive years progress, but this shouldn't directly affect libido much until after menopause or surgical removal of the ovaries. Indirectly, varying estrogen levels can occasionally affect sexual function even before menopause. For example, if premenstrual symptoms or irritability become more pronounced, or vaginal atrophy causes you to associate intercourse with physical discomfort, sex drive can certainly suffer. *Estrogen therapy* to counteract these problems will be discussed in the pages ahead.

ACT 2: AROUSAL

Arousal is your physical response to stimulation—the process of warming up during foreplay, becoming physically primed for intercourse. The arousal process, including vaginal engorgement and lubrication, normally occurs at a slower pace as years go by. Before menopause, women can usually adjust to this change quite easily, relying on nothing more sophisticated than a warm bath, perhaps a glass of red wine, and longer foreplay. But after menopause, a lack of estrogen in the vaginal tissues makes the process of arousal a much greater challenge. Atrophy can lead to progressive vaginal dryness, thinning, irritation, itching, and even narrowing of the vagina. The skin of the vagina actually becomes less flexible, causing friction during intercourse. To make matters worse, atrophy of the urogenital tract may increase your risk for bladder and vaginal infections. Any or all of these changes can ultimately dull your desire, slow your arousal, and make intercourse downright uncomfortable. The use of vaginal estrogen creams or tablets—to restore the normal thickness, blood supply, and lubrication to the vaginal skin—can work wonders. Use water-soluble lubricants liberally, and keep yourself well hydrated, since dehydration dries the skin of the vagina just like anywhere else.

ACT 3: ORGASM

The inability to reach orgasm can be caused by a lack of sufficient stimulation but can also result from specific medications or disease states. Be sure to review your overall medical history with your doctor while considering a few easy tips.

- *Location, location.* It's one of the most important elements not only in real estate but also in sexual pleasure. Think about your physical surroundings, the answer to minimizing inhibition. Are you and your partner taking some time to set the mood and to allow the arousal phase to occur? A warm bath, some well-placed aromatherapy candles, and slow foreplay can go a long way. As years go by, you'll need more time for arousal—and orgasm—to occur. And contrary to popular belief, up to two thirds of women do not have orgasms during intercourse.

Also pay attention to the anatomic places where your stimulation is maximized down below. Some partners need help learning how to find this location and deal with it properly. If you've had no luck teaching your partner after a glass or two of wine, well . . . try champagne.

- *Get estrogenized, or at least lubricated.* A healthy estrogen supply increases blood flow to the genitals, promoting engorgement of the areas responsible for orgasm. The use of estrogen-containing vaginal creams or pills may help, though their full effects may not be seen for months. Simple lubricating gels can provide a substitute if you're not interested in using estrogen, or if you can't use it for medical reasons. Although it won't enrich atrophic vaginal skin like estrogen, it will provide temporary lubrication for intercourse, which may further stimulate your own natural secretions. Only water-based products should be used.

- *Local estrogen products.* Estrace or Premarin (cream), Vagifem (tablets); your physician will determine the appropriate dosage.

- *Water-based lubricants.* K-Y jelly, Astroglide, Replens, Liquid Silk, Gyne-Moistrin, Slippery Stuff

- *Exercise for better sex.* Because the levator muscles contract during orgasm, building them may cause the intensity of orgasm to increase. By improving the tone of your levator muscles, pelvic-floor exercises can help you develop better control over your sexual tension. Well-toned muscles may also help to eliminate any urine leakage that might occur during intercourse— relieving fear of accidents, boosting self-confidence, and improving your ability to relax and let go.

ESTROGEN: A KEY INGREDIENT FOR SEXUAL FUNCTION

Whenever estrogen levels decline—whether from natural menopause, surgical removal of the ovaries, or breast-feeding—the vagina and bladder may become thin, dry, and atrophic. These are among the most common changes affecting sexual arousal and overall sexual function. Local estrogen-containing creams, vaginal pills, or rings can replenish the vaginal skin, restoring its thickness and moisture. Estrogen is one of the most important treatments for menopausal women coping with diminished sex-

ual satisfaction. The cream should not, however, be used as a lubricant
during intercourse, since absorption into the male organ can occur.

THE ROLE OF TESTOSTERONE . . . AND OPRAH!

Did you know that testosterone is actually a part of *your* chemical
mix? It's the basic fuel of libido, arousal, and orgasm, and it also provides the building block for one type of estrogen in the female body.
By menopause, somewhere around 50 percent of testosterone production is lost; after surgical removal of the ovaries, the decline is
more dramatic. But even for women with working ovaries who
haven't yet reached menopause, symptoms of androgen deficiency
may occur as early as the late thirties. The use of oral contraceptives
may also occasionally contribute to a mildly testosterone-deficient
state. A decline in testosterone activity can place a slow, indefinite
chill on sexual desire.

In October 1998, Oprah Winfrey and guests on her show shared
some spicy news with the female world, a hormonal shot heard round
the world on daytime television: the use of testosterone propionate
cream for improving female libido. Androgen replacement has been
known for quite some time to increase sexual desire and arousal,
helping to improve a flagging libido more effectively than estrogen
alone. Relatively new, however, is the variety of ways this hormone
can be used—including oral pills, or as a cream for application to the
genitals or elsewhere.

FORMS AND DOSES

Determining the safest and most appropriate role for testosterone
in treating decreased libido or arousal has proven to be a difficult task.
Very high doses of androgens will increase the sex drive of almost any
woman, but these levels would be unsafe. The smaller doses used for
replacement have demonstrated a rather unpredictable effect. Only
your doctor can judge your safest and most effective dose.

- *Injection.* Muscular injections have been shown to increase the
  intensity of desire, arousal, and fantasy, as well as the frequency
  of sexual activity and orgasm.

- *Cream and gel.* Applied directly to the labial, vaginal, or clitoral areas by some women; once you see improvement, you may want to switch to oral form. It remains unclear whether there are long-term side effects and at what dosages they're likely to occur. More research is needed to guide the proper use of these products.

- *Oral therapy: Combination estrogen and testosterone.* Oral testosterone therapy has become increasingly popular in recent years. For women without functioning ovaries, the estrogen included in these combination pills may, at least in theory, balance the potentially bad cardiovascular effects of testosterone. But in reality, the side effects of long-term testosterone usage are unknown, and certain estrogen-progesterone combination therapy may also pose significant risks if taken on a long-term basis (see "Estrogen and Other Hormones," chapter 12). Therefore, the dosage and duration should be carefully discussed with your doctor. There are only a few approved products in the United States: Estratest and Estratest HS (Solvay Pharmaceuticals); and Premarin with Methyltestosterone (Wyeth-Ayerst).

- *Skin patches and implants.* Testosterone skin patches (transdermal) are available for men, but there is no such product approved for women. The main theoretical advantage of taking testosterone through the skin, rather than by mouth, is to avoid its chemical breakdown in the gastrointestinal tract. Implants for beneath the skin (subcutaneous) are another emerging option but are not yet available for women.

SIDE EFFECTS

The challenge of testosterone replacement is achieving the good effects without running into potentially serious side effects. They range from cosmetic—such as deepening of the voice, acne, increased facial hair, hair loss (male pattern baldness)—to clitoral enlargement and alterations in cholesterol profiles marked by lowering of good cholesterol (HDL) and elevation of bad cholesterol (LDL). Especially if you're using a noncommercial cream or gel, the amount of active medication you're receiving can vary widely from dose to dose. Be sure to work closely with your doctor to keep your regimen safe.

OTHER ELIXIRS
DHEA

Dehydroepiandrosterone is a relatively weak steroid hormone (androgen) that's widely prevalent in fountain-of-youth supplements. Your own body's production of DHEA reaches its peak in your mid-twenties, then slowly tapers off; commercial DHEA, in contrast, is extracted from plants. Although research has been scarce, one three-month study of DHEA supplementation failed to show any improvement in libido or mood. It also hasn't been found to help prevent heart disease in women, despite initial hopes. Concern has been raised over its possibly lowering HDL levels. DHEA has not received FDA approval for medical use and is not recommended at this time.

Viagra: Not Just for Men Anymore?

As many women watched the born-again response of their male partners to this arousal-enhancing little blue pill, it didn't take long for the collective question to arise: "Hey, what about me?" Unfortunately, based on results of the first Viagra-for-women study conducted at Columbia Presbyterian Center in New York, women receiving a twelve-week course of the medication were no more likely to report improved sexual function than those who took placebo during the same period. Undoubtedly, more data on the use of Viagra for women will emerge; for now it appears to have no established role.

PAINFUL INTERCOURSE: UNDERSTANDING AND ALLEVIATING IT

Painful intercourse for the postreproductive woman can signal a number of possible underlying causes. The discomfort can be deep or superficial. It can arise from any number of structures, including the labia, perineum, levator muscles, bladder, urethra, vagina, cervix, or uterus. It may relate to vaginal dryness or atrophy, chemical irritation, infection, endometriosis, ovarian cysts, or fibroids. The list goes on, and sorting through all the possibilities may take effort, but it's worth it. Find a doctor interested in sticking with you and your problem until a solution is found. In the meantime, a few tips may help.

- *Think lubrication.* Inadequate lubrication is probably the most common reason for painful intercourse. Some medical conditions (including long-standing diabetes) and medications (including certain antibiotics, or the breast-cancer drug tamoxifen) may cause decreased lubrication. Water-soluble lubricants (K-Y jelly, Replens, Astroglide) can often provide the solution. Avoid oil-based lubricants (baby oil, petroleum jelly), since they can linger in the vagina and promote infection.

- *Fight atrophy.* Atrophy of the vulva and vagina can lead to itching, irritation, and narrowing of the vagina, making sex difficult or impossible. This can be due to a temporary decline in estrogen supply for women who are breast-feeding, or a permanent decline for those who are past menopause. Ask whether vaginal estrogen—in the form of creams, tablets, or rings—might be for you (see chapter 12).

- *Avoid vaginitis (yeast, bacterial vaginosis).* Vaginitis is another common source of burning or pain with sexual activity, and one that can be fully treated or prevented (see chapter 12). Avoid treating recurrent or persistent yeast without seeing the doctor first, since other conditions can mimic a yeast infection, and the wrong treatment may aggravate your symptoms. Bacterial vaginosis, for instance, is an often overlooked source of vaginal irritation and discharge that will not improve with antiyeast treatment, but it can be easily treated with a different type of medication.

- *Take care of the vulva.* Vulvar irritation can result from exposure to chemicals, perfumes, soaps, powders, and clothing materials. If you become sore or overly sensitive, eliminate these potential irritants (see chapter 12).

- *Recognize a painful bladder.* Cystitis can cause pain during intercourse, whether it's arising from a bacterial infection or another inflammatory condition. If your doctor identifies infection, inflammation, or abnormal tenderness of the bladder, treatment of the bladder problem may significantly improve your sexual function.

- *Understand and treat vaginismus.* *Vaginismus* refers to an involuntary tightening or spasm of the vaginal and pelvic-floor muscles, making penetration painful and sometimes impossible. Although it may relate to past sexual trauma or abuse, childbirth alone may account for enough stored memory of pain—indeed, trauma—to trigger the problem. The pain or sensitivity that accompanies healing of an episiotomy or spontaneous laceration of the perineum can lead to postpartum apprehension over just inserting a tampon, let alone having intercourse. In some women, this guarding of the pelvic area may persist well beyond the postpartum period, and tightening of the vagina and pelvic-floor muscles becomes a reflex in the bedroom.

Mind-body approaches may sometimes help to reduce both mental and physical stress. Your doctor or nurse or a pelvic-floor physiotherapist may utilize biofeedback to show you how to relax the pelvic-floor muscles during vaginal dilation. Sexual apprehension stemming from problems of past or present relationship strain or abuse may ultimately respond best to counseling or therapy. Referral to a sexual therapist is sometimes advised in this case.

A Kegel routine may help when used alone, or when enhanced by biofeedback (see Appendix A). Developing the strength and tone of the pelvic-floor muscles will help you to more effectively identify and relax them during intercourse.

As with any other muscle spasm, your levators can get tense and sore. Pelvic-floor massage may help to release that tension and improve vaginismus. Some pelvic-floor physiotherapists have a focused interest in pelvic-floor massage. Pelvic-floor electrical stimulation (see Appendix A) may be used either in the doctor's office or at home to accompany this therapy.

LEAKING, BULGING, AND SEX: WHEN INCONTINENCE OR PROLAPSE ENTERS THE BEDROOM

A loss of bladder or bowel control, or advanced pelvic prolapse, can dim just about any woman's sexual spark. Not unlike impotence in males, these problems may diminish not only your physical pleasure but also your self-confidence, presenting a real challenge to sexual identity.

- *Relaxed vagina or perineum.* We've discussed perineal relaxation and the reasons why the vagina and pelvic-floor muscles can become stretched out after childbirth. This can lessen a woman's feeling of fullness during intercourse, or diminish the ability to reach orgasm. The loss of sensation may be enough to cause frustration for a partner, too. It's unknown whether episiotomies make this postreproductive anatomic change more likely.

  Pelvic-floor exercises can help to restore vaginal muscle tone, but results may not be seen for several months. And sometimes exercises are simply not enough to rehabilitate and restore tissues that were stretched and weakened. *Perineorrhaphy* refers to surgically tightening the muscles of the perineum and vaginal opening—the same ones that might relax after childbirth—something like a delayed episiotomy repair. Decreasing the caliber of the vaginal opening may produce a fuller sensation with intercourse.

  Before signing on for this type of surgery, be sure to understand its risks, benefits, and limitations. Just because your perineum and vagina are restored closer to their prechildbirth virginal state doesn't guarantee that life between the sheets will transform from ice-cold to torridly passionate. And though the risks are low, any vaginal operation carries a small chance of scarring, pain, or nerve injury. So be sure there aren't other, less anatomic problems contributing to your sexual dissatisfaction, such as relationship stress, diminished libido, or insufficient foreplay.

  Outline clear goals and realistic expectations. Elective operations have their appropriate place in gynecology, but your decision to enter the operating room should never be made lightly.

- *Tender prolapse bulge.* A prolapsed cervix or uterus may create an uncomfortable thump during deep penetration, as if something is in the way. Similar symptoms can occasionally indicate an ovarian cyst, fibroid, or other abnormality in the pelvic area, so be sure to have this symptom checked out before making any assumptions on your own.

- *Coital incontinence.* The leakage of urine or stool during intercourse or foreplay is a condition that many women are reluctant to discuss, and it's more common than most physicians suspect.

One study found that among 324 sexually active women with incontinence, 24 percent experienced leakage during intercourse; among them, two thirds had leakage with penetration, and a third had leakage with orgasm. Incontinence can have a major impact on sexual function. For some women, diminished sexual pleasure—caused by a growing fear of embarrassment and an inability to let go and enjoy the moment—is one of the most troubling secondary effects of incontinence. One study recently found that women with urinary incontinence had fewer sexual thoughts and fantasies.

Other studies have shown that women with urge incontinence tend to suffer the greatest impact on their sexual health. A European study involving 447 women and men with overactive bladder found that for over a third, their bladder problem was a major reason for sexual abstinence. Avoidance of intercourse, and intimate relationships in general, was surprisingly common among individuals with urge incontinence.

Frequent leakage may also cause irritation of the vulvar area and vaginal opening, leading to diminished sexual function for purely physical reasons. Fortunately, coital incontinence is almost always remediable, if you understand its source.

Leakage during penetration often indicates stress incontinence due to a floppy or thin urethra (see chapter 8) and pelvic-floor muscle weakness. As the bladder is bumped during intercourse, the sudden pressure increase may be too much for the weak urethra to hold back. To prevent this kind of leakage, you may wish to:

- Empty your bladder before intercourse.
- Start a pelvic-floor exercise routine (see Appendix A). Extra muscle tone around the bladder and urethra can make the urethral valve more effective.
- Wear a large contraceptive diaphragm, which will provide a stronger floor for the bladder and urethra.

 Leakage during orgasm can signal an overactive bladder in some cases and stress incontinence in others. As the nerves around the pelvis go a bit haywire, an involuntary bladder contraction can result, leading to a sudden uncontrollable urge or even silent leakage of urine. You might want to try:

- Antispasmodic medication, taken an hour or two before intercourse (oxybutynin, Tofranil).

- Healthy voiding habits (bladder drills) and avoiding potential dietary irritants (bladder diet) (see chapter 8).

DEALING WITH SEXUAL CHANGES DURING AND AFTER MENOPAUSE

The transitions of menopause, whether relating to mood, to sense of well-being, or to sexuality, affect each woman in a unique way. Some studies have suggested that diminished desire and sexual function can be expected to accompany "the change," whereas others have found no such association. For some women, sex may become even more enjoyable with the freedom from fear of unwanted pregnancy, or from motherhood, or from the grind of a full work week. For others, hormonal swings, irregular periods, and hot flashes may take their toll on sexual desire, moods, and overall sense of well-being. One Australian study found that among women followed through their menopausal transition, 61 percent noticed no change in their sexuality, 7 percent reported an increase, and 32 percent noticed a change for the worse. Surveys in the United States reveal similar trends, with around 39 percent of menopausal women reporting a decreased interest.

What if, despite those better-than-even odds, you're among the women who *have* noticed decreased function after menopause? We've already discussed a number of basic strategies to get you started on the right path. But above all else, one rule may be most important: use it or lose it! Whether it's biceps, triceps, or washboard abdominal muscles, most parts of the body follow this universal rule. Your pelvic and vaginal areas are no exception: if they're not properly exercised, their tone and function will slowly but surely fade. Narrowing, dryness, irritability, and pain become common with a lack of sexual stimulation. One study published in *The Journal of the American Medical Association* showed that women over fifty who had intercourse at least three times each month had less vaginal atrophy than women who were less sexually active. Another study looking at vaginal skin cells under the microscope also found that sexually active women experience fewer atrophic changes than similar women who are not sexually active. Sexual activity, in other words, actually prevents vaginal atrophy.

Moral of this story? Keeping your postreproductive body in shape sometimes takes a strong commitment between the sheets!

PART 4

YOUR SYMPTOMS ARE STILL TROUBLING YOU

WHAT'S THE NEXT STEP?

ᔥ 12 ᔥ

Maintaining Your General Health to Minimize Symptoms

TIPS ON HORMONES AND MENOPAUSE,
YOUR GYNECOLOGIC HEALTH, AND HIDDEN
TRIGGERS OF PELVIC-FLOOR PROBLEMS

*B*y now you've learned a great deal about the most common pelvic-floor conditions that might affect your postreproductive body, and the specific ways to treat them. But if you're coping with troubling symptoms down there—whether it's incontinence, pelvic discomfort, bladder irritation, or vague symptoms that are tough to figure out—more general medical and gynecologic conditions may be playing a role. For example, in your postreproductive body, the symptoms triggered by vaginal infections and irritation may be far less familiar or typical than they once were. Bladder infections may present themselves in new and unexpected ways, becoming more common or exacerbating existing pelvic-floor symptoms. The changes of menopause may have a ripple effect throughout the urinary tract and pelvic floor. Commonplace gynecologic problems of many different types may feel peskier to your postreproductive body than they did before.

By familiarizing yourself with the following tips, you'll help to minimize some of the most common hidden triggers of pelvic-floor symptoms.

Tip #1: Prevent Vaginal and Vulvar Symptoms

YEAST INFECTIONS

Vaginal itching and burning are the most well-known symptoms that lead young women to suspect a yeast infection. But as the years go by, yeast infections might reveal themselves through less typical clues.

- *Urinary burning, urgency, and frequency.* When vaginal yeast infections involve the tissue around the urethral opening, urinary symptoms (rather than vaginal ones) may be the most severe complaint. Even though it arises from a vaginal infection, this so-called urethral syndrome can feel like cystitis.

- *Urge incontinence.* If a bad yeast infection irritates the urethra enough to trigger bladder spasms, leakage from an overactive bladder may actually worsen.

- *Sexual discomfort.* Intercourse can trigger a yeast infection, leading to rawness and discomfort during intercourse. The usual cause is irritation of the vaginal skin and a change in the vaginal acid balance caused by the male ejaculate, not an actual infection transmitted from one partner to the other. Nevertheless, if intercourse remains a constant trigger and all other means of prevention have failed, some clinicians will recommend treating a male partner with oral medication for up to fourteen days, in case he has a yeast infection and is transmitting it to you.

PREVENTION

A handful of tips may help to reduce the odds of having to cope with yeast infections and the symptoms they trigger.

Avoid Unnecessary Antibiotics

The vagina and perineum have their own balanced ecosystem, inhabited by both good and bad types of bacteria. Antibiotics taken for any reason can disrupt this ecosystem by reducing the population of good bacteria and providing yeast with more opportunity to flourish.

Keep Dry and Cool

The temperature and texture of your vulvar and vaginal skin plays a large role. Trapped moisture makes yeast feel right at home. Staying dry and cool down there is the most basic prevention.

- *Dress wisely.* Avoid tight clothing, nylons, and other noncotton undergarments that don't breathe. Remove wet bathing suits ASAP. After showers and baths, if towel drying still leaves you damp, try a cool hair dryer on your bottom area. During your period, use a tampon instead of a menstrual pad.

- *Cornstarch.* A simple, very inexpensive absorbent powder, very gentle on the skin. Be wary of medicated powders. They may keep you dry, but their additives can occasionally irritate sensitive skin.

- *Lactobacillus acidophilus.* Lactobacillus is the most common good bacteria found in the vagina. When its population is strong, there is little room for yeast to thrive. Some women supplement each time they have intercourse, swim, or take antibiotics, to rebalance the vaginal ecosystem and possibly help to prevent vaginitis. If you already are suffering from a yeast infection, however, taking acidophilus is unlikely to offer a cure.

  One 1992 study suggested that eating eight ounces of yogurt each day reduced the risk of yeast vaginitis after six months. Be sure that the yogurt contains acidophilus and not too much added sugar. Acidophilus-containing milk, miso, and tempeh are also available, as are acidophilus vaginal cream and suppositories, although it's unclear whether these are any more or less effective than the dietary form. You can also take acidophilus in oral tablets and powders.

TREATMENT

Most yeast infections can be handled with an over-the-counter medications or a homespun remedy. But before starting any treatment, be sure to run it by your doctor.

Boric Acid

Vaginal tablets, suppositories, or even ointments containing boric acid are a time-tested remedy for yeast infections. The treatment works without the use of antifungal medication by simply helping to rebalance the vaginal pH. It may occasionally cause a mild burning sensation or general discomfort in the vagina. You can also try Aci-Gel, an acidic vaginal gel available through the pharmacy.

Douching

For most women, douching is not necessary and may actually *cause* problems. But for some women, they can provide periodic relief.

- *Vinegar.* Although an occasional vinegar (acetic acid) douche can help to lower pH, control a heavy discharge, and calm early yeast infections, douching too often will disrupt the vaginal ecosystem and increase your risk of a yeast outbreak. The usual mix is two tablespoons of white vinegar with a quart of water. It's best to check with your doctor before douching on any sort of regular basis.

- *Peroxide douche.* Hydrogen peroxide—the same brown-bottled substance you've used to clean wounds—is naturally produced in the vagina by lactobacilli, and it helps maintain a healthy vaginal pH that is resistant to infection. A teaspoon of 3 percent hydrogen peroxide in a cup of water can be used for occasional douching, but only if approved by your physician.

Antifungals

Over the past several years, many of the common antifungals have become available over the counter.

- *Vaginal creams and suppositories.* You'll find a whole pharmacy aisle devoted to these products, now available in one-, three-, and seven-day forms. Some of the more common ones are miconazole (Monistat), clotrimazole (Gyne-Lotrimin, Mycelex), butoconazole (Femstat), tioconazole (Vagistat), and terconazole (Terazol).

- *Pills.* Fluconazole (Diflucan), ketoconazole (Nizoral), nystatin, amphotericin B.

BE SURE IT'S YEAST

Some women will self-treat for years with antifungal creams and tablets only to find it was something else! Other conditions can mimic typical yeast infections. Have a close exam by your doctor to find out for sure.

THE OTHER COMMON TYPES OF IRRITATION

Not all that itches, burns, or irritates the vaginal area is yeast. A few other common conditions may also trigger a confusing array of symptoms in that region. Whenever vulvar itching, bleeding, discomfort, or burning becomes a bother, tell your doctor.

- *Bacterial vaginosis.* "BV," or gardnerella, occurs when certain bacteria in the vagina multiply. It causes a thin gray discharge and is occasionally responsible for vaginal itching and burning. A fishy odor may increase after intercourse or after washing with certain alkaline soaps. It's found in 12 to 25 percent of women visiting health clinics, and a recent study found that douching may increase the risk of developing BV. Treatment consists of a prescription medication, either an oral pill or vaginal gel, for five to seven days.

- *Trichomonas.* "Trich" (sounds like "trick") is a sexually transmitted organism (actually a protozoan) that causes a yellow-gray odorous vaginal discharge and sometimes painful urination. It can be cured with a single dose of medication or a series of smaller doses over several days. Unlike yeast and BV, trichomonas can be transmitted sexually between partners, so all sexual partners should receive treatment to prevent reinfection.

- *Diaper rash.* Sometimes it's not just an issue for the kids. Postreproductive women with any type of incontinence—stress, urge, or mixed—may find that when urine contacts the skin, it can leave the vulva looking red, raw, and angry. This type of chemical rash usually occurs in predictable areas: outside the urethra, across both labia, and often extending onto the groin and inner thighs.

    To treat diaper rash, separate the outer vaginal lips (labia) when urinating, and gently rinse with cold water afterward to keep urine away from the external skin. Avoid the constant use of deodorant pads to allow the skin to breathe and prevent chemical irritation. You can also try a barrier cream. These rather thick, opaque creams are useful for blocking contact between the skin and urine and are intended for use on the outer vulva and groin. Zinc oxide is the least expensive generic alternative. Other barrier ointments have been designed and marketed specifically for incontinence-related irritation (Carlesta, Desitin, Balmex).

- *Cosmetic irritants.* The vulvar skin can also become irritated by a long list of nice-smelling and beautifully packaged health and hygiene products. Eliminate the source of irritation and you'll feel better.

   Choose toilet paper, pads, and panty liners that are unscented, colorless, and ideally, hypoallergenic. Avoid bubble baths, scented or colored soaps, perfumed or talcum powders and fabric softeners, and try not to lather up or shampoo while you're soaking in the tub. Watch out for spermicidal foams, creams and jellies, and condoms or diaphragms made of rubber. Despite the many varieties of powders, perfumes, and feminine hygiene available in the pharmacy aisle, remember one basic rule when it comes to this part of your body: simple is best!

   Also keep in mind that wiping, scrubbing, or scratching will make a contact dermatitis worse. Let the shower stream gently rinse this part of your body; if you lather, do it softly. Pat the area with a towel or unscented tissue, and air-dry as much as possible.

VULVODYNIA AND VESTIBULITIS

These disorders with the strange names, also referred to as vulvar syndromes, are far less common than the basic inflammatory conditions, affecting only a very small percentage of women. But those of you who have been diagnosed with one of them can attest to the uncomfortable array of vaginal, pelvic, bladder, and sexual symptoms that they cause, and also to the profound effect they can have on a woman's quality of life.

Vulvodynia refers to pain localized around the vulva (outside of the vagina); vestibulitis refers to chronic irritation, tenderness, burning, and rawness around the inner labia, vaginal opening, and urethra. Because the bladder, rectum, pelvic floor, and sexual organs are all supplied by the same power grid of nerves, these vulvar problems can sometimes trigger confusing symptoms nearby.

Some women notice that their vulvar condition flares after childbirth; others after an episode of cystitis, or after taking medication for a presumed yeast infection, or after starting a new hormone therapy. Some women's problems will arise with certain foods or beverages, or using certain perfumes or detergents, or wearing certain fabrics. Although some of these vulvar syndromes run in families, it remains a mystery whether any true genetic links exist. Treatments range from modifications in diet and sexual habits to vaginal steroids, estrogen therapy, pain-blocking medications, and local anesthetic injections.

Tip #2: Control and Prevent Bladder Infections

Bladder infections are the pits. Almost any woman can vividly describe the signs: burning, strong-smelling or cloudy urine, and the overwhelming constant urge to urinate. Adult women of all ages are prone to cystitis, largely because of a short urethra allowing bacteria relatively easy access into the bladder. But why dwell on this condition in a book focused on your postreproductive body?

Even if you've sworn by your ability to identify bladder infections in the past, it's common to find that typical cystitis symptoms aren't so typical anymore. Rather than the burning and bladder pain that tend to accompany bladder infections during your twenties and thirties, symptoms during the decades that follow—such as increased frequency of urination, worsening of incontinence, or just feeling crummy—may provide the tip-off that an episode of cystitis has begun.

Also, certain features of your postreproductive body may increase your risk for cystitis. Prolapse, for instance, can make hygiene around the urethra more difficult to maintain. Cystoceles can result in an ever-present pool of urine in the bladder, another setup for cystitis. And urogenital atrophy—drying and thinning of tissues around the bladder, urethra, and vagina—introduces yet another risk for infection if you're postmenopausal or have had your ovaries surgically removed.

Prevention

Most women experience bladder infections infrequently. With the help of their doctor, they'll take a course of antibiotics until the infection clears, then forget about their bladder until a problem arises once again. But if infections become more frequent, then you should develop a preventive approach. With the help of a few basic tips, your risk of becoming infected in the first place can be dramatically reduced.

Empty Regularly

The simple act of emptying your bladder is an important defense against bladder infections. Staying well hydrated encourages a good flush of urine on a regular basis, leaving bacteria fewer opportunities to cling to the bladder wall and cause infection. Drinking three to four pints of liquid each day, and voiding around every three and a half hours, is a reasonable goal.

Empty After Sex

Intercourse is the single most important risk factor leading to bladder infections in women. Up to 75 percent of bladder infections in younger women can be traced back to the bedroom, with more vigorous sexual activity leading to higher infection risks. Sexual activity shifts bacteria (usually E. coli) from their normal location around the anal area to around the urethra and bladder, where they shouldn't normally be found. Whether an infection will then develop depends, at least in part, on how long these bacteria are allowed to stick around. Urinating shortly after intercourse—a healthy flush, not just a dribble—should be your habit within fifteen to thirty minutes of intercourse. It's one very simple way to reduce bacterial numbers before they have the opportunity to multiply.

Keep Clean

- *Clean sex.* If recurrent infections are a problem, make a habit of showering before intercourse. Avoid irritation of the urethra by altering your positions. Keep well lubricated, and avoid using condoms that leave you feeling raw.

- *Wipe right.* Wiping the wrong way after urination—from back to front—shifts more bacteria from the anal area into direct contact with the urethra, and it may increase your odds of developing bladder infections. Always wipe from front to back after urination.

- *Prolapse and pessaries.* Even when they're fitting right and working well, pessaries can cause a fairly heavy vaginal discharge, which can make both vaginal and bladder infections more common. Careful hygiene, and periodic removal of the pessary at bedtime, will help to minimize this problem.

Acidify the Urine

Following a bladder diet—including cranberry, prune, and other juices discussed in chapter 8—is sometimes all that's needed to keep the urine acidic and resistant to bacterial growth. If diet isn't enough, oral supplements can help. Ascorbic acid, or vitamin C, is available in regular and buffered tablets and can help to acidify the urine alongside its other potential health benefits. Methenamine is another urine acidifier that, taken two or three times daily, can help to suppress the germs leading to bladder and kidney infections.

TREATMENT
Flush It Early

Early bladder infections can sometimes be chased away without the help of antibiotics by simply rinsing the bladder clean of bacteria with a good flush. At the earliest sign of infection, try drinking two to three glasses of water at once, followed by a large glass over each of the next three hours. Don't, however, reach for the cranberry juice. At this stage, you're *treating* an infection, not *preventing* it, and the acid-rich cranberry juice may feel to your irritated bladder lining like salt being rubbed into a wound. It's a good idea to call your doctor's office and ask whether a test will be needed, even if your symptoms seem to improve.

Bladder-Soothing Remedies

A few tips can be useful for simply relieving your symptoms. Since they don't actually cure the infection, always call your doctor so that definitive therapy can also be started without delay. Also, if you have a heart or other medical condition, check with your doctor before starting any of these therapies. Because some contain the basic salts of sodium and potassium, they're not suitable for everyone.

- *Baking soda.* You already know how this household substance can whiten your teeth and freshen your fridge, but baking soda, or sodium bicarbonate, can also help to relieve bladder burning by reducing its acidity. Mix one teaspoon of baking soda into one of the glasses of water you're using for the flush.

- *Rolaids or TUMS.* These can have an antacid effect in the bladder, just like baking soda, producing the same soothing effect.

- *Potassium citrate.* This is similar to sodium bicarbonate and sometimes better tolerated.

- *Aspirins for the bladder.* These tablets contain chemicals that soothe the symptoms of cystitis. Although they won't cure the underlying infection, they're often prescribed alongside antibiotics for symptom relief.

- *Phenazopyridine hydrochloride* (Pyridium). A urinary-tract pain reliever that reduces burning, pain, urgency, and frequency.

- *Methenamine (Urised).* A prescription medication that turns the urine bluish-green. In addition to its mild antibacterial effect, it can also have an antispasmodic soothing effect on an irritated bladder.

- *Uristat.* Available over the counter for the temporary relief of bladder symptoms. May be useful while you're waiting to see the doctor or for antibiotics to take effect. Turns the urine reddish-orange.

- *Flavoxate (Urispas).* An antispasmodic, sometimes handy for symptom relief.

Antibiotics

If you develop a full-fledged bladder infection, you'll probably need a course of antibiotics. Up to 80 percent of typical infections can be treated with a single dose, though a three-to-seven-day course is usually prescribed for assurance. Dozens of antibiotics are available for the treatment of cystitis, and your doctor will need to prescribe the drug of choice based on allergies, previous infections, and whether you're pregnant or breast-feeding. Your pill will most often come from a short list of favorites.

- *Trimethoprim-sulfamethoxazole (Bactrim, Septra)*. This sulfa drug is available in generic form and is very effective for most bladder infections.

- *Nitrofurantoin (Macrodantin, Macrobid)*. As effective as tri- methoprim but a bit more expensive. Macrobid is a microcrys- talline form, more expensive but less likely to cause nausea.

- *Quinolones (Ciprofloxacin, Norfloxacin, Ofloxacin, Floxin)*. Very effective but expensive and often reserved for more stub- born or complicated infections. Should not be used by breast- feeding women.

- *Penicillin and cephalosporins*. Penicillin and cephalosporins are often chosen during pregnancy because of their long safety record.

RECURRENT BLADDER INFECTIONS AND PROPHYLACTIC ANTIBIOTIC THERAPY

Recurrent cystitis is defined by more than three infections during a single year and affects around 15 percent of women at some point in their lives, sometimes despite all of the preventive efforts. This condition can present not only a pattern of very frustrating symptoms but also a risk of kidney damage if left untreated over time. Your doc- tor may recommend the prophylactic use of antibiotics to prevent recurrent infections from keeping you down.

This strategy involves keeping a supply of mild oral antibiotic pills at home and taking them before bladder infections occur. Since only low levels of bacteria (rather than a full-blown infection) are being treated, small pediatric doses are usually enough. Prophylactic antibiotics can be taken via either the *coital method* or the *daily method*.

The coital method involves taking a mild antibiotic right before or after intercourse. The idea is to mop up bacteria from the bladder when they're in greatest number. This method works well if your bladder infections occur predictably after intercourse.

The daily method entails routinely taking a baby dose of antibiotics each and every day. The daily method is preferred over the coital method if your infections occur unpredictably, unrelated to sexual activity. After six to twelve months of therapy, your doctor will usually decide whether to keep you on the preventive pills for a longer span of time. Some women stay on a daily antibiotic for many years.

Herbs That May Prevent Infections

- *Cranberry extract.* As mentioned, a safe and simple way to achieve cranberry-juice protection, without all the fluids and calories.

- *Grapefruit-seed extract.* Another substance with possible antibacterial effects in the vagina and urinary tract, though one study indicated that chemical preservatives within the extract—rather than the grapefruit itself—might account for this effect.

- *Golden seal.* A popular herb, claimed to be one of nature's antibiotics.

- *Echinacea.* Available in costly drinks and supplements stacked at arm's reach in the supermarket checkout aisles, echinacea has been claimed to help prevent respiratory infections and urinary tract infections. Despite the fact that it's perceived as mild and harmless, there is little in the way of science to prove that it works.

- *Others.* You'll find a number of herbs mentioned for the relief of bladder and pelvic symptoms. *Be careful*—not all herbs are alike. Comfrey, for instance, is mentioned as a bladder tonic, but it has been linked to serious liver damage and should not be used. Other herbal remedies may be perfectly harmless and worth a try. Always check with your doctor first.

KNOW THE LIMITS OF SELF-TREATMENT

Home remedies can often work beautifully. But they should never be substituted for a prescribed medication without your doctor's permission. If you suspect that you have frequent bladder infections, remember that there are other conditions—such as bladder stones, tumors, diverticula (small outpouched areas of the urethra or bladder), and inflammation—

that can feel just like typical episodes of cystitis. Some of these conditions can become serious if they're overlooked, especially if you're pregnant or have diabetes. Rather than relying on your own assumptions, see the doctor so you can both be sure.

KNOW WHEN *NOT* TO SELF-TREAT

Remember, not all antibiotics are safe for pregnancy, breast-feeding, and certain medical conditions. *Never* take antibiotics without consulting your doctor first. Always notify the doctor when you suspect cystitis that:

- Occurs during pregnancy.
- Is accompanied by a fever or pain in your back or side.
- Isn't improving with treatment.
- Keeps coming back. Overusing antibiotics can lead not only to vaginal yeast infections but to serious problems with bacterial resistance (specific bacterial types that no longer go away with antibiotics) over the long run.

Tip #3: Evaluate Your Health and Lifestyle

A number of activities and ailments, conditions and habits, that may at first seem far removed from your lower body can have a definite impact on incontinence and other common postreproductive problems. Before you march onward to the realm of pills, devices, and perhaps even surgery, consider these other factors that might be playing a role.

WORK AND EXERCISE

Physical fitness is central to the way virtually every part of your body feels and functions, and these areas of your postreproductive body are no exception. Will certain activities strain your pelvic supports and make incontinence or prolapse more likely to develop over time? If you're dealing with incontinence, prolapse, or other postreproductive symptoms, what's the right activity for you? Will high-impact aerobics cause stress incontinence to progress from mild to severe? Should you stop jogging to prevent your small cystocele or mild uterine prolapse from getting worse? Unfortunately, there's little science to guide our recommendations. One study comparing high-impact and low-impact Olympic athletes found that the degree of physical impact had no obvious influence on the risk of developing stress incontinence. The effects of more moderate recreational stress, such as jogging, aerobics, muscle training, karate, horseback riding, or weight lifting, remain unknown. In the absence of conclusive research, consider a few commonsense tips.

Stay Active, But Know What to Avoid if Symptoms Arise

We've discussed how evolution has left the female pelvic floor quite vulnerable to physical forces within the abdomen and pelvis, and the similarity between female pelvic prolapse and hernias in men. So it should come as no surprise to hear that a routine filled with heavy exertion may cause prolapse and incontinence to occur more rapidly. On rare occasion, even one particularly strenuous set of activities—like several days of heavy lifting during a move, or a summer of intense work in the garden—can have a noticeable effect.

On the other hand, it's common for women with prolapse and incontinence to get out of shape as they begin to avoid situations that might make their pelvic symptoms feel worse, or leave them feeling more vulnerable to accidents. Among 290 regular exercisers surveyed in one gynecologic practice, 20 percent of those with urinary incontinence reported that they stopped exercising because of this problem. Patients with advanced prolapse often follow a similar pattern. Allowing your physical fitness to decline is the worst possible effect that a pelvic-floor condition can have on your life. Your risk for a number of far more serious problems, such as heart disease, osteoporosis, stress, and even depression, will only increase. More specifically, for women choosing surgery to address their pelvic-floor problem, obesity means a higher risk that the operation will fail to provide a cure over the long run, due to the stress of excess pounds on the pelvic-floor supports. What's the best advice if you're already dealing with postreproductive symptoms? *Stay active* while keeping a few sensible tips in mind.

- *Think low-impact.* It's important to appreciate the way physical impact is absorbed by your body and the effect it can have on existing pelvic-floor problems over the long run. Particularly if you're coping with prolapse, beware of high-impact activities such as martial arts, weight lifting, crunches, horseback riding, and heavy aerobics, if they're exacerbating your symptoms down below. Focus on exercises that strengthen your midbody, pelvic area, and thighs until you're evaluated by a physician.

- *Yoga.* Provides a great low-impact routine, strengthening the thighs, back, and trunk while improving posture.

- *Walking, biking, water exercise, swimming.* Great workout options that create minimal pelvic stress.

- *Abdominal exercise.* Certain muscles in the abdominal wall may contribute to the function of your pelvic floor; as a result, abdominal muscle training might play a role in rehabilitating a dysfunctional pelvic floor. For starters, try fifteen sit-ups each morning, and over time, increase to thirty. That simple routine may give you that six-pack abdomen you always wanted while also preventing pelvic-floor problems.

  Bridges are done while lying faceup on a mat or soft surface. They help to strengthen the midbody from the buttocks to the abdominals. With your knees bent, try slowly lifting your body, keeping only your heels and shoulders on the floor. With practice, try increasing your lift time from five seconds to a full minute; to increase the difficulty, more your feet farther away from your hips. Pelvic tilts are another popular low-impact abdominal strengthener during pregnancy and afterward (see chapter 4).

- *Say good-bye to heavy hauling.* Keep exercising and stay as fit as you can, but if you're dealing with significant prolapse or incontinence, bid farewell to the joys of lifting heavy boxes, rearranging furniture, or hauling oversize bags of gardening soil, at least until you're evaluated by the doctor.

- *When you* need *to do heavy work, do it* right. If you do find it necessary to lift a heavy object, brace your pelvic floor with a Kegel squeeze, and exhale as you lift. Holding your breath will only increase the pressure on your most important pelvic supports. A few ounces of prevention—by modifying your activities and learning to brace your pelvic floor—may help keep you out of trouble down the road.

GENERAL MEDICAL AILMENTS

VASCULAR PROBLEMS, HIGH BLOOD PRESSURE, AND HEART DISEASE

Swelling of the feet and lower legs during the daytime—in some cases caused by heart conditions, large varicose veins, or certain medications—can lead to an abnormally high output of urine at night. This nighttime flooding (*diuresis*, in medical terms) is a result of fluid draining from the swollen lower extremities back into the bloodstream and eventually through the kidneys.

Some medications for high blood pressure may relax the urethra and bladder neck, sometimes enough to make incontinence worse. If you're on a medication for blood pressure or a heart condition, or a diuretic (water pill), ask your doctor whether it might be contributing.

RESPIRATORY CONDITIONS

Control asthma, and consider a flu shot. Many women can testify that a bad bout of bronchitis can push mild incontinence symptoms into a much bigger problem. Over time, a chronic cough may increase the wear and tear on your pelvic-floor supports, setting the stage for worsening prolapse, incontinence, and overall problems related to the pelvic floor. Chronic obstructive pulmonary disease (COPD), a lung condition often caused by smoking, is associated with urinary incontinence rates of up to 66 percent, and also more nighttime voiding.

DIABETES

Long-standing diabetes can cause a number of urinary problems, including bladder weakness, urinary retention, and overflow incontinence. When diabetes is poorly controlled, excess glucose may be excreted through the kidneys, causing an elevated urine output. Careful glucose control will benefit a number of bodily organs, including your bladder.

NEUROLOGIC PROBLEMS

Stroke, multiple sclerosis, Parkinson's disease, and other neurological problems can result in overactive-bladder symptoms, urge incontinence, urinary retention, and overflow incontinence. Although these diseases are chronic, they are often manageable in many ways, and extra attention to pelvic-floor symptoms can make a big difference in quality of life.

OBESITY

Being overweight puts you at higher risk for incontinence and prolapse by stressing the pelvic-floor supports. As an extreme example, one interesting 1992 study from the Medical College of Virginia evaluated urinary symptoms among obese women, before and then after surgically induced weight loss (stomach stapling). The study showed significant improvement in urinary symptoms after weight loss. Of twelve women who complained of incontinence before surgery, all but three resolved afterward. In Norway, the EPICONT study involving nearly twenty-eight thousand women revealed obesity as a clear risk factor for urinary incontinence. In other words, losing weight may sometimes prove to be the only therapy you need for your postreproductive problem.

WHAT YOU WEAR

Yes, even your wardrobe might affect the way your postreproductive body feels. Synthetic materials, for instance, can irritate the urethra and vagina and trigger pelvic symptoms. Wear cotton instead of nylon undergarments. If urinary or vaginal infections are a problem, avoid wearing tight clothing. Girdles or corsets, which squeeze the abdomen tightly, might actually strain the pelvic supports if worn regularly. If you're coping with pelvic-floor symptoms or recovering from surgery, these garments are probably not your best choice.

Tip #4: Quit Smoking

You know all about the effects of smoking on your heart, lungs, and blood vessels, and you've heard everything there is to hear about the links between cancer, strokes, and cigarettes. Why mention smoking in a book on postreproductive problems involving your pelvic area? Smoking also spells bad news for women with prolapse, incontinence, and other bladder symptoms. One study found that if you currently smoke or did so in the past, your risk of urinary incontinence is up to twice that of a nonsmoker, and your risk of pelvic prolapse may also be higher. The Norwegian EPICONT study also found higher rates of severe incontinence among smokers.

One major reason is the chronic smoker's cough. Whether it arises from asthma, bronchitis, emphysema, or the host of other smoking-related problems, a smoker's cough delivers a constant stress test to the pelvic floor and vaginal supports. Over time, this not only creates a higher risk for stress incontinence and prolapse but also decreases the chance of a surgical repair holding up over the long run.

Smoking can also mean trouble for an overactive bladder or urge incontinence. That's because nicotine can trigger contractions of the smooth muscle within the bladder wall, and it can also irritate the bladder lining. One British study of more than three thousand women confirmed that cigarette smoking does significantly increase the risk of an overactive bladder. A study from Virginia found that current and former smokers are over twice as likely to report stress incontinence as compared with nonsmokers. There must be quite a few restrooms in Marlboro Country for all them wranglers and cowgirls.

If you're a smoker who has thought about quitting, consider your postreproductive symptoms yet another good reason to do so. Cutting the habit is one great way you can help preserve the health of both your upper and lower body over the years, and perhaps even prevent a trip to the operating room.

Tip #5: Manage Menopause Masterfully

By now you've seen volumes of medical hype and endless demographic blurbs written on "the change." Behind all of the hype is an undeniable fact: the largest group of women in human history will pass through menopause over the next few years. Since many of these women will live as many years without functioning ovaries as they did with them, the physiological changes associated with menopause are taking on ever-increasing significance in women's health. You're probably well aware that the hormonal changes accompanying the end of menstruation affect your body in ways both big and small, ranging from simple hot flashes to an elevated risk for heart disease and osteoporosis. Less commonly known is that the same drop in estrogen can play a major role in bringing out postreproductive symptoms for the first time, or making existing problems feel worse.

- *Vaginal symptoms.* Urogenital atrophy is the most significant consequence of low estrogen levels when it comes to your genital area and urinary tract. During the decades after menopause, some degree of vaginal atrophy is nearly universal. Fortunately, not everyone will be bothered by it, but many are. As previously mentioned, a lack of estrogen can lead to vaginal dryness, causing irritation and even infections. For some women, these are the very first signs of reaching menopause. For others, bothersome vaginal changes don't arise until years or even decades later.

- *Sexually.* Vaginal atrophy is a common reason for painful sex. The earliest change is usually vaginal dryness, causing friction during intercourse; later, the vagina may actually become narrower.

- *Urinary symptoms.* Stress incontinence and/or urge incontinence might emerge, along with weakening of the tissues around the vagina, bladder, and urethra. An estrogen-deprived bladder lining may cause urinary frequency and urges to void throughout the daytime and night. Urogenital atrophy from low estrogen levels can increase your risk for bladder irritation, overactive-bladder symptoms, and even infections. If you noticed one or more of these problems after menopause, local estrogen therapy may provide an effective preventive strategy. In the section ahead, you'll learn about estrogen creams, vaginal rings, and tablets.

"IS INCONTINENCE ASSOCIATED WITH MENOPAUSE?"

That was the title of a recent Australian study involving nearly 1,900 women. It concluded that although incontinence is highly prevalent among women in midlife, the end of ovarian function might not be the key biological risk factor. More than the hormonal change, other factors— such as obstetrical history, body weight, and prior gynecologic surgery— may simply manifest themselves as problems at this time in midlife.

ESTROGEN AND OTHER HORMONES: THEIR IMPACT ON PELVIC SYMPTOMS

Estrogen is a vital ingredient for your pelvic area. The urethra, bladder, vagina, and pelvic floor are all incredibly rich with receptors (sites on the cells where hormones attach) for this most famous female hormone. When estrogen is in abundance, the skin, connective tissues, and blood vessels throughout these areas are well fed, well lubricated, thick, and strong. When estrogen is in short supply, after menopause or surgical removal of the ovaries, the lining of the vagina and bladder can become thin, dry, weak, and irritated—in other words, atrophic. Good vaginal bacteria (*lactobacilli*) may also become less abundant, making some women prone to infection with bad bacterial types or yeast. Urogenital atrophy is a remarkably common cause of vaginal, bladder, and sexual symptoms among postreproductive women.

When estrogen is replaced, all of these areas of your lower body respond with improved blood flow, thickness, and strength. Estrogen replacement can improve the condition of your pelvic-floor supports and relieve some of the symptoms associated with atrophy in the vagina, urethra, and bladder. But which types will actually work best, and what regimen is healthiest for you?

A Hormone-Rich Diet
Plant Estrogens
Natural estrogens can be found in more than three hundred plant products and ordinary foods, referred to as *isoflavones* or *phytoestrogens* (*phyto* means *plant*). They've attracted great interest in the past several years, largely over the hope that they might provide a natural way to relieve hot flashes and menopausal symptoms, prevent heart disease and bone loss, and even reduce the risk of breast cancer by providing a more balanced supply of weak estrogen types compared

to hormone pills. Much of this optimism arose from the observation that Asian women, who consume at least five times more certain phytoestrogens than Western women, seem to have a lower risk of all these problems. Most of the potential benefits have yet to be scientifically proven. Nevertheless, phytoestrogens can't hurt you, and hormone-rich foods can be found in some unexpected places.

- *Soy.* Isoflavones from soy are one of the richest sources of dietary estrogen. Try soy milk (Silk) on cereal. Soybean products (such as roasted soy nuts, soy flour, or boiled soy beans) can deliver high isoflavone content; be aware, however, that soy oil and soy sauce will not. Imitation soy meat (Boca burgers, Soy Dogs) and snack bars are abundant in grocery aisles and do contain isoflavones but are often disappointing to the tastebuds. Tofu is made from soy milk and comes in several forms, ranging from soft to very firm, suitable for cooking, roasting, and frying. Tempeh is fermented soybean, rich in isoflavones and useful as a meat substitute.

- *Certain yams.* The Mexican wild yam is a highly estrogenic food. Be sure not to confuse it with regular yams or sweet potatoes, neither of which contains significant phytoestrogens.

- *Flaxseed.* A seed with high estrogen content that can be added into baked goods.

- *Kidney and lima beans, chickpeas, seaweed, lentils.* Common isoflavone sources.

- *Chinese cactus.*

How effectively these plant estrogen sources might ease a specific postreproductive problem—for instance, improving vaginal lubrication, soothing an overactive bladder, or enhancing sexual function—remains uncertain. A small 1990 study of postmenopausal women showed that six weeks of a high soy and flaxseed diet caused increased vaginal lubrication that lasted for two weeks after resuming a regular diet. Currently, the National Institutes of Health is sponsoring research to evaluate the true effects of these substances on a broad range of menopausal symptoms. Even before all the questions have been answered, adding these foods to your diet in moderation may be worth exploring. Try a soy-rich diet for three to six months and see if you notice a change.

Nina Shandler's book *Estrogen the Natural Way* contains hundreds of estrogen-rich recipes from pancakes to soup, and a good discussion of their potential benefits to your heart, bones, and overall health.

What About Herbal Estrogen?

Several herbs and supplements may have effects similar to estrogen. But again, don't assume that they are understood in great detail or that we know their long-term risks. One basic problem of herbal products is that they aren't held to the same scientific scrutiny as mainstream pharmaceuticals. Their strength can vary widely, and their effects may (just like regular medicines) vary substantially between individuals.

- *Dong quai.* This well-known herb contains phytoestrols, a weak estrogen source that may (at least in theory) promote hormone production in your body. It has been claimed to help counteract vaginal atrophy, but according to my search of the medical literature, no such evidence yet exists. May be taken as tablets or in the form of a tincture.
- *Soy protein.* A phytoestrogen source, just like dietary soy.
- *Wild-yam extract.* Another natural phytoestrogen supplement, in dried extract form.
- *Red clover.* An herb with significant estrogen content in the form of isoflavones—enough that in the 1940s, Australian sheep grazing on red clover were found to be infertile. They were, in essence, consuming a natural oral contraceptive, with estrogens not unlike those in a regular birth-control pill. Among humans, it's taken as a pill, capsule, or tea containing the red-cloverleaf extract.
- *Black cohosh.* A centuries-old wildflower used by Native Americans, touted as a remedy for vaginal dryness and menstrual and menopausal symptoms. Europeans have advocated black

cohosh as an estrogen alternative (marketed as Remifemin) for menopause symptoms and hot flashes, and sales in the United States have become substantial. Just like the other herbs on this list, the verdict is still out regarding safety and efficacy.

HERBS AREN'T FOOD . . . THEY'RE DRUGS!

As you peruse the aisles at the vitamin shop in search of a natural remedy for your postreproductive problem, be aware of some basic facts about the herbal industry, and some potential pitfalls. Though it's true that herbs and other natural products have provided the raw material for countless modern medications, there's a great deal that's simply not known.

- In most cases, the effectiveness and proper doses are not very well established.
- Both the benefits and the potential risks are often unclear. Herbs and supplements may have widely variable production standards, which can make it hard to pinpoint the dose entering your body. Safety *is* an issue. Serious side effects are quite possible, and the regulatory status of these substances is often poorly defined. Especially if you have a history of breast cancer, uterine cancer, or abnormal blood clotting, consult with your doctor before taking an estrogenlike herb. As with hormone pills and patches, certain estrogen precautions may apply.
- Herbs mixed with some medications can, on rare occasion, create dangerous cocktails that can even be life-threatening. Be sure to check with your doctor before starting something new.
- Watch the sugar content if you're diabetic, and the salt content if you have high blood pressure. And if you're pregnant, absolutely, positively *never* take these products without your doctor's permission.
- Stick with brands recommended by your doctor or pharmacist, and avoid products that make outrageous or overly broad claims. If it sounds too good to be true, it almost certainly is.

Estrogen and Other Hormones in Their Many Medical Forms

In July 2002, the medical world was rattled with some surprising news. According to a study of more than sixteen thousand post-menopausal women taking part in the Women's Health Initiative, the use of combined conjugated equine estrogen and progestin (marketed as Prempro) caused more harm than benefit with respect to heart disease, strokes, and venous blood clots (a potentially dangerous condition) as compared with women taking a placebo pill. Although combined hormone therapy appeared to reduce hip fractures and colorectal cancer, these benefits were clearly outweighed by the increased cardiovascular risk. As a result, this portion of the Women's Health Initiative was halted, and women on this type of combined hormone replacement are discontinuing their long-term use of this therapy in great numbers. At the very least, any woman taking this particular hormone replacement on a long-term basis should review the best approach for prevention with her doctor, in light of this most recent data.

Types of Estrogen Therapy

Type #1: Systemic Estrogen—Pills and Patches

Systemic medications are those that enter your bloodstream and travel throughout your whole body. For estrogen, this refers to pills or skin patches, prescribed either with the short-term goal of relieving symptoms like hot flashes or insomnia; or, more commonly, the long-term protection against heart disease and weakening of bones (osteoporosis). Other potential benefits around the body may exist, from the skin to the brain, but at this point, they are not fully understood.

- *Pills (Premarin, Estratab, Estrace, Ogen, femhrt, Activella, Ortho-Prefest).* This is the most commonly prescribed form of systemic hormone replacement, used with the intent of providing protection against heart disease and osteoporosis. Although some of the estrogen that enters the bloodstream through these pills will eventually reach the vagina and pelvic tissues, it's most often not enough to fully relieve symptomatic atrophy.

EMPOWERING PATIENTS:
THE POWER OF HIGH-QUALITY RESEARCH

The Women's Health Initiative provided a few important lessons. First, that one particular type of combined hormone replacement (Premarin with Provera) was *not* the preventive panacea it had hoped to be—a surprise ending for a long chapter in women's health. Second, the Women's Health Initiative emphasized the power of carefully performed research. A single randomized placebo-controlled study had more scientific impact than dozens of less well-designed studies that had come before it. With the results of one good trial, several decades of debate were abruptly settled, to the benefit of millions of women. Wouldn't it be nice to see randomized trials looking at other questions in women's health—for instance, determining the best labor strategies and pushing positions? High-quality research trials are expensive indeed, but as we've learned from the Women's Health Initiative, they're worth their weight in gold.

• *Patches (Estraderm, Climara, Alora, Vivelle, FemPatch, Esclim).* These are the second most common form of synthetic estrogen. Medicated stickers applied to the trunk, buttocks, or abdomen, they are changed once or twice weekly. The available patches deliver estradiol, the most potent type of estrogen, and may reduce the odds of side effects caused by pills. Newer patches are thin, strong, and barely visible.

Is Systemic Estrogen Right for You?

Whether or not to begin using systemic (pill or patch) estrogen replacement therapy has proven to be a perplexing medical decision for many women. Are the symptoms of menopause pathological conditions that should be treated with medications, or natural transitions that should be met with simple changes to diet and lifestyle? Is hormone therapy an unnecessary manipulation of a natural event, or an example of preventive medicine at its finest—right up there with childhood vaccinations and Pap smears, increasing your odds for an increasingly long and healthy life? The basic biological dilemma revolves around the fact that estrogen affects the whole body, in both desirable locations (heart, bone, brain tissue, muscle, and fat) and undesirable ones (breast and uterus). While estrogen (when not combined with certain progestins) may offer some protection against osteoporosis and perhaps heart disease, it may also increase the risk of breast cancer. The ongoing estogen-only portion of the Women's Health Initiative will hopefully provide answers to these questions in the coming years. In the meantime, does it suit your health goals to take this medication today, accepting its potential risks, to possibly prevent certain diseases decades from now? The pros and cons of taking systemic hormones after menopause remain central questions in women's health and are the subject of an ongoing debate that's worth discussing with your doctor.

Our questions regarding systemic hormone therapy are much more limited in scope. Can estrogen in the form of a pill or patch provide relief of incontinence, pelvic prolapse, sexual dysfunction, or any other postreproductive problems? If estrogen pills and patches do help to improve the bladder symptoms of urinary incontinence, the benefit is probably subtle. Some studies have found mild benefits to bladder control. Another study on hormone usage (the HERS trial)—as an aside to the main analysis concerning cardiovascular effects—raised concern that taking oral estrogen along with progesterone may even worsen incontinence for some women.

What about sexual function? For reasons both physical and psychological, systemic hormone replacement will provide benefit to some women. But in most cases, little improvement will be seen in the way of vaginal atrophy, often the biggest culprit leading to sexual troubles. Local estrogen therapy (vaginal creams and vaginal tablets) are the more effective route in this respect, and they can be used right along with oral estrogen for women whose vaginal atrophy is causing sexual, urinary, or other pelvic problems.

THE MANY FACES OF MEDICAL ESTROGEN

Though the term *estrogen* may sound like it refers to just one chemical, it's a family of hormones derived from several different sources and consisting of several different types.

- *Conjugated equine estrogens (Premarin).* Extracted from the urine of pregnant horses, containing several estrogen types.

- *Estradiol (Estrace).* The most potent estrogen type, mirroring the estrogen produced most abundantly by your ovaries before menopause. The estradiol contained in Estrace is derived from plant sources.
- *Plant-derived estrogens (Cenestin, Gynodiol, Estratab, Menest).*
- *Raloxifene (Evista).* The breakthrough designer estrogen that has attracted enormous attention over the past several years. Belonging to the SERM (selective estrogen receptor modulator) family of medications, it was developed with the hope of selectively providing all the benefits of estrogen while avoiding any increased risk of breast and uterine cancer. While raloxifene seems to offer protection for the heart and bones, it's unclear whether its urogenital benefits—in other words, the prevention of atrophy in the vagina and bladder—are as potent as standard estrogen's. Ongoing research trials should provide this answer in the near future.

Type #2: Local Estrogen Therapy—Creams, Gels, Tablets, and Rings

Local hormone replacement refers to creams, tablets, and devices that deliver estrogen straight to the target areas in your pelvis. Unlike systemic pills and patches, they tend not to enter the bloodstream very much, but by targeting symptoms of atrophy right at the source, they may provide even more relief. For instance, regularly using vaginal cream results in bloodstream levels of estrogen that are only a quarter of those reached with oral estrogens. This means that much higher doses can be delivered directly to the urogenital area, with far less chance of an undesirable effect elsewhere. If your vaginal, urethral, and bladder tissues have become thin, pale, or dry from atrophy, you may benefit from local estrogen therapy in one of a few available forms.

- *Vaginal estrogen creams (Estrace, Premarin, Ortho-Dienestrol, Ogen).* Vaginal estrogen cream is a very effective treatment for vaginal and urinary symptoms resulting from atrophy. It's inserted at bedtime with a measured applicator. Estrogen cream slowly but surely makes atrophic tissues thicker, better lubricated, and less prone to infection. Like all forms of local estrogen therapy, full effects may take six to twelve months to achieve. Estrogen cream comes in two forms in the United

States: Premarin (conjugated equine estrogens) and Estrace (micronized estradiol). Estrogen gel exists in Europe, but it has not been FDA-approved in the United States. When used once or twice weekly, these creams raise blood estrogen levels minimally, which means that no protection can be expected for the heart or bones. On the other hand, if taken in high enough doses, estrogen in the vagina can enter the bloodstream in significant quantity and will carry risks similar to estrogen taken as a pill or patch.

- Insert the cream at bedtime to minimize leakage while you're upright and active.
- Load the applicator by screwing it onto the opening of the tube. Fill the tube with the dose prescribed by your doctor.
- Lie on your back and fold up your knees; or stand with one foot on a chair.
- Insert the loaded applicator slowly, like a tampon, and press in the plunger. Don't insert any farther than is comfortable.
- Applicators are rinsed with warm water (not hot or boiling) and reused.

- *Vaginal tablets.* Some women may prefer inserting a tablet, rather than cream, into the vagina. Similar local estrogen effects can be achieved.
  - Vagifem tablets come in preloaded disposable applicators.
  - Oral estrogen tablets can also be used for vaginal insertion, with your doctor's guidance regarding the correct dosage.
- *Estrogen rings (Estring).* This small Silastic ring has been designed for insertion into the vagina, like a small diaphragm, releasing estrogen over a span of three months at a very low but continuous dose. Every three months, it's removed and replaced with a new ring. Great for women seeking the most hands-off approach to local estrogen therapy.

Local estrogen therapy might improve the following problems:

- *Overactive bladder and urge incontinence.* Several clinical trials have shown that estrogen applied directly to the genital area can improve urinary urgency, daytime urinary frequency, and night-time voiding. Although several studies have tried to show an effect of estrogen therapy on reducing the amount of actual urine leakage, the results have been mixed and inconclusive.

- *Stress incontinence.* Vaginal estrogen treatment can help to improve stress incontinence by improving blood flow and making tissues around the urethra and vagina thicker and healthier. Although only one in ten of mild stress incontinence cases will be cured with estrogen therapy alone, at least 30 percent of them will be improved.

- *Urinary tract infections.* Estrogen can help to prevent bladder infections in some women with signs of vaginal atrophy due to low estrogen levels, since the same changes associated with decreased estrogen (thinning and drying) tend to also affect the urethra, increasing its susceptibility to bacterial infection. Intravaginal estrogen in particular has been shown to decrease recurrent infections among postmenopausal women.

- *Painful intercourse.* Vaginal atrophy is a major cause of painful intercourse after menopause, or dyspareunia, due to poorly lubricated and irritable vaginal skin. Estrogen replacement is a common remedy.

- *Pelvic prolapse.* One 1995 study from the University of Southern California concluded that vaginal estrogen can decrease the need for surgery to repair prolapse by strengthening the vaginal skin and its connective-tissue components. We cannot conclude on this one study, however, that local estrogens help with mild prolapse.

WILL VAGINAL ESTROGEN CAUSE SIDE EFFECTS?

Low doses of vaginal estrogen are unlikely to cause any serious side effects; however, occasional breast pain or enlargement, vaginal itching, headaches, or nausea can occur. Higher doses may cause vaginal bleeding, a symptom that's extremely important to report to your doctor. With the doses typically used, most women notice no side effects whatsoever—one major reason why vaginal estrogen therapy is a great preventive strategy.

SYSTEMIC VERSUS LOCAL HORMONES

The increasing array of local estrogens in today's pharmacy allows women to treat their urogenital symptoms while minimizing the entry of estrogen into the bloodstream. Local replacement is free from most of the risks and side effects of estrogen therapy and is often the most potent form used in urogynecology. Before taking the leap into hormone therapy, take time to discuss your goals with a doctor, and assure yourself that you're choosing the type and dosage that best suit your needs.

THE "OTHER" HORMONE: PROGESTERONE

When taken alone, estrogen causes the inner lining of the uterus to become overgrown, and over time, this can lead to malformed or even cancerous cells. If you still have a uterus and begin estrogen therapy, taking a progestin (synthetic progesterone) keeps the uterine lining in normal condition and nullifies the risk of uterine cancer. Unfortunately, progestins quite often cause side effects, including mood changes, weight gain or fluid retention, and breast tenderness. For better or worse, they should have no noticeable effect on the postreproductive problems that we've discussed.

- *Medroxyprogesterone acetate (Provera, Cycrin).* The most commonly used progestin for hormone replacement. Very effective but likely to cause side effects.

- *Micronized natural progesterone (Prometrium).* Natural progesterone in the form of tiny particles engineered for even absorption into the bloodstream.

- *Norethindrone acetate (Aygestin, Micronor), norgestimate (Ortho-Prefest).* Mild synthetic progestins common in oral contraceptives; also useful for hormone replacement, especially if other progestins have caused bothersome side effects.

- *Vaginal cream or gel (Crinone).* Yet another alternative for women who develop side effects to oral progestins.

- *Single combination packs (Prempro, Premphase, CombiPatch, femhrt, Ortho-Prefest).* A number of HRT products include both an estrogen and progestin. As with all hormone therapy, their use over the short term and long run should be carefully discussed with your doctor.

OPTIMIZING PREVENTION AND IMPROVING YOUR FUNCTION AT ANY AGE

Whether you're thirty-five or sixty-five, there are always opportunities to explore connections between your pelvic-floor symptoms and other aspects of your health and lifestyle. Minimizing your gynecologic problems, understanding the occasional link between general medical ailments and pelvic-floor symptoms, and managing menopause masterfully all may have an impact on your postreproductive symptoms. As you sort through pelvic-floor symptoms for the first time, keep these important connections in mind.

❧ 13 ❧

Seeing the Doctor

WHERE TO GO, WHAT TO EXPECT, HOW TO PREPARE

Of the 10 million Americans with urinary incontinence, more than half have had no evaluation or treatment.

—National Institutes of Health,
1988 consensus conference

I consider my problem to be quite severe. It's affected all my activities, even intercourse, ever since I had a baby. I'm too young to be going through this!

—Thirty-two-year-old, during her
first office visit

So, now you have a new understanding of the likely roots of your problem, and you've decided, despite all the tips for getting started on your own, that it would be best to see a doctor. *Good job.* By the time most women seek medical help for incontinence, it's after an average of seven years of leaking. Very frustrating years, without a doubt. Those with sexual dysfunction or prolapse will also endure years with symptoms, detracting from what should be active stages of their lives. Unfortunate but totally understandable. These are personal problems, after all—ones that just about anyone would prefer not to discuss. Many women simply find excuses: "This happens to everyone after having kids. What gives *me* the right to complain?" "As long as I don't jog or play tennis, I'm fine. I'll just become a walker." "This is way too embarrassing—I'm going to cancel that appointment again." According to national data, only one in five women with the symptoms we've discussed will see a specialist.

268

Nearly every woman with one of these postreproductive problems can enjoy a better quality of life by refusing to suffer in silence and seeking help sooner. You've hopefully gained an awareness of your physical changes, and you might even have taken steps to treat yourself at home. But if your symptoms are still a bother, and you'd like to find relief so you can channel your energies toward more exciting areas of your life, it's time to seek some professional advice.

Types of Providers

Believe it or not, many doctors are either too busy or simply not familiar with treating these postreproductive problems. Others don't encounter them often enough to recognize their impact on quality of life. Still others, surprisingly, are too embarrassed to ask patients about them. But many professionals are very interested, and your first task is to find one of them. Once you've brought incontinence, prolapse, or other postreproductive pelvic symptoms to your doctor's attention, you may be referred to a specialist in female pelvic-floor disorders.

- *Urogynecologists* first train in obstetrics and gynecology, then devote their specialty training to advanced gynecologic surgery and the lower urinary tract. They provide the full range of surgical and office treatments for pelvic prolapse, incontinence, and other disorders of the pelvic floor. In addition, their gynecological training spans the management of female reproductive and menopausal health care.

- *Urologists* complete residency training in both male and female urology. Some then go on to complete further specialty training dedicated to female problems.

- *Nurses and nurse practitioners* often play a key role in office care; they will participate in some of your visits and testing procedures, such as biofeedback and urodynamics.

- *Pelvic-floor physiotherapists* are physical therapists specializing in pelvic-floor disorders, providing an array of noninvasive treatments such as pelvic-floor stimulation, massage, and biofeedback.

- *Gastroenterologists and colorectal surgeons* may be called upon to help treat fecal incontinence in the office and/or operating room.

Whomever you choose to see, make it somebody who's prepared to offer you a reasonable range of alternatives. Even if the doctor believes strongly in surgery for your problem, did you have the opportunity to at least discuss why physical therapy or nonsurgical therapy is not a good option? How many surgical procedures does your doctor perform each year? During your search for a provider, take the time to ask the opinions of your other doctors, friends, and colleagues, in order to find the professional whose outlook matches yours, with whom you'll hopefully have a sense of rapport and trust.

YOUR MEDICAL HISTORY

At the doctor's office, you'll be asked to answer dozens of questions in the form of written questionnaires and face-to-face discussion. Your doctor will be reconstructing in detail when your symptoms first occurred, how they've progressed, and what seems to provoke them. Before the first visit, you may be asked to complete a voiding diary that logs every voiding and leakage episode over a period of one to four days. If you've already charted your own Voiding and Symptom Diary (see Appendix B), bring it in to show your doctor.

Before your visit, try to make a file of medical, surgical, or obstetrical records and a list of your medications, including over-the-counter pills and herbal supplements. Your doctor will be interested in medical conditions and daily habits that place you at risk for pelvic symptoms, and any medications that might affect your lower body. Don't assume that any aspect of your medical history is irrelevant, since seemingly unrelated medical problems can sometimes create a higher risk for prolapse, incontinence, and other pelvic-floor symptoms. For instance, asthma, emphysema, and irritable bowel may play a role. Diabetes or congestive heart failure may affect your urine production at night. More unusual conditions, such as connective-tissue disorders, may affect the strength and resilience of tissues all around the body, including the pelvis. Your doctor should know of any prior surgeries, especially urologic, gynecologic, or abdominal. Any extensive injuries to the vagina, rectum, or bladder, forceps, deliveries, long labors, or very large newborns will be of special interest.

Finally, your lifestyle at home and work will probably be discussed. Patterns of heavy lifting, smoking, diet, and exercise will be evaluated as potential risk factors for pelvic-floor problems. Conversely, you may be asked about the impact of any postreproductive symptoms on your work, recreation, fitness, and overall enjoyment of life.

BEFORE-YOUR-FIRST-VISIT CHECKLIST

1. Write down your questions.
2. Complete your Voiding and Symptom Diary (see Appendix B).
3. Bring copies of any past surgical and medical records, including testing results and laboratory reports.
4. Bring a list of medications and dosages, including over-the-counter pills.

YOUR PHYSICAL EXAMINATION

Diagnosing your postreproductive problem requires a detailed physical examination in focused areas.

NEUROLOGICAL EXAM

A brief neurological exam will usually focus on the sensation, strength, and reflexes in both your legs and genital area, since neurological function in these areas mirrors that of the pelvic floor (they are supplied by the same sacral nerves). The neurological exam is particularly important if you have overactive bladder symptoms or retention of urine due to incomplete emptying, since on rare occasion, these problems may have a neurological cause.

THE PELVIC

Your pelvic examination will not be so brief. It will focus on all of the supports around the vagina, bladder, rectum, and pelvis. Using a speculum, the doctor will separately evaluate the upper, lower, sides, and top supports of the vagina while you're asked to bear down forcefully. This is your doctor's opportunity to diagnose all of the conditions we've discussed: cystocele, rectocele, enterocele, and prolapse of the uterus or vaginal vault. By straining as if you were giving birth, the increased pressure will provoke your maximum state of prolapse for the doctor to see. Often a separate evaluation is done in the standing position. Though somewhat awkward, the standing exam causes the prolapse to bulge out even farther, making it easier for the doctor to see and diagnose the full extent of your problem.

Q-tip Test

Remember the importance of upper vaginal wall supports and the floppy urethra? Your doctor may perform a Q-tip test to evaluate whether this is part of your problem. This involves placing a lubricated sterile cotton swab into the urethra and measuring its movement while you're straining. It feels just like a small catheter being inserted, then removed a moment later.

Kegel Squeeze

Your doctor might test your pelvic-floor contraction strength using an examining finger and guiding your technique as you squeeze. This will allow for a quick assessment of your levator muscles and the control you have over them.

Stress Test

As you've learned, accidental squirts or dribbles of urine during a cough, sneeze, change of position, or strain usually indicate stress incontinence. As part of your initial evaluation for this symptom, you may be asked to cough or strain while your doctor looks for sudden leakage from the urethral opening. If leakage occurs, the doctor may then support the upper vaginal wall around the urethra with a small instrument or with two fingers. If you stay dry with a cough when the urethra is supported in this manner, your stress incontinence is probably due to a floppy urethra (see chapter 8).

"HEY DOC, WHY ARE YOU TAPPING ON MY KNEES?"

If you finally made that first appointment with the urogynecologist only to find that the doctor bypasses the speculum and reaches instead for the reflex hammer to tap on your kneecaps, don't worry. You didn't walk into the wrong office! Certain clues to your pelvic-floor symptoms may, in fact, come from as far away as the knees and ankles. What's that all about?

The same bundle of nerves arising from your lower spine supplies both your pelvis and your legs; as a result, identifying a neurologic problem in one of these areas can be the first tip-off that there's a problem in the other. That's why reflexes, strength, and sensations in your legs may be examined when you're evaluated for certain pelvic symptoms.

Even more interesting are the ways in which these rather unlikely connections have enabled certain treatments. Pacemakers implanted near the lower back, for instance, can stimulate the sacral nerves and alleviate a number of troublesome pelvic-floor symptoms; amazingly, when these pelvic pacemakers are working effectively, they'll trigger a muscle contraction in both the pelvic-floor muscles and the big toe! Acupuncture and stimulation treatments around the foot and leg, believe it or not, have also been utilized with modest success for the treatment of the overactive bladder and are still being investigated.

CATHETERIZED URINE SPECIMEN

At your first office visit, a urine sample will usually be obtained through a small urethral catheter around the size of a cocktail straw.

- *Urine culture.* A portion of this urine will be sent to an outside laboratory for culture. This is the definitive test for ruling out a bacterial infection. The result is usually available in two to three days.

- *Urinalysis.* This is a dipstick test of urine done right in the office, with immediate results, to look for evidence of infection or other substances not normally found in the urine (bacteria, white blood cells, blood). It cannot definitively confirm an infection.

- *Postvoid residual.* This is one of the most important initial office tests. It determines not how much you void but how much you leave behind. Urinary retention means a volume greater than fifty to one hundred milliliters (roughly three ounces) left inside your bladder after urinating. Retaining small amounts of urine is rarely of concern; more severe retention, however, can indicate a definite abnormality and usually warrants a more detailed investigation. A handheld ultrasound machine, rather than a catheter, is sometimes used to measure postvoid residual.

Uroflowmetry

You may be asked to urinate into a specialized toilet seat rigged with a large funnel that spills your urine into a measuring sensor. This is *uroflowmetry*, a device that measures the rate of urine flow out of your bladder, the total time for urination, and the pattern of your void. Uroflowmetry is an initial test for detecting an obstructed or weakened urinary stream.

Cystometry

Cystometry is an office test that measures the bladder's ability to fill to normal capacity (around twelve to twenty ounces of urine) and retain urine. The test involves slowly filling your bladder through a catheter while observing the pressure within the bladder. An abnormal rise in bladder pressure can indicate spasm of the bladder muscle. Cystometry can provide a quick and simple means for diagnosing an overactive bladder.

Urodynamics Testing

Depending on your incontinence or prolapse symptoms, *urodynamics* may be recommended to determine the exact nature of your problem and the most effective treatment. Urodynamics examines the function of the bladder, urethra, and pelvic-floor muscles all at once. The test enables your doctor to play detective when symptoms become confusing. For instance, leakage provoked by a cough may reflect either weakness of the urethra (stress incontinence) or the triggering of a sudden involuntary bladder contraction (urge incontinence), and to the naked eye, these two conditions can appear identical. They can be distinguished with the help of urodynamics, allowing for proper treatment decisions.

Urodynamics is performed in an odd-looking chair with small catheters and wires. One small (spaghetti-size) catheter will be placed into your bladder, and another will be inserted into either the vagina or rectum. Your bladder will then be slowly filled until it reaches its maximum capacity. Afterward, the function of your bladder and urethra are measured as you force a cough or strain. You should expect the feeling of a very full bladder, but no pain. The doctor will analyze any leakage that occurs by studying the pressures within these various anatomic areas at the moment of leakage. Was it stress incontinence from a floppy urethra, or a thin urethra, or both? Was it an overactive bladder or mixed incontinence?

At the end of the urodynamics test, you'll be asked to empty your urine into a special collection device. This voiding phase of the test will help your doctor to recognize problems with bladder function due to prolapse or other causes. Video urodynamics combines pictures of the bladder with computerized pressure readings; some specialists prefer it.

Urodynamics may sometimes be recommended even if your only complaint is a prolapse bulge, with no incontinence problem. If you have a large prolapse bulge repaired, there is a 30 to 80 percent risk of stress incontinence arising after surgery. Some women experience worse stress leakage while wearing a pessary even before their testing. Potential stress incontinence, as this is called, occurs because unsupported prolapse bulges tend to bend or kink the urethra, creating, in effect, an artificial valve that keeps you dry. To avoid the frustration of potential stress incontinence after a prolapse repair, urodynamics allows the doctor to plan a combined surgery that addresses prolapse and incontinence at the same time.

CYSTOSCOPY

To evaluate certain bladder symptoms, your doctor might recommend *cystoscopy* (*cysto* is the Greek root for *bladder*). The test is performed through a catheter-size telescopic camera, in either the office or the operating room, allowing your doctor to look directly into the bladder and urethra. During a five- to ten-minute procedure, the doctor checks for a handful of important conditions.

- *Inflammation.* An irritated bladder and/or urethra is sometimes responsible for urinary symptoms, even a loss of bladder control. Interstitial cystitis is one type of noninfectious irritation that can be seen with office cystoscopy.

- *Tumors and polyps.* Benign growths in the bladder or urethra can occasionally be the source of symptoms. Fortunately, malignant growths are rare.

- *Diverticulum.* An outpouching of the bladder or urethral wall that can cause infection and irritation during and after urination.

- *Fistulas.* These are abnormal connections or holes that can develop between the bladder or urethra and the vagina or bowel, sometimes leading to very severe or constant leakage of urine. They can be caused by prolonged pressure of the fetal head during a very extended childbirth, when the layers of tissue that separate these structures become badly damaged. In the developed world, where protracted labors are rare, fistulas due to childbirth are exceedingly uncommon; they can, however, occasionally result from pelvic operations, including hysterectomy. The risk is also increased by forceps delivery. The only remedy is surgical repair to close the hole.

- *Bladder stones.* Various types of stones can develop all through the urinary tract. When they exist in the bladder, urinary frequency, urgency, and infections may result.

- *Foreign body.* On rare occasion after pelvic or vaginal surgery, a stitch, staple, mesh, or graft can erode into the bladder or urethra and cause irritation. Finding any of these foreign bodies during cystoscopy may help to plan for their removal.

Intravenous Pyelogram (IVP)

This test is performed in the radiologist's office, where a special intravenous dye creates an outline of the kidneys, ureters (tubes connecting the kidneys and bladder), and the bladder itself. An IVP is most commonly recommended when your doctor suspects the presence of a stone, narrowing, or other problem in the upper part of your urinary tract.

SPECIAL TESTING FOR ANAL INCONTINENCE

- *Anal sphincter testing (electromyography/EMG).* This test measures the function of the anal sphincter nerves and muscles, using electrodes similar to an EKG's stickers.

- *Anal ultrasound.* A very slender probe is inserted rectally and used to create pictures of the anal sphincter muscles. Ultrasound can reveal obstetrical injuries that may be responsible for a loss of fecal control.

- *Manometry.* Pressure measurements of the lower colon and rectum are used to evaluate the function of these structures, using specially designed balloons able to record pressure.

- *Barium enema.* After air or opaque fluid is infused into the rectum, X rays of the pelvis and abdomen create a picture of the bowel.

Now, That Wasn't So Bad, Was It?

From meeting the doctor to the examination and various types of testing, a complete urogynecology evaluation might entail a series of office visits and feel like a strange new world. Even when you come in with one symptom, it's very common to find more than one underlying postreproductive problem. For instance, urinary incontinence may be diagnosed as mixed (stress and urge), or a bulging cystocele might be accompanied by potential stress incontinence (leakage that becomes apparent only when the prolapse bulge is supported during testing).

The tests outlined in this chapter are your doctor's best tools for appreciating the big picture and offering you the most complete long-term relief. As you move along with your evaluation, keep your doctor's treatment goals, and your improved future quality of life, in mind.

☙ 14 ☙

Preparing for Pelvic Reconstructive Surgery and Optimizing Your Recovery

CHOICES, EFFECTIVENESS, RISKS, RECUPERATION, AND WHAT TO DO WHEN THINGS DON'T FEEL FIXED

The only "minor" surgery is one performed on somebody else!
—Wise woman

I'm playing in a softball league this summer for the first time in three years. It wasn't much fun when I was always soaking wet by the third inning.

—Forty-six-year-old after
incontinence surgery

Five Key Questions to Ask Before Your Operation

So you've decided, "Enough with pessaries, gadgets, and pills—fix me!" If that's the case, rest assured—there's a very good chance that a very good surgical correction is waiting for you, one that may dramatically improve your lifestyle if it's been diminished by urinary or fecal incontinence, prolapse, even sexual dysfunction. Despite the countless medications, exercises, and innovative devices available to treat your postreproductive problems, many women each year bite the bullet and decide to have surgery. Up to 11 percent of the general female population will make this choice during their lifetime for prolapse and incontinence alone. In order to find the best operation for you, and to enter into it with the most realistic expectations, you'll

278

need to sort through an array of choices. Not all operations are alike, and not all surgeons will not give you the same advice. Before signing on, make yourself an informed consumer.

Let's assume that you're frustrated with leakage when you cough, sneeze, and exercise—a straightforward case of urinary stress incontinence. You might have heard through the grapevine that surgery can offer wonderful results with high rates of success, and a quick return to work, exercise, and a full daily routine. But which method of surgery is right for you? The vaginal, laparoscopic, or open abdominal route each has its own risks, benefits, results, and recovery time. The repair of a cystocele, rectocele, or other prolapse bulge could involve anything from ordinary stitches to man-made mesh or even cadaver-tissue grafts, and each technique has its own track record. How will the success of these surgical alternatives compare not only for tomorrow but for ten or twenty years in the future?

When it comes to having surgery for a postreproductive problem, you'll often face a broad range of alternatives. Though these conditions all relate to weakness and relaxation within the fairly confined region of the pelvic floor, there are a surprising number of ways to rebuild strength and support; this means many choices and countless questions. Amid all of the testing, talking, and fear of the unknown, let's focus on a few key questions that will help you to arrive at your own best choice of surgery.

QUESTION #1: WHY HAVE SURGERY?

Though postreproductive problems may severely threaten your lifestyle, they're almost never life-threatening. Even pelvic-prolapse bulges that may look rather dramatic are rarely medically urgent in the way a bowel hernia might sometimes be, so in most cases, surgery is not a requirement, it's a choice. When it comes to choosing surgery for prolapse or incontinence, take your time and make your decisions with a few simple thoughts in mind. Surgery might be a good option if:

- *You're bothered.* Incontinence, prolapse, or vaginal relaxation that does not cause symptoms usually does not need to be fixed just for the sake of restoring your anatomy back to a picture-perfect state. Ask yourself how these problems are affecting your life. How much do they detract from your physical activity, social routine, and intimacy? For some women, even a great deal of leakage, bulging, or a change in sexual functioning may have little effect on happiness; for others, minor accidents or small physical alterations may make it impossible to enjoy exercise, work, travel, or sex.

- *You've explored and know your options.* By now you've learned about the many nonsurgical alternatives for the most common postreproductive problems; before having surgery, explore any that sound attractive. Some women consider life far too busy for exercise routines, devices, pessaries, magnetic chairs, or injections, and they choose the quick fix of surgery right from the start. Others will do anything and everything to avoid the operating room and will embark on a stepwise approach even if it involves committing to a daily effort or combining several therapies. In this day and age of countless options, there's only one rule that applies to all women in choosing a treatment plan: to each her own!

- *You're informed and feel comfortable with what you've learned.* Take whatever time you need to clearly understand the procedure your doctor is recommending, including the typical recovery and potential complications. No matter how simple a surgery is intended to be, your recuperation can always turn out to be more difficult than expected. If you're still uneasy, ask if you can speak with a patient who has undergone the procedure.

- *Is prolapse surgery ever medically urgent?* Not often, but on very rare occasion, it becomes medically important to proceed with surgery for a postreproductive problem. This operation is no longer truly elective. The most common example is when severe prolapse causes blockage of urine flow from the kidneys to the bladder. In this predicament, watching and waiting can eventually lead to kidney damage.

QUESTION #2: IS NOW THE RIGHT TIME?

Though you may choose to call upon family, friends, or others for opinions and advice, the final decision to have an operation is yours alone. It's your body, and the recovery after surgery, whether smooth or rocky, will be yours alone to cope with. How will you know when the time is right?

- *Think about your family planning.* Are you absolutely certain that your childbearing years are behind you, or are you still keeping family-planning options open? Many operations for incontinence and prolapse are best delayed until childbearing is complete, to minimize the risk of weakening the repair and needing yet another operation in the future. If you do plan to have more children, using a pessary or continence device may provide temporary relief until the time is right for surgery. However, if symptoms become severe, surgery may sometimes become a consideration even if you do want to have a future pregnancy. In this case, be sure to plan an operation that will preserve your fertility and ability to withstand pregnancy, and discuss how its long-term success might be affected by a future pregnancy and delivery. Many operations will allow you to have a baby afterward, but all of the issues need to be discussed.

- *Consider your life stage and support network.* If you still have young children at home, will you be able to avoid lifting them during your recovery? Is there somebody who can help carry those grocery bags from the garage to the kitchen counter, or shovel snow off the front steps? Young mothers are often advised to delay having pelvic surgery until their youngest child is a toddler. By then the whole family should understand—or at least *may* understand—and can cope with the fact that Mom won't be cleaning, carrying, or lifting at full steam for a little while.

- *Examine your health.* Later in life, your general health will begin to weigh into your surgical decisions. If you're a good candidate to safely undergo surgery today, will you be as fit several years down the road? Your immune system, mobility, and overall cardiovascular status all factor into the way you'll bounce back after an operation; unfortunately, all of them diminish with age.

- *Have you tried the pessary test?* If you're undecided over surgery for pelvic prolapse, especially if your pelvic symptoms have been vague—such as a little bulging, a bit of pressure, or occasional pain—try wearing a pessary over a period of days or weeks. With the pessary inside, was your vaginal bulging, rectal pressure, or lower abdominal discomfort less severe at the end of each day? Were you able to empty your bladder or bowels more completely? Did your overall quality of life feel improved? When big questions are still blowing in the wind, try the pessary test. You can't fail this exam, and it just might shed some much-needed light on your presurgical choices, such as which symptoms surgery might alleviate and which it might not.

QUESTION #3: WHAT ARE MY CHOICES OF ANESTHESIA?

Although the risks associated with modern anesthetic techniques are quite low, discuss your options before surgery and feel comfortable with your choice.

- *General anesthesia.* You're put fully to sleep, and a breathing tube is inserted during the operation. For open abdominal and laparoscopic operations, a general anesthetic is almost always necessary. For vaginal procedures, you'll often have the opportunity to choose between the following other options.
- *Epidural and spinal.* Injection of anesthesia into the spinal area, which results in temporary numbness of the lower body. *Epidural* involves the placement of a tiny catheter into the area around the spinal column, which is left for the duration of surgery. *Spinal* refers to a single injection of anesthesia, intended to last until the end of surgery.
- *Local anesthesia.* Injection of anesthetic (such as novocaine) into and underneath the skin. Local injections can be used throughout the body, including the vaginal skin and abdominal area. However, their use is generally limited to operations involving only small incisions.

QUESTION #4: WHICH OPERATION IS BEST?

If you ever decide to quiz two different pelvic surgeons on the very best operation for your postreproductive problem, be prepared—

you'll probably hear three different opinions. Surgery for incontinence and prolapse can be performed in a variety of ways, perhaps more than for any other area of the body. Some centers specialize in vaginal operations, others in the laparoscopic approach, and still others swear by open abdominal repairs as the gold standard.

You should be aware of the pros and cons for each surgical alternative. Ask the following questions:

- Which operation has been around the longest?
- Which will get you back to work and exercise most quickly?
- Will minimally invasive procedures using small laparoscopic or vaginal incisions be as reliable as a traditional open approach over the long run?
- How did your doctor arrive at the decision to perform this particular operation or specific technique? When you ask about other alternatives, is your doctor defensive in explaining his or her choice, or confident and enthusiastic that it's simply the best for you?
- What is your surgeon's level of expertise? Just as important as the operation you choose is the surgeon who performs it. Don't assume that all surgeons are doing the same procedures with the same level of experience. Some specialists perform three hundred surgeries each year, while others enter the operating room only once or twice a month, yet both may be excellent surgeons.

QUESTION #5: ARE YOU PREPARED TO OPTIMIZE YOUR RECOVERY?

Within the hustle and bustle of today's medical marketplace, there's a fast-track approach to postoperative healing. Hospital stays range from only a few hours, following laparoscopic and certain vaginal operations, to perhaps two or three days for open techniques. Gone are the days when postoperative hospital stays lasted a week, each patient backed by a cadre of nurses, candy stripers, hospital trays, and housekeeping. Recuperation after a pelvic operation, not unlike most other types of surgery these days, occurs mainly at home, among friends and family. It requires a good amount of work and the right attitude on your part.

BACK IN THE SADDLE, BUT NO GALLOPING

However enticing a quick return to normal life may seem, there are a few realities of the recovery process. Even in a new millennium filled with fast food, fast computers, and a back-in-the-saddle approach to recovery, healing follows its own lazy pace. Above all else, keep one very humbling statistic in mind: up to 30 percent of women who undergo reconstructive surgery for pelvic relaxation or incontinence will eventually have two or more future operations to fully correct their problem. Keep yourself out of this unenviable club by learning how to protect your new anatomy while resuming a healthy level of activity after surgery.

You'll Be Tired

Even minimally invasive operations involve a recovery process, and as anyone who has undergone surgery can attest to, healing makes you tired for at least several weeks. Don't fight it. Many women won't feel 100 percent in terms of energy and drive for three to six months and even beyond.

Use Your Body Wisely

The following tips should help to maximize healing while keeping you in shape.

- *Exercise smart.* Yes, on rare occasion, a surgical repair can come undone after a stressful activity. Protect your lower body more carefully than usual for the first few postoperative months. Avoid lifting objects or children heavier than ten pounds, and don't partake in weight-bearing exercises during that initial recovery period. Avoid aerobics, weight lifting, swimming, and biking until your doctor okays them. Brisk walking and other nonstraining exercises should be fine. Some surgeons advise their patients to never again engage in a strenuous job, lift over twenty pounds, or participate in regular high-stress exercises. The majority of surgeons, however, place no major restrictions on your lifestyle after the first two to three months. Discuss your specific surgery and lifestyle afterward, with your doctor.

- *Pelvic-floor exercises.* Also a fine idea, even if they're not a real workout in the traditional sense. Building strong pelvic muscles will not only help you feel better but will also help to preserve pelvic function in a number of ways (see Appendix A).

- *Avoid pelvic stress.* The idea is to avoid large pressure increases in the abdomen and pelvis. If you must lift something heavy or suddenly exert yourself, exhale rather than holding your breath, and brace your pelvic floor instead of straining. Driving is usually not recommended for the first two to four weeks, for two reasons: first, because soreness may decrease your ability to quickly brake, increasing your odds of a fender bender. Second, because reaching for the pedals may strain the pelvic supports during their most fragile state of healing.

- *Listen to your body.* If whatever you're doing hurts, pulls, pulsates, or pinches, stop or find another way to do it.

AVOID THE BIG C's—CHRONIC COUGH AND CONSTIPATION
Chronic Cough

Whether it's from smoking, asthma, or bronchitis, repetitive coughing can present major stress to pelvic supports trying to heal. Call your doctor if you develop a bad cough, especially if it's accompanied by colored sputum or a fever. High-potency cough syrups (containing codeine or an equivalent) may occasionally be necessary. Your doctor may prescribe antibiotics if he or she suspects bacterial sinusitis or bronchitis.

Constipation

You've already learned about this archenemy of a healthy pelvic floor. After surgery, straining to move your bowels can directly stress the areas of healing, particularly if your surgery involved the repair of a rectocele or relaxed perineum—and that's the *last* thing you need after making it over the hurdle of your operation. A few basic tips should keep you regular:

- *High-fiber diet.* The same Bowel Diet discussed in chapter 10 will hold you in good stead after surgery.
- *Stool softeners.* Colace, Metamucil, or a generic stool softener should be strongly considered for the first twelve weeks, unless your stools are soft and regular with a careful diet alone.
- *Occasional laxative.* If stool softeners aren't enough, try an occasional oral laxative or suppository (Dulcolax, glycerine, Fleet). Seek your doctor's advice, especially before using stimulant laxatives (see chapter 10).
- *Walking, exercise, hydration.* The importance of these factors can't be overlooked for maintaining normal bowel activity. Sometimes starting a walking routine or other exercise program is all you need to get your bowels back to normal after surgery.
- *Minimizing narcotics.* Narcotic pain medications (codeine, hydrocodone) will slow your bowels. The sooner you're off them and switched over to nonnarcotic pain pills (ibuprofen, acetaminophen), the better.

REMEMBER THE BIG E—ESTROGEN!

If you've passed through menopause or had your ovaries removed, vaginal estrogen—in the form of creams, vaginal tablets, or an insertable vaginal estrogen ring—can improve the health of the vaginal skin and promote healing after surgery. In most cases, use of these products should be postponed until at least a few weeks after surgery, when the vaginal and perineal incisions have closed. Check with your doctor about whether local estrogen therapy might be the right choice for you.

KEEP IT SIMPLE DOWN THERE

After surgery, treat your perineum and vagina just as you would after childbirth—*gingerly.* Avoid scrubbing, douching, and using perfumed or colored hygienic products. Also avoid vaginal creams or anesthetic jellies until your doctor says they're okay. After most pelvic operations, you'll be instructed to avoid intercourse and insert nothing in the vagina, including tampons, for six to twelve weeks.

TIPS FOR PREPARING BEFORE SURGERY

- *Optimize your weight.* Let's face it: few of us would be motivated to shed pounds before having an operation, let alone keep them off. But on occasion, extraordinary individuals do manage to slim down before pelvic surgery. These women enjoy not only the pleasure of looking trim but also reduced odds of their prolapse or incontinence returning over the long run. An optimal body weight means less strain on the pelvic floor, less stress on your surgical repair, and a lower risk of pulmonary and anesthetic complications during the operation and recovery period. A 1997 study from Mexico found that among 148 women, those who were obese had twice the risk of surgical failure after incontinence surgery.

- *Stop smoking.* Quitting within even a few weeks of surgery will improve the function of your lungs and lower your risk of complications. Over the long run, avoiding a smoker's cough will reduce your chances of surgical failure due to chronic strain on the structures and supports of the pelvic floor.

- *Stop taking aspirin.* Aspirinlike products can interfere with blood clotting and should most often be discontinued a week before surgery. Check with your doctor about whether this applies to you.

- *Medical clearance.* Usually includes a full physical examination, electrocardiogram, chest X-ray and blood tests. Your primary-care doctor may be asked to perform a head-to-toe checkup before your surgery.

- *Bowel preparation.* Occasionally, patients may be asked to self-administer an enema or take a strong laxative at home the day before surgery.

- *Pretreating with vaginal estrogen.* For postmenopausal women with signs of vaginal atrophy, vaginal estrogen in the form of a cream, tablet, or ring may be recommended in the weeks before surgery. By improving the thickness and strength of the vaginal skin, estrogen may increase your chances for surgical success.

YOUR PRESURGERY CHECKLIST

As you decide on surgery for your postreproductive problem, make a list of questions and topics to discuss with your surgeon. Here are a few that may be useful:

- Is this procedure old or new?
- What type of incision will I have? What type of scar?
- How long will the procedure take?
- How long will I be in the hospital, off work, and out of the gym?
- What are the chances of a complete cure? During what time period do most failures occur?
- How does my minimally invasive option compare to its older gold-standard alternative?
- What new problems might arise after the surgery?
- Do my vaginal tissues have enough estrogen supply to optimally heal?
- What choices of anesthesia will I have: general, epidural, spinal, or local?
- Will you use my own ligaments and tissues for this repair, or do you plan to use a piece of graft or mesh? If so, where will it come from, and what are the risks?
- Will I have any long-term activity restrictions?
- Will this be covered by insurance?

Five Common Concerns After Surgery

I was forty-four years old when I had a vaginal hysterectomy and repair of my cystocele and rectocele. Now it's six years later, and I've begun to notice pressure inside my vagina after I've been standing at work. Worse than that? I'm wearing pads again, because bending, coughing, and sometimes even just walking have been making me leak. Last week, though, was the real killer. While the doctor was doing my Pap smear, she told me that it looks like I've prolapsed again. What have I done wrong—and more importantly, what can I do? I feel like a helpless case.

—Mara, e-mail correspondence

CONCERN #1: "MY PROBLEM'S STILL THERE"

Any type of prolapse or incontinence surgery can fail, even the best procedure performed by the best surgeon. The numbers are still encouraging for most pelvic-reconstructive operations, with odds for success ranging from 65 percent to over 90 percent in the first one to five years. Why, though, might a surgery fail?

THE WHOLE PROBLEM WASN'T FIXED

Failure can result from not repairing all of the defects that were present in the pelvic-floor supports: for instance, choosing to leave behind a partially prolapsed uterus while fixing a large cystocele or rectocele. Experienced surgeons will go to great lengths to identify all areas of prolapse at the time of surgery, including small enteroceles (small-bowel hernias behind the upper vagina), which can often be challenging to find.

YOU HAVE A NEW PROBLEM

In other cases, even after a perfect prolapse repair, the forces of gravity may begin to bear down on other, newly exposed nearby organs. This may predispose you to a totally new prolapse bulge. You might increase this risk by resuming heavy physical activity too soon after surgery, stressing the repair before full healing has occurred. Getting back on your feet after pelvic surgery is a good thing, but pushing too hard is not. Until your healing is truly complete, follow the rules and restrictions of your recovery plan for long-term success.

YOU'RE LOOKING FOR TOTAL PERFECTION

A surgery may *seem* to have failed because of unrealistic expectations for success. While it's true that around 85 percent of women are significantly improved after surgery for stress incontinence, becoming completely, totally, and utterly "Sahara Desert dry" is far less likely. You may still have an accident every now and then, but hopefully much less often than before.

YOU HAVE ANOTHER PROBLEM

Persistent symptoms after surgery may continue due to a problem your surgery was *not* meant to fix, such as an overactive bladder.

Most often these separate conditions can be effectively relieved with medications, physical therapy, or perhaps simple office treatment. If you head into the operating room with several postreproductive problems, the expectation of rolling out of the operating room "good as new in every way" can be a setup for disappointment. Fortunately, the vast majority of women who enter surgery with realistic expectations will be very pleased with their results.

CONCERN #2: "I'M DONE WITH SURGERY . . . AND STILL LEAKING!"

There may be nothing more disappointing after surgery than returning to activity only to notice leakage. Suddenly, the relief of having your operation behind you can be replaced by a sense of failure, even guilt. "Did I lift something too heavy? Do I have a hopeless case?" Don't panic or throw in the towel. Leakage after surgery usually boils down to one of a few common causes, and they're all treatable.

Overactive Bladder

Any woman choosing an operation for stress urinary incontinence should understand that after surgery for stress incontinence, an overactive bladder can develop in 6 to 20 percent of those who never had one before surgery. Among women who had an overactive bladder before their operation, 75 percent can expect it to persist. Only around one in four women entering surgery with mixed incontinence will have the good fortune to experience relief of their overactive bladder after their stress incontinence is surgically repaired.

The underlying message behind all of these statistics? Don't panic if your bladder still misbehaves after surgery. If an overactive bladder causes leakage after your surgery for stress incontinence, begin with a bladder diet and bladder drills (see chapter 8); with more time for healing, many cases will resolve on their own. If the problem persists, then medications or physiotherapy, using biofeedback or pelvic-floor stimulation, may be needed.

Type 3 Incontinence

Sometimes the walls of the urethra are simply too thin to form a good seal, even after its floppiness has been stabilized (see "Floppy

Urethra" and "Thin-Walled Urethra," chapter 8). A relatively simple procedure performed right in the office—*periurethral injections*—can often achieve dryness. The newer tension-free operations for stress incontinence are also demonstrating reasonable odds of success in some of these cases (see chapter 8).

VAGINAL DISCHARGE

Vaginal discharge after surgery is very common as tissues heal and stitches dissolve. During the first several weeks after vaginal surgery, the discharge can be heavy enough to be mistaken for leakage of urine.

CONCERN #3: "MY BLADDER'S NOT EMPTYING RIGHT!"

Pam was thirty-eight years old when she underwent a vaginal sling procedure for a long history of urinary stress incontinence. The surgery itself was a breeze—she was walking that evening, home the next day, and in much less pain than she'd anticipated. There was only one problem: two weeks later, she still couldn't urinate more than a few drops of urine on her own. She had learned to insert a self-catheter before the operation, and every few hours, she used it to drain a healthy amount of urine. But without the catheter, she just couldn't empty. She called the office, very concerned. "What happened to my bladder?" she asked. "Did something go wrong?"

URINARY RETENTION: WHAT IS IT, AND WHAT CAN BE DONE?

An inability to completely empty your bladder, causing urinary retention, can occur after many different types of pelvic surgery—including those that directly involve your bladder or urethra, and even those that involve just the nearby structures and supports. Mild retention is not a big deal, usually resolving on its own within a period of days or weeks, and often not even noticed by the patient. A persistent total inability to void is rare. The good news is that the newest operations for stress incontinence are generally less obstructive to the bladder. Nevertheless, the problem is still relatively common. If you're dealing with retention and waiting for normal bladder function to return, some basic tips may help to speed the process.

- *Minimize pain and swelling.* After any type of pelvic surgery, pain and swelling can make it difficult to empty both your bladder and bowels by overloading the delicate bundle of nerves surrounding your pelvis and bladder. This is the most common reason for voiding difficulties right after surgery. Although the phenomenon can occur after abdominal surgery, it's a great deal more likely following vaginal surgery, due to urethral swelling and perineal pain.

- *Maximize relaxation.* In order to pass urine, the urethra and surrounding pelvic-floor muscles need to relax as the bladder simultaneously contracts. Focus on fully relaxing all of the muscles you'd tighten during a Kegel routine. Whistle, hum a tune, or run the faucet. To relieve the tension caused by dangling legs, use a stepstool if your feet don't reach the floor while you're sitting on the toilet. For women who have difficulty fully relaxing their pelvic floor and bladder neck, muscle relaxants like Valium, or urethral relaxers like Hytrin or Minipress, can help. Finally, although it may seem logical to strain, avoid the temptation. After certain procedures, straining makes emptying more difficult and may put your stitches in jeopardy.

- *Urethral dilation.* In some cases, your doctor can loosen the urethral supports by inserting small dilators in the urethra. This is an office procedure.

- *Urethrolysis.* If your difficulty with emptying persists, or if you are able to urinate only in awkward positions even after all of your healing is complete, it might become necessary to surgically release the tension of your repair. This is called *urethrolysis*, which involves simply cutting enough sutures or sling material to loosen up the bladder neck and urethra a bit. It's successful in up to 85 to 90 percent of cases, very often without disrupting the ability of the original surgery to keep you dry. In most cases, you can do it as an outpatient under local anesthesia, but doctors usually wait several weeks or even months before considering this option.

- *If you're having a problem, don't deny it . . . treat it!* Dealing with bladder problems after surgery is frustrating. In order to understand your problem and get you back to normal, your doctor may want to perform a urodynamics test to be sure that you're entering your operation with healthy voiding—meaning the presence of a strong bladder-muscle contraction, and the ability to relax your pelvic floor during a void. Postoperative roads often have bumps and unexpected turns. Always try to face them squarely, and focus on the long-term destination of better health and function that lies ahead.

USING A CATHETER

Whatever the cause, if your bladder is not empting the majority of its contents after surgery, you'll need to learn how to use a catheter, a small strawlike device made of flexible rubber that will allow you to empty and prevent your bladder from overfilling during the healing process. There are three basic options.

Self-Catheterization

This involves inserting a tiny catheter through the urethra and into the bladder on your own. If you're able to insert a tampon, it's just about that easy. However, it requires a bit of learning and practice before your operation.

- Wash your hands before and after catheterization.
- Dip the catheter's tip into lubricating jelly (plain water-soluble, or anesthetic jelly prescribed by your doctor). Don't touch the catheter tip to anything else before insertion.
- Spread the labia, and find your urethra. You can wear rubber gloves if you're concerned about long fingernails scratching or irritating this sensitive area. Sit, and use a mirror to directly visualize the urethral opening. Or use an index finger to locate the vaginal canal. Your urethral opening is a smaller opening that lies just about a half inch above your inserted finger.
- Insert the catheter into this opening, and advance it (angling up toward your belly button) about an inch or two until the urine starts flowing. Stop inserting once you see a steady urine flow.
- After emptying, wash the catheter with warm soapy water and allow it to dry. Store the catheters in a Ziploc bag.

The advantage is that you're bag-free and tube-free at all times between voids. You can try to void on your own at any time, which will allow you to keep day-to-day tabs on your bladder's progress. But if you have poor coordination or mobility, or if you can't get used to the idea of inserting something into your body, self-catheterization may not be for you.

Foley (Transurethral) Catheter

The Foley is a regular catheter inserted into the urethral opening and held inside the bladder by a small inflated balloon at its tip. While the catheter is in place, it is attached to a small, concealable bag that straps around the leg or belly during the daytime; at night, it can be hooked to a larger-sized bag for continuous drainage during sleep. The Foley catheter is easy to place, and it drains the bladder on a continuous basis. But you can't urinate through the urethra without removing the catheter, and as a result, you can't monitor your bladder's daily progress, and your ability to fully void on your own. As you wait for bladder function to fully return, the Foley may need to be removed and replaced at the doctor's office several times, to evaluate your ability to void.

Suprapubic (SP) Catheter

This catheter is placed through the actual wall of the bladder, through a tiny incision in the lower abdominal area. Like a Foley, the suprapubic catheter can also be hooked to a small or large drainage bag. Unlike a Foley, the urethra itself is free of any catheter. The SP is typically more comfortable than a Foley catheter. You're able to attempt voiding at any time, through the urethra, by simply clamping the suprapubic catheter shut and allowing the bladder to fill. If you're not able to empty at that time, you simply unclamp the suprapubic catheter and resume drainage. As with self-catheterization, this allows you to keep daily tabs on your bladder progress. The SP's disadvantage is that it requires a tiny abdominal incision. After catheter removal, urine will drain from this incision for one to two days before it permanently closes. A pad or dressing is worn over the incision during this period of time.

HANGING IN THERE

The average time you'll need to catheterize is difficult to predict. A substantial number of women need only a day or two of bladder rest; for the newer, tension-free procedures, many women are able to resume voiding right after surgery and can avoid the inconvenience of catheterization altogether. The average time for recovery from stress incontinence procedures tends to range between one and two weeks, but some women will require more time before resuming normal bladder function. Needing to catheterize forever is an extremely rare complication of bladder surgery.

- *Don't overfill.* Distending the bladder to large volumes will stretch the muscle and make it temporarily weaker, perhaps extending the number of days you'll need to catheterize.

- *Try to be patient.* Stay focused on the long-term result that led you to have surgery. Waiting can be a frustrating process for both you and the doctor, but allowing the bladder a bit more time to heal is often the most effective therapy of all.

- *Keep in contact.* Stay in touch with your doctor or the office nursing staff, and call about any obvious changes. If you ever notice very cloudy urine, bladder pain, flank pain, or fevers, then an evaluation or a course of antibiotics may be warranted in order to prevent a more severe infection. If you're unable to empty and you feel like your bladder has become uncomfortably full after surgery, call your doctor or head for the nearest emergency room.

- *Live your life!* During your days or weeks of catheterization, don't let it slow down your overall recovery. Walking, shopping, and socializing with friends and family *should not* wait for the return of full bladder function. Resuming an active life is the best thing you can do for yourself after surgery.

CONCERN #4: "I'M TIRED, UNCOMFORTABLE, AND FEEL LIKE I'VE BEEN HIT BY A TRUCK"

Many women after pelvic reconstructive surgery are surprised by how quickly they bounce back to relative comfort. Although the first few days can be trying, by the time they visit the doctor's office a few weeks after surgery, the majority of women already feel themselves turning the corner. But not all women.

It is important for your surgeon to evaluate persistent pain. Only he or she can determine whether your pain is routine, or reason to be concerned. At the very least, your doctor will be able to help you maximize your pain relief. Fortunately, after most minimally invasive operations, persistent pain tends to be the exception, not the rule. Fatigue, on the other hand, is more the rule than the exception. There's something about surgery, however it's performed, that takes the wind temporarily out of your sails. If you need more help at home, call a friend. If working full days at the office is a struggle, try half shifts for a few transitional weeks. Your energy level *will* return, but there's little you can do to hurry the process.

- *Abdominal surgery.* Operations involving open abdominal incisions will require several weeks for healing, and several months for return of your full energy.

- *Vaginal operations.* Healing after vaginal surgery involves surprisingly little pain in most cases, and the return to activity is usually quite rapid. However, pain and tenderness around the perineum may last for weeks or even months, to some degree.

- *Laparoscopic procedures.* These Band-Aid operations are known for allowing a quick recovery. However, unlike abdominal and vaginal procedures, upper abdominal and shoulder discomfort are common during the first few days after laparoscopy, due to small amounts of gas left behind in the abdomen. One fairly consistent benefit of recovering from laparoscopy: you should feel progressively better with each passing day. If you notice that your recovery starts to move in reverse, call the doctor.

CONCERN #5: "SEX ISN'T WORKING RIGHT"

Though you'll need time to heal, you should always be able to return to a satisfying sex life after pelvic surgery. For women who have been uncomfortable or inhibited due to vaginal relaxation or incontinence, correction of these problems may *improve* sexual function for a few reasons: first, directly through relief of the physical problem. For instance, women who have had a hysterectomy for prolapse may notice an improvement in sexual pleasure, as the cervix is no longer bumped during penetration. Second, sexual function may be enhanced indirectly—for example, due to the elimination of anxiety and inhibition that once accompanied fear of accidents during intercourse. That's right—surgery might even enhance your sex life!

On the other hand, new sexual problems can sometimes arise after surgery, and they need to be specifically addressed. Changes in vaginal anatomy, postoperative scarring or pain, decreased libido: which of these should you worry about? A better understanding of how surgery will affect the various areas down there might help to clarify the issues.

THE OUTER GENITALS

The clitoris, most directly responsible for female sexual pleasure, is almost never directly affected by surgery for incontinence or prolapse.

THE OVARIES

No matter how extensive your pelvic operation, if you're premenopausal and the ovaries are left intact, their production of sex-related hormones should remain unchanged. With removal of the ovaries (oopherectomy) in premenopausal women, hormonal changes may lead to vaginal dryness, hot flashes, and even mood swings. All of these low-estrogen changes can affect sexual desire and function. You should discuss with your doctor starting hormone replacement, or dealing with menopausal symptoms via nonhormonal strategies.

THE UTERUS

A great deal of interest has been focused on sexual function following hysterectomy. Are there reasons to be concerned? During arousal, the uterus normally elevates and congests with blood; during orgasm, small uterine contractions occur. Some women are aware of these physical events and others are not, and the importance of them to each woman's sense of pleasure is highly variable. Though some women might notice the absence of uterine contractions and other secondary sexual sensations after hysterectomy, very few perceive it as a negative change.

One report from the Maryland Women's Health Study, published in *The Journal of the American Medical Association*, suggested that women after hysterectomy often experience an increase in their sexual pleasure, desire, and function. In this study, both the frequency of sex and overall libido were increased after hysterectomy, and the rate of painful intercourse declined from 40 to 15 percent.

Interestingly, a Scandinavian study of more than a hundred women found that after removal of the uterus, partners with a good relationship before surgery had a 61 percent chance of enjoying improved sexuality afterward. Those with a poor presurgery relationship had improved sexuality only 17 percent of the time. Perhaps, in the end, true love really does conquer all!

THE VAGINA AND PERINEUM

The perineum is a highly sensitive area, critical to sexual function. If you had a perineal incision for the repair of a rectocele or a lax vaginal opening, try following the same basic tips outlined in chapter 7 for episiotomy healing, starting with ice packs on your bottom. The vagina itself is an amazingly forgiving part of the body—quick to heal and almost always left with no visible scars. The majority of stitches used for pelvic reconstruction are absorbable and disappear on their own. However, as mentioned earlier, a graft of synthetic mesh, or permanent stitches, may be used in some cases. Rarely, these materials may poke through an adjacent area of vaginal skin that hasn't fully healed, causing an erosion; pain during intercourse (for either partner) or a heavy discharge with spotting are the most common signs. For some, part or all of the permanent surgical material must be removed for proper healing to occur.

YOUR NEW SIZE AND SHAPE

By definition, the anatomy of the vagina after surgery will always be different than before, and these differences will be most pronounced after the repair of advanced pelvic prolapse. Pelvic surgeons take great care to avoid any changes that might make intercourse difficult or painful. A goal of surgery is to improve sexual function by normalizing the vaginal anatomy and perineal tone. Nevertheless, occasionally the width or depth of the vagina may be left too narrow or short to allow for comfortable intercourse. Don't worry—this can almost always be effectively addressed. The first task is localizing the problem. Narrowing can occur at the perineum, along the vaginal walls, or up at the vaginal apex. Your doctor can make this assessment during a simple examination once you have fully healed. Treatment involves stretching the tissues, slowly but surely, back to the desired size and shape. The dilation can be performed by self-massage or gentle and well-lubricated intercourse; alternatively, silicone dilators can be used to gradually stretch the vaginal tissues. Estrogen creams are sometimes useful during this process, to keep the vaginal skin well lubricated and pliable. As evidenced by the physical changes of childbirth, when the vagina stretches more than ten centimeters wide and later shrinks to a fraction of that size, these tissues are among the most malleable in the whole body.

POOR LUBRICATION

Dryness is the enemy of lovemaking, and it must be ruthlessly combated. After surgery, you'll need plenty of lubrication to avoid friction against healing areas that can remain hypersensitive for many months. Try copious quantities of plain water-based lubricants such as K-Y, Slippery Stuff, Astroglide, or Liquid Silk. Also, as we've discussed, the use of vaginal estrogen for postmenopausal women—in the form of tablets, creams, or an insertable ring—is often the best way to improve lubrication and skin tone.

As with healing after childbirth, the return to comfortable sex after vaginal surgery may occur sooner or later than you had expected. Intercourse should be avoided for six to twelve weeks, as determined by your doctor, while the incisions heal and stitches dissolve. When you finally give it a try, choose positions that put you in control of the angle and depth of penetration.

The Cutting Edge: Will New Procedures Make Surgery Obsolete?

Wide open, phenomenal, meteoric. There aren't enough adjectives to describe the growth that's taking place within this niche of women's health. The number of innovations under development is astounding, including a number of fascinating minimally invasive alternatives to major surgery. As you keep abreast of all that's new, temper your enthusiasm with a healthy dose of skepticism. After all, over the past several decades, a number of procedures have looked very appealing in the short term but have revealed limitations a few years down the road. Only through careful research will we find the needles within this haystack of medical innovation. Among the many emerging therapies are:

- *Radio-frequency therapy.* This outpatient technique uses painless microwave rays to actually tighten up, or shrink-wrap, the fascia in the vaginal walls. This restores strength to the vaginal walls and support to a floppy urethra, and early results have shown some effectiveness in curing stress incontinence. The long-term benefits and risks will need to be assessed over time.

- *Implantable gizmos.* Tests are under way for injectable microstimulator devices (such as the RF Bion), designed to stimulate the pelvic nerves and muscles. A tiny chip is injected beneath the vaginal skin using local anesthesia, requiring no incision. Can you imagine?

- *Botox.* Yes, the same injectable antidote for the common wrinkle is also being tested for various bladder problems. Stay tuned.

- *Acupuncture.* Speaking of needles, can acupuncture be used to improve incontinence and bladder overactivity? The answer is not so clear. Some people feel that actual sites and meridians located around the back of the lower leg, or on the lower back, can directly soothe the sacral bundle of nerves surrounding the bladder; others feel that a general release of endorphins and brain chemicals may improve urinary control. One study demonstrated improvements in overactive-bladder symptoms within a group of women; others since then have been unable to confirm a beneficial effect. Acupuncture and traditional Chinese medical treatments—including moxabustion, hot cups placed over the skin—are being studied at some centers.

- *Percutaneous tibial nerve stimulation (SANS).* This novel therapy is a loose variation of acupuncture, focused on a site near the foot. A thin needle is inserted just above the ankle, right next to a chain of nerves leading up to the pelvic-nerve circuit. Once or twice weekly, electrical stimulation is delivered through the wire. Amazingly, it can work, at least for overactive-bladder symptoms. Short-term improvements have been seen, but unless treatments continue, the effects disappear. An even more futuristic variation is currently being tested: it involves the use of a laser light pen to stimulate the same suspected acupuncture point without any needles at all. Whether it will cure symptoms remains to be seen.

The Stage Is All Yours

NAVIGATING THE POLITICS, ECONOMICS, CULTURE, AND ETHICS OF CHILDBIRTH

Disease varies from place to place, less because of climate or geography than because of the way work and reproduction are organized and carried out in those places.

—Jurshen, 1996

Medical and social prejudices against women sidestepping their biblical sentence to painful childbirth are still with us.

—Feminist professor of English,
British Medical Journal, 1999

Want to make some mischief? Try logging on to your computer, finding a women's-health chat room on the Internet, and typing these words: "A woman should have the right to choose how she delivers her own baby!" Give it a day, or maybe two, and then check back in.

You won't believe the number of responses you receive.

Voices from both sides of the debate will claim with equal conviction that they represent the true interest of women. One side maintains that cesarean delivery is an artificial disruption of a natural event, and that offering this choice is meddling with a female body that knows how to give birth. The other side believes that not offering women free choice in the labor room is a denial of personal autonomy, an intrusion into one of life's most intimate medical decisions. Political correctness is an elusive target when it involves such an emotionally and politically charged subject.

As doctor, my goal has been to provide you, the patient, with enough information to establish your own voice in the debate, and to understand how this handful of often overlooked female problems can be caused, treated, and hopefully prevented. Our understanding of these topics is by no means complete. Even the best research study will often introduce more questions than answers. Nevertheless, new and exciting answers have been emerging, and I'd argue that the woman who is truly informed based on our best existing knowledge, and is exposed to all sides of the debate, has had her autonomy and intelligence respected in the highest regard. She is able to speak for herself rather than depending on others, and she is more fully in control of her own body. According to at least one recent survey, the overwhelming majority of women are ready to have their own voice. Eighty-three percent expressed a desire for information regarding the postnatal risk of prolapse and incontinence; 94 percent wanted to be more actively involved in making decisions regarding forceps, cesarean section, and other obstetrical interventions. I hope these chapters have achieved their goal of informing at least some of you among that silent majority.

But however vital the role of medical information and scientific research may be in determining the best approach to childbirth, our understanding of these topics would be incomplete without one inescapable and elemental fact: reproductive choices will never be made on the basis of science and medicine alone. It's impossible to fully understand your childbirth experience and postreproductive body without at least some appreciation of the economics, politics, personalities, and even ethics behind the baby business. So in these last few pages, let's step back from the microscope we've used to understand the nerves, muscles, and inner workings of your pelvic anatomy and take a telescopic view of factors that lie beyond the realm of science. Although these players on the stage of childbirth may remain unseen, their influence on your reproductive choices, and the physical effects that sometimes follow, can be potent.

The Ethics of Childbearing and Informed Consent

"Why wasn't I told about all this stuff *before* I had my baby?"

Whether facing a food label or surgical-consent form, today's consumer wants to know everything pertaining to risks, benefits, and side effects—all the ingredients of decisions, big and small. Informed consent is the ethical and legal principle that safeguards each person's right to know and choose in the medical world. It's a standard that requires a particular form of communication between doctor and patient: the disclosure of basic risks and benefits of any procedure that's about to be performed, and a discussion of the alternatives that are reasonably foreseeable at the time of consent.

For millennia, giving birth required few decisions, big or small. No ovulation kit, ultrasound, amniocentesis, or epidural, and only one reasonably foreseeable way out for the newborn: one that too often proved itself to end tragically for baby, Mom, or sometimes both. Along with the last few ticks of the historical clock, the miracles of antibiotics, blood transfusions, and safe surgery began to quickly erase the fear of death from the labor room. Today fewer than four hundred women die from childbirth-related complications each year in the United States. The new era of childbirth is no longer one of fear, but one of decisions, technological options, and ultimately, ethics. Suddenly, there are more ways for a mother to give birth, more factors entering into her physician's medical judgment, and more attitudes and beliefs behind each woman's image of the ideal child-birth. And we, as patients and doctors living in this privileged era, enjoy the luxury of debating the most appropriate role for a constant stream of technological innovations.

With all of childbirth's many choices, are the standards of informed consent being met? Without question, over the past few decades, women and their partners have become informed and active participants in many key areas—for instance, choices surrounding contraception and fertility, pain control, and fetal testing. Yet arguably, when it comes to the effects of childbirth on each woman's body and the problems that can follow, truly informed participation is often lacking. Though episiotomy may arise as an issue before or during labor, other issues more important to the pelvic floor generally do not. What about all of those muscles, nerves, and supports of the deeper pelvic floor? What about the effect of obstetrical choices on a woman's future risk of incontinence, prolapse, or sexual dysfunction? What about the potential effects of forceps, fetal size or position, the length of labor and pushing, the decision over vaginal birth after cesarean, or elective cesarean birth? These and other factors, as you've learned, may have reasonably foreseeable consequences to a woman's health. In the future, our discussions and disclosures during pregnancy and childbirth probably will weigh more carefully these basic connections between childbirth and female function afterward, between obstetrics and gynecology.

The emergence of postobstetrical problems into the spotlight of women's health raises other ethical issues that are no less challenging. Consider one in particular: the right to choose between vaginal and cesarean birth. Should cesarean delivery be considered an elective procedure—a luxury, like cosmetic surgery, to freely choose—or a matter of medical necessity? If a healthy, low-risk woman is allowed to choose a cesarean, has her obstetrician abdicated his or her own responsibilities and been reduced to the role of technician?

On what basis can women be denied the right to choose? Is it the view that vaginal childbirth, and all that may follow in its aftermath, is inherently more natural than a surgical birth? Or is it because cesareans are simply too expensive to offer on demand?

What about the woman who refuses vaginal delivery to eliminate the small but serious risk of a previous cesarean scar rupturing, versus one determined to prevent the incontinence or prolapse that her mother endured, or yet another who simply wants to avoid the physical or emotional effort of a vaginal birth?

What is the proper role of an elective cesarean birth in preventing later problems that are not ones of life and death but rather of quality of life?

To what degree women will be permitted free choice in these matters will remain a subject of debate for years to come, and it's wrong to start drawing blanket conclusions until we have more definitive answers. In the meantime, it's not wrong to start talking. Each woman is entitled to balance the pros and cons of medical decisions involving her body, including the route of delivery, the management of labor, even forceps and episiotomy, considering their possible aftereffects. The female body surely does know how to give birth, and it should always be encouraged to do so. But informing a woman what to expect while she's expecting is not enough—she should also know what to expect afterward, not only days but years later. In this age of free-flowing information between patients and doctors, the maternal repercussions of childbirth should be freely disclosed and no longer overlooked.

WISDOM—OR WARNINGS—FROM THE MEDITERRANEAN

In Italy, the law protects each woman's right to choose between vaginal and cesarean delivery. Over the past two decades, cesarean rates have drastically increased to at least 33 percent, among the highest in Europe. Rates are highest in private hospitals where the technology is more readily available, and they also vary widely by region, indicating that a culture of cesarean delivery has evolved within certain areas. Are Italian women enjoying a personal choice to which they're entitled, or does their experience reflect a misallocation of resources that other countries should avoid? The issues are complex, and simple answers are hard to find, but understanding the experiences of other countries and cultures may help us make better decisions of our own.

Economics: The Bottom Line of Labor and Delivery

Once upon a time—right up until the 1980s—medicine was a fee-for-service profession. Like all other surgeons, obstetricians were paid for nearly every procedure they performed; and cesarean delivery was recognized by physicians as one that was particularly safe, convenient, quick, and also profitable. There were few built-in incentives—cultural, economic, legal, or otherwise—for doctors to push for vaginal births. To no one's great surprise, cesarean rates skyrocketed from roughly 5 percent in the 1960s to rates exceeding 22 percent in the United States and Canada today.

Health-care economics still influence the way babies are delivered in the industrialized world, though many of the basic trends have reversed. Along with the emergence of cost-conscious managed-health-care plans such as the HMO, cesarean delivery began to appear awfully expensive at the bottom line of the accountant's ledger, with its steep operating-room charges and longer hospital stays. Obstetrical statistics became powerful bargaining chips among physicians, hospitals, and insurance providers, with the new emphasis on *reducing* the number of cesarean births. The validity of these new-age cost calculations have been met with their share of criticism; some experts argue that crucial costs, such as that of time spent on the labor floor, are regularly left out of the analysis. One study, recently presented at the American College of Obstetricians and Gynecologists' annual scientific meeting, calculated that the per-patient cost of elective cesarean delivery was only 2.3 percent higher than that of attempted vaginal delivery. The high costs of nursing in the labor room, and of failed vaginal delivery, appeared to account for the overall cost of the two strategies being nearly equal. Nevertheless, departments and hospitals began to receive praise for maintaining target rates of vaginal delivery in nearly any form—spontaneous, forceps and vacuum-assisted, even vaginal births after cesarean. Enormous insurance contracts could, for some institutions, be jeopardized by cesarean rates exceeding the target; some went so far as to prohibit their physicians from presenting alternative treatments viewed as less cost-effective. Merely discussing the alternative of elective cesarean with patients would violate company code and, in some instances, put the physician's job in jeopardy.

Although gag rules are no longer legally permitted, insurance coverage may still have an influence that reaches—directly or indirectly—into the labor room. One Harvard study showed that mothers with private, fee-for-service insurance had higher cesarean rates than mothers covered by HMO plans and also those who were uninsured. An Australian study of one hundred and seventy thousand women showed that privately insured women were more likely than those with government insurance to undergo cesarean, forceps delivery, and episiotomy. In Chile, privately insured women had cesarean rates of 59 percent compared to 28 percent for those who were publicly insured. In the Campania region of Italy, the cesarean rate in private birthing units exceeded 55 percent, a rate 1.3 times higher than that of public facilities in the same area. Determining the overall pros and cons of these trends throughout the world is a complicated puzzle.

Our economic understanding of women's reproductive health, and the cost-effectiveness of various childbirth strategies, cannot be considered complete until the postreproductive conditions we've discussed are included in the financial formulas. These gynecologic problems of incontinence, prolapse, and pelvic-floor dysfunction cannot be rationally separated, medically or economically, from their potential obstetrical causes. Put more simply: even if promoting vaginal delivery shrinks short-term costs, the same strategy may increase the number of pelvic-floor disorders we'll pay for over the long run—creating financial, physical, and emotional costs that may far exceed the initial savings. According to a 1997 study based on the National Hospital Discharge Survey database and average Medicare reimbursements, the direct costs of pelvic-prolapse surgery that year were $1 billion. As the authors of the study emphasized, that figure did not even include the costs of evaluation, diagnostic testing, and office therapies; the indirect costs, such as lost work time and child care; or the millions spent each year on absorbent products.

As a fuller understanding of pelvic-floor disorders emerges, and their impact on a rapidly expanding postreproductive female population is appreciated, the links between childbirth events and postreproductive health—indeed, the bridge between obstetrics and gynecology—will become clearer. With that transition in women's health, the economic bottom line of labor and delivery will be calculated not only according to costs incurred in the maternity suite but also according to those that can accumulate during the postreproductive years. Indeed, we're learning that the true costs of childbirth must be viewed with a wide lens over a woman's lifetime. Regardless of future financial calculations and miscalculations, fads and trends, only one bottom line is sure to indefinitely persist: the ways we choose to experience the miracle of childbirth will never boil down to economic formulae alone.

Politics, Policies, and Personalities

You will find, as a general rule, that the constitutions and the habits of a people follow the nature of the land where they live.
—Hippocrates

Just like the foods you choose to eat and the car you decide to drive, your perceptions of childbirth are filtered through multiple layers of your surroundings—family, friends, culture, marketing, advertising, and even politics.

YOUR GOVERNMENT

Politics and policies certainly may influence obstetrical culture and practice, though their presence is not always apparent on the surface of society. Consider, for instance, the landmark Healthy People 2000 program supported by the World Health Organization and the Department of Health and Human Services. Among its many stated goals, one was to reduce the nationwide cesarean delivery rate from over 20 percent to a target of 15 percent by the year 2000—in order to spare resources and reduce unnecessary intervention. Replacing cesareans would be more assisted deliveries (forceps or vacuum) and more vaginal deliveries among women with prior cesareans. This is a goal that was well intentioned but not free of controversy. Perhaps most vocally, the notion of a blanket policy to reduce this cesarean rate drew public criticism from several leaders in obstetrics, who viewed the plan's stated goals as paternalistic, authoritarian, and too strongly driven by economic forces rather than the well-being of mothers and babies. More research into the safety of the program, and a look at its true costs, would be needed before concluding an optimal cesarean rate, according to Dr. Benjamin Sachs of Harvard University Medical School. Even if further research proves that cesarean rates can be reduced to this level without detrimental effects on newborns, the question remains: what about their moms? As Healthy People 2000 evolved into its current form, Healthy People 2010, the target cesarean rate of 15 percent has not been reached, but the policy continues to have an impact. Bolstered by the Healthy People goals, the performance and quality of physicians and even hospitals is often judged, for better or worse, largely around one loaded question: "What's your cesarean rate?"

YOUR PART OF THE GLOBE

Childbirth is an interesting mirror of society all around the globe, and what may be state-of-the-art in your corner of the world may raise questions elsewhere. Consider affluent areas in the United States, for instance, where women and their partners often go to great length to achieve a natural childbirth experience; then compare these trends to Latin America, where the wealthiest countries have some of the highest rates of cesarean birth in the world. Over the past thirty years in Brazil, the cesarean delivery rate in certain communities has sky-rocketed from around 20 percent to over 80 percent. Within this culture that places great emphasis on sexuality and aesthetics, cesareans are viewed as less traumatic to the mother's genitalia, even a status symbol. For a variety of reasons, including patient pressure for cesareans on demand, physicians have become less inclined to wait through a full labor and delivery. It's a trend that Brazil's own health minister recently described as "barbarous," and one the government has itself recently begun discouraging by offering incentives for vaginal birth. The experience in Brazil represents an extreme by any measure. But clearly, in all corners of the world, the way we have babies is determined by far more than medical science alone.

THE MEDIA

Alas, the most global and powerful filter of modern life: the media. Always portraying a story that we'd love to believe, but one that never quite fits our reality. For instance, on daytime soaps and prime-time melodramas, television and Hollywood perpetuate an image of the glowing parturient puffing through the final push, the story always ending with a baby's cry.

Or how about those commercial breaks during which millions of dollars are spent on advertisements for absorbent products, portraying menopausal women as attractive, content, and comfortable while wearing pads and diapers on the tennis court, the beach, and at work—leaving you to wonder, "What drug are they really on?" After all, for most women, pads and diapers are not an acceptable solution over the long run.

Perhaps most confusing of all, the Internet. Filled with sites and chat rooms disparaging any type of medical intervention during childbirth, and others at the opposite extreme indiscriminately mocking the notion of natural birth, it's a realm that's overdosed with politics and often underdosed with reliable facts. In a world teeming with targeted marketing, and a cyberspace rich with electronic pulpits for anyone with an opinion to preach from, it's important to realize how deeply some of these words and images can permeate your consciousness. Sometimes they can even get in the way of good old common sense.

A Few Golden Rules for the Postreproductive Woman

If you're a boomer or younger mom who was convinced that "those problems" your mother dealt with are still inevitable milestones of womanhood, I hope this book has convinced you otherwise, and that any knowledge you've gained will help you to navigate the road to better health. As the science, surgery, and medicine surrounding postreproductive problems continues to rapidly expand, keep a few pearls of advice in mind and you'll do just fine.

RULE #1: POSTREPRODUCTIVE PROBLEMS MAY BE COMMON, BUT THEY'RE NOT NORMAL OR INEVITABLE

For better or worse, female prolapse and incontinence have yet to attract a spokesperson as mainstream as Bob Dole for Viagra. One wonders, if curing female pelvic-floor disorders were as profitable as stomping out male impotence, how quickly these issues would emerge from the shadows into the mainstream medical agenda. Make no mistake: female pelvic, bladder, bowel, and sexual function are no less important to your overall wellness than erectile dysfunction is to your male counterpart's—and perhaps no more inevitable. By now you've learned about countless ways to find relief, ranging from exercise, diet, and medications to nearly incision-free surgery, magnetic energy waves, and pelvic pacemakers. If your symptoms are making your life feel less full, there will be no blue-ribbon prize for suffering in silence. Be sure to seek help, in some form or another.

RULE #2: DON'T GIVE UP UNTIL YOU FIND RELIEF

With rare exception, there's always another treatment out there for you to try. Postreproductive women's health and urogynecology are works in progress, rapidly expanding with a steady stream of innovations coming down the pike. Even if you gave up in the past after finding no relief, check back with a specialist. Very likely, there will be something new for ameliorating, preventing, or at least coping with the major changes that can follow childbirth. Be persistent, remain your own best advocate, and don't give up until you find relief.

RULE #3: STAY INFORMED

Women these days are barraged with facts and figures concerning the hottest health topics, like hormone replacement, osteoporosis, breast cancer, and heart disease. There seems to be a never-ending supply of latest studies on these problems and their prevention, many head-lined in mainstream newspapers and magazines. There is also much to keep abreast of on the less mainstream female conditions. Stay informed, and keep giving these areas of your body the attention they deserve.

RULE #4: ELECTIVE SURGERY IS ELECTIVE!

We're fortunate to live in an age when surgical procedures have become less invasive and more effective than ever before. But even if you've found the most skilled surgical hands in the world, a decision to enter the operating room should never be taken lightly. After all, there will never be a surgical procedure that can guarantee a perfect cure, and there will always be the small risk of an unforeseen com-plication or a rockier postoperative road than you expected. If you're more uncomfortable with the potential aftereffects of elective surgery than remaining in your current situation, you don't need to have it!

A Few Golden Rules for the Woman Looking Ahead to Childbirth

For the younger woman looking ahead to the wonders of pregnancy, labor, and delivery—whatever politics, personalities, and emotions surround your childbirth planning—remember a few basic rules, and don't forget that you're the star player of an eternal drama on a stage that belongs to *you*.

RULE #1: YOUR BODY ALWAYS MATTERS . . . EVEN DURING CHILDBIRTH

Bringing a newborn safely into the world will always take highest priority, at any stage of pregnancy and childbirth. By sheer instinct, we'd gladly sacrifice our own comfort for that of our baby, such is the profound transition to the awesome role of parent. But it's time to incorporate into the planning for pregnancy, labor, and delivery some discussion of how your body might feel and function afterward. Rather than viewing childbirth as an inevitable physical sacrifice, think of it as an opportunity to experience one of life's most profoundly beautiful events, while gaining a better understanding of your body and planning ahead for many years of your own health, control, and intimacy. Promoting health in the most intimate areas of your body, maintaining control over your most basic bodily functions, and preserving your sense of youth and sexuality—these goals deserve a place in your health planning. Your one and only body does matter during childbirth, and for a long lifetime afterward.

RULE #2: MAKE INDIVIDUALIZED CHILDBIRTH CHOICES

Each pregnancy has its own fingerprint created by a unique mom and newborn, making each and every labor and delivery a completely unique event. As a result, blanket obstetrical strategies will, in the end, be to the detriment of some. Although every birth is a miracle, on a physical level, they're not all equal. In some cases, a prolonged labor, a forceps extraction, or an extensive perineal injury during vaginal birth may be more physically traumatic for both mother and baby than a cesarean section. For others, the opposite will be true. Unfortunately, the conventional wisdom characterizing vaginal delivery as better in almost any circumstance may be more a product of politics, economics, and culture than of the medical realities of childbirth. Don't let politics and other people's beliefs dictate the way in which you and your doctor decide to proceed.

RULE #3: BE FLEXIBLE, LIKE A WEDDING PLANNER

It's wonderful when labor is picture-perfect, but sometimes it's not meant to be, and the best-laid plans can require some quick reshuffling. So prepare as you wish, and hope for the best, then *let go*. As with your wedding day, if it starts to rain on the ceremony, be sure to have the physical and emotional flexibility to change your plan. Rainy weddings, after all, can produce some of the most beautiful marriages. By this stage, you should trust your doctor's or midwife's outlook on the whole journey; if the road begins to suddenly change before your eyes, take your hands off the wheel and allow them to drive. Rest assured, it will still be a wonderful day.

RULE #4: NEVER, EVER SKIMP ON SAFETY

Whether you've chosen delivery by a doctor or midwife, at a hospital, birthing center, or home, put safety first. Align yourself with a provider who is either capable of managing a labor that becomes complicated, or able to quickly transfer responsibility to a backup provider. When labor complications occur, they often strike in a quick and devastating way, and the priorities and mood in a labor room can shift in a matter of moments. There are plenty of practitioners— whether obstetricians, midwives, or family doctors—who can keep the priorities of childbirth clear and provide a safe version of the birthing experience you're seeking. Again, like a wedding, childbirth can be simultaneously fun to plan, wonderful to experience, and kept in perspective.

ONE LAST RULE: DON'T FEEL LIKE YOU FAILED IF IT DIDN'T ALL GO AS PLANNED

At the end of the day, only two things matter: a healthy baby and a healthy mom. By the time you're watching him or her stumbling through first baby steps—not to mention strutting down the graduation aisle—the intensity and importance of the labor drama will have long since faded.

Beyond the Crossroads

Along the road of life, childbirth is the most fascinating intersection between medical science, public health, ethical choice, economics, and pure emotion. Keeping informed in this area of women's health will help to ensure that your decisions are not steered by economics, politics, or personalities alone, but also by an understanding of benefits and risks, and informed choice.

Our views on childbirth are approaching a crossroads, and women's health is nearing a fundamental change. As women live longer and more active lives, we will need to face the long-term repercussions of childbirth to the pelvic floor more squarely. As you've learned, they are often problems that attest to the extraordinary physical demands of pregnancy, labor, and delivery. Beyond the crossroads, decisions in the labor room will be reconsidered not only in medical terms but also with respect to economics, politics, and ethics. A healthy baby *and* a mother's physical health will define success, and these significant health issues will no longer be casually accepted as normal. As women insist on more research into the physical consequences of their childbirth choices, we will gain a greater understanding of which pelvic-floor problems relate most closely to pregnancy, delivery, or both. Most importantly, we'll improve our ability to prevent them. Beyond the crossroads—for obstetricians, urogynecologists, midwives, family doctors, and women of all viewpoints—lies a new and more complete vision of women's health care.

Kegel Exercises, Biofeedback, and Other Techniques to Strengthen Your Pelvic Floor

My mother had this same problem and finally had an operation that didn't work at all. Is there anything I can do to avoid all of that?
—Liz, age forty-seven, mother of two

Whatever your age and wherever you may be along your reproductive timeline, maintaining the strength and health of the pelvic floor is a key strategy for minimizing pelvic-floor symptoms. A healthy pelvic floor can help to prevent all of the major problems discussed in the previous chapters—incontinence, sexual dysfunction, and in some cases, even pelvic prolapse. That's why, right at the outset, even before you consider the wide array of more problem-specific treatments, you should devote some time and energy to improving the condition of your pelvic floor.

Learning Perfect Kegel Exercises: Working Out Your Pelvic Floor

Your pelvic floor won't bulk up during a regular workout on the StairMaster, and well-toned levator muscles will rarely, if ever, attract flirtatious glances at the beach. But learning how to give your pelvic muscles a workout of their own can be the least expensive and most effective way to prevent and treat a number of postreproductive problems before ever setting foot inside the doctor's office. And there's nothing more attractive than that.

Kegel exercises (rhymes with *bagel)* first aim to increase your awareness of the muscles around the vagina, perineum, and bladder, then strengthen and tone them. In some Eastern cultures, pelvic-floor exercises have been taught as a rite of passage to young women during their transition to adulthood. In the Western world, they were introduced in the 1940s for treating stress urinary incontinence by their inventor, Arnold Kegel, a gynecologist who reported remarkable improvement in up to 93 percent of women. Kegel observed that pelvic muscle weakness was not exclusive to women with a previous vaginal delivery, but vaginal birth was the precipitating cause of muscle weakness for a great number of women. Over the decades since their introduction, Kegels have been successfully used for not only stress incontinence but also a handful of other postreproductive problems resulting from alterations in the pelvic-floor musculature.

- *Stress incontinence.* By toning the sling and shelf of the levator muscles, pelvic-floor exercises can compensate for a floppy or thin urethra and significantly improve stress incontinence. Success is reported for around 50 percent of women with stress incontinence, making it the most popular reason to begin a pelvic-floor exercise routine.

- *The overactive bladder and urge incontinence.* Kegel exercises can help to prevent overactive-bladder symptoms in several ways. First, as part of a bladder retraining regimen (see chapter 8), they can help to decrease the frequency of urination and number of nighttime voids. Second, because contracting the pelvic-floor muscles tends to relax the bladder, learning to quickly flex them can provide you with a tool for nipping unexpected bladder spasms in the bud. For treating urge incontinence, overall success rates of around 41 percent have been reported, with three good scientific trials showing improvement over controls. At the very least, developing your pelvic-floor muscles can help you hold it in and make it to the bathroom during close calls.

- *Anal incontinence.* If you developed anal incontinence after vaginal delivery, Kegel exercises may increase your chances of regaining control over your bowels. One study demonstrated a strong preventive effect: among women who had experienced rectal injuries during delivery, pelvic-floor exercises lowered the risk of anal incontinence from 21 to 7 percent one year later.

- *Sexual dysfunction.* Kegel exercises may be useful for various postreproductive sexual symptoms, including loss of sensation, painful intercourse, and the inability to reach orgasm. Strengthening and toning the muscles of the perineum and vagina may maintain vaginal sensation and fullness during intercourse, which can diminish after childbirth. For other women, the pelvic-floor muscles become overly tense and sensitive, like any other muscle cramp in the body. In that case, Kegel exercises (perhaps along with pelvic-floor physiotherapy or massage) might restore a more normal tone to the pelvic muscles and improve their ability to relax.

- *Prenatal prevention.* Your first pregnancy is the ideal time to learn the art of pelvic-floor exercises, if you haven't already. As mentioned in chapter 4, incorporating Kegel exercises into your prenatal routine can be a natural fit.

FINDING YOUR KEGEL MUSCLES: STARTING WITH THE STOP TECHNIQUE

Even if you're familiar with the basic idea of Kegel exercises, odds are you're probably not aware of the proper technique. First, you'll need to locate the right muscles. The simplest way to start is the stop technique.

The stop technique is done while you're emptying your bladder on the toilet. After you've been urinating for a few seconds, try interrupting your stream of urine with a strong squeeze of your vaginal muscles, then relax. Were you able to stop or at least slow the stream? If so, you've just found your Kegel muscles.

Try it one or two times more while you're sitting, and this time shift your focus to avoiding any tightening of your legs, buttocks, or stomach muscles. Your goal should be to isolate the muscle groups of the vagina and pelvic floor. Straining these other areas will not only divert your mental and physical energy but can also generate high pressures in the bladder and encourage the urethra to open—working against your Kegel muscles and causing them to fatigue. If you're not sure whether your stomach and inner thigh muscles are relaxed, try placing one flattened hand against each, so you'll feel any accidental tightening of these non-Kegel muscles during your workout routine. When you've got it right, you should feel a squeezing and lifting sensation within the vagina, and a tightening around the anal area.

Got it? That muscle you've just tightened—the same that you'd use in the car when forced to wait just one more exit—should be the *pubococcygeus*—probably the most important Kegel muscle. Another muscle you may contract is the *bulbocavernosis*, located beneath the outer lips of the vagina and responsible for tightening up the vaginal opening. You may also feel the deeper pelvic-floor muscles contract.

Once you've used the stop technique to find these pelvic-floor muscles, be sure *not* to continue using it as part of your actual workout routine. Regularly interrupting your urine stream can harm your bladder and even your kidneys over the long run.

Now empty your bladder, and try tensing these muscles while you're lying on your back with your knees bent and feet flat on the floor, or sitting in a chair. Keep breathing while you do three to four repetitions in a row, with a short rest after each squeeze. Go slowly, as if your pelvic muscles were a freight elevator lifting a heavy load. Remember to avoid the temptation to squeeze your buttock, thigh, or stomach muscles.

If you had no luck locating your Kegel muscles with the stop technique, try lying down and squeezing tightly around a finger or tampon inserted into the vagina. Imagine that you're trying to prevent the tampon or finger from slipping out, or that you're trying to hold back a bowel movement. These muscles span your pubic bone and tailbone. Feel for a tightening or lifting sensation in that area.

If you've never exercised your pelvic muscles before, or if they lost much of their strength after childbearing, you might not have the ability to find them on your own; it may be difficult to even sense the appropriate muscles. If that's the case, you're not alone. It's been shown that only around 50 percent of women can identify and effectively contract the correct muscles after verbal instruction, and that around 25 percent of them will develop ineffective or even counterproductive techniques. But don't despair—learning pelvic-floor exercises might still be possible using special techniques and devices that you'll learn about later in this appendix (see "Biofeedback" and "Vaginal Cones").

LESSON FROM THE FAR EAST: YOGA FOR THE PELVIC FLOOR

It is claimed that certain yoga poses work out your pelvic floor in a way similar to the Kegel routine, though they've never been scientifically tested. *Aswini mudra* is one such pose that you might want to ask an instructor about. It begins in the sitting position, with a straight spine. The pelvic, vaginal, and sphincter muscles are tightened, as with a strong Kegel squeeze, while the rest of the body is relaxed. The pose is maintained for several breaths, then relaxed. With time and practice, extend the time of each pose, and let your urogynecologist know if it brings you any relief.

THE WORKOUT: MAKING THE WORLD YOUR PELVIC GYMNASIUM

Once you've managed to find your Kegel muscles, it's time start a workout routine. First, choose a comfortable place where you can make some frightening facial grimaces without the least bit of shame. You can sit, stand, or lie down. Some women prefer lying faceup, with knees bent and feet flat on the floor and perhaps a small pillow tucked beneath the lower back. Body positions don't make a critical difference in most cases, though you will most likely find certain ones help you to isolate the pelvic muscles, both mentally and physically, while keeping the rest of your body relaxed. For most women, standing is significantly more difficult than sitting or lying down with knees bent.

WEEK 1
With your legs slightly apart and your stomach and chest relaxed, gradually squeeze your Kegel muscles until they're at maximum

tightness, for three to five seconds. You should feel tensing around the anal and vaginal areas, and lifting of the whole area in and up. Focus on the vagina, urethra, and perineum, and once again imagine you're driving in a car, this time with a full bladder and two exits to go. If you feel your thighs, belly, or buttocks tightening, focus on relaxing these muscles. Then completely relax everything for ten seconds, and feel the tension release. After the ten-second rest, start with another three-to-five-second squeeze.

Repeat this up to ten times, or until you start feeling the muscles fatigue. When did your muscles start to fatigue? If it was after only three repetitions, then that's your starting point for the first week—try doing those same three repetitions twice a day. If you were able to complete ten truly strong squeezes during your first session, then you've started with a significant amount of pelvic-floor strength and can move on to a more aggressive routine of ten contractions, twice daily. If you're developing muscle soreness, skip a session and cut the number of repetitions by half for the next day or two. Each Kegel session should take you no more than five minutes.

WEEKS 2 AND 3

After the first week, increase your number of ten-squeeze sets. Anywhere from two to three sets each day, spaced at least twenty minutes apart, should be your goal. Try to increase the strength of your contractions each day until they're rock-hard from start to finish.

WEEKS 4 TO 6

Increase your squeeze time to a full ten seconds for each repetition, if you haven't already reached that goal. Try to hold it just as strongly from beginning to end. Along the way, as you increase your exercise challenge, alternate your positions among lying, sitting, and standing for individual sessions. Try standing with your legs apart, which tends to be the most difficult position. You can also experiment a bit with the speed and duration of your Kegel contractions. Try some quick-flicker squeezes: rapidly contract and then completely release after only two seconds instead of the usual ten-second slow-hold clenches that you first learned. These flicks will both reinforce your familiarity with the correct muscle groups and increase your ability to produce a strong, quick contraction using your fast-twitch muscle fibers. Flicks can provide a useful insurance policy against leakage during moments of sudden physical stress (see "Pelvic-Floor Bracing," below).

When you're able to hold a strong contraction for ten seconds, repeating ten times, then you've reached the basic training goal. Continue with two or three sets of ten to twelve contractions—in other words, a range of twenty to forty daily squeezes—to maintain your strength. Try keeping it up at least three to five days each week. Congratulations! You're buff.

KEEPING A PELVIC-FLOOR EXERCISE LOG

A simple daily log will help you keep track of your progress with pelvic-floor exercises.

    How many sessions today?   _____

    How long was each session?   _____

    How many squeezes or repetitions per session?   _____

    How many seconds was each squeeze?   _____

"HOW WILL I REMEMBER?"

Patients often ask what's the right time and place to do their Kegel exercises, and the answer is surprisingly simple: any regular routine that you'll actually keep up with and not abandon, is the right one. It's no different than opening that membership to your neighborhood gym—you'll have to realistically fit a pelvic-floor exercise routine into the rest of your busy schedule. As any gym member can testify, even with the best intentions today, good workout habits are tough to maintain through tomorrow and beyond.

The most reliable way to remember your pelvic-floor exercises is to link them to other daily routines. Since you can perform these exercises in nearly any place or position, your potential links are limitless. Try linking your exercise sessions to the same time of day or night that you're nursing your baby, watching a TV sitcom, or riding the bus. If you commute to work by car, try Kegeling at red lights. If you ride the train, squeeze at the stops. If you're a golfer, try a few flicks each time you're waiting at the tee. Boring board meetings, bus stops, and chair lifts work equally well. One patient told me she'd performed a ten-minute pelvic-exercise routine at her kitchen table every morning for over ten years, while drinking her Folgers coffee and watching the *Today* show—now, that's a patriotic American scene! As you make the world your pelvic gymnasium, just be sure to breathe and pay attention to your facial expressions. After all, the only real danger of Kegel exercises is accidentally displaying a bizarre-looking facial twitch or grimace during an important meeting, job interview, or romantic candlelight dinner for two.

EXPECTATIONS: WILL KEGEL EXERCISES REALLY WORK?

As with any other exercise program, pelvic-floor exercises will improve your symptoms only if you keep up with them regularly, and only if you're patient. It often takes between six and twelve weeks to see significant results after beginning a Kegel routine, sometimes with a shorter time to improvement seen for urge symptoms. So, if you haven't noticed improvement after a few months, don't throw in the towel quite yet.

The best results are often achieved when a nurse, doctor, or therapist supervises your first several workouts. Ongoing and structured pelvic-floor exercise programs—in other words, a series of regular office visits or group exercise sessions—are even better, with much higher rates of success and dryness. Cures may be attainable for over 30 percent of women, with improvement of symptoms for 60 to 70 percent. With only brief instruction, on the other hand, less than 20 percent of women will succeed. Two very important points: don't spend more than ten minutes with your exercise routine, and don't perform hundreds of contractions just for kicks. First, because overworking your pelvic-floor muscles is not of benefit; and second, because you'll be likely to burn out. A slowly-but-surely approach will increase your odds of long-term success. Two or three sessions each week may be enough, especially if it's a routine you'll actually stick with.

While pelvic-floor exercises can work well for mild urinary incontinence and prolapse symptoms, they rarely provide a solution for more severe cases. You'll be unlikely to transform constant leakage into total dryness with exercise alone; and if a thin-walled urethra is causing your incontinence, the odds of a cure from exercises alone are even steeper. You also won't significantly improve prolapse that's already bulging outside your body. But when done correctly and regularly, pelvic-floor exercises can always play a part in preventing and controlling early bladder, pelvic, and sexual symptoms. Best of all, they have no side effects, require no prescription, and won't cost you a dime.

PELVIC-FLOOR BRACING

What about those times you can't avoid straining, coughing, or lifting heavy loads? Bracing the pelvic floor can at least help you reduce the risk of stressing it during those activities. Bracing—also referred to as *the knack* by some pelvic-floor specialists—means quickly squeezing the pelvic muscles a split second before the moment of physical exertion. By tightening and reinforcing the levator shelf and sling at just the right time, bracing counteracts the pressure working against the pelvic supports.

If nothing else, bracing during moments of physical stress should help you to reduce leakage. One study from the University of Washington showed that with a deep cough, women taught the knack could reduce their cough-related leakage by nearly 80 percent, as compared with women who didn't use the technique. For other women, bracing may even help to slow the progression of prolapse by strengthening the levator-muscle shelf that supports the pelvic organs, and reducing the downward bulge of these organs through the pelvic opening. Once you've developed a strong Kegel contraction, try to make pelvic-floor bracing one of your healthy habits.

SEEING A PELVIC-FLOOR PHYSIOTHERAPIST

Most urogynecology doctors and nurses know a great deal about pelvic-floor muscle training and can help get you to maximum strength. But women seeking the most natural approach may want to call upon a pelvic-floor physiotherapist. They have the training and the time to discuss and utilize a variety of techniques such as massage, pelvic-floor stimulation, and postural training. A physiotherapist may also work through nuances of pelvic-floor exercise not covered in the doctor's office. For instance, some pelvic-floor physiotherapists may focus on strengthening abdominal muscles rather than relaxing them. Toning the transverse abdominals may, for instance, restore function to levator muscles that haven't responded to routine Kegel exercises.

BIOFEEDBACK: ZEN BUDDHISM
MEETS THE PELVIC FLOOR

The roots of biofeedback lie in Eastern meditation techniques. It was observed that with practice, individuals were able to gain control over bodily processes that typically weren't under voluntary control, such as pulse or body temperature. Pelvic-floor biofeedback is an office method based on that principle, providing you with feedback during your pelvic-floor exercises. By allowing you to see what you're doing down there, biofeedback helps you to focus on muscle groups that you're probably not accustomed to sensing, making your Kegel exercises stronger and improving their impact. Electrode (electromyography) stickers are placed over the abdomen; a tamponlike sensor is inserted into either the vagina or rectum; and each is attached to a computer. On a visual or audio monitor, you'll see when you've contracted the correct pelvis muscles and when you've flexed incorrect muscles, such as your stomach or legs. At each session, you can visually assess how strong your contractions have become and how much progress you've made since the last visit. Home devices are available for women interested in long-term use of this therapy. A low-tech but effective alternative involves the nurse or doctor simply examining the muscles as they're flexed, and giving verbal feedback.

When used as directed, biofeedback can improve many aspects of pelvic-floor function, including bladder and bowel control, pain syndromes, even sexual functioning: in other words, the same handful of benefits that can stem from an effective Kegel routine.

One study of a structured biofeedback program optimistically showed reduced leakage episodes among 81 percent of women using biofeedback and pelvic-floor exercises, versus 69 percent using overactive bladder medication and 39 percent who received no treatment. Another, more recent study of women over age fifty-five showed a 70 percent reduction in leakage episodes using either high-tech or low-tech biofeedback techniques.

According to one study of a three-visit biofeedback series over a six-week period, up to 75 percent of participants considered the method effective, though only around 20 percent or so were objectively shown, with office testing, to have improved bladder control. After biofeedback, the bladder may often feel better and more in control, even if the doctor can't always prove that a cure has been achieved.

Fecal incontinence can also be treated with biofeedback, with improvement reported for 50 to 90 percent of women. Special fluid-filled balloons are used to create the sensation of rectal fullness during these sessions, providing the patient with something to squeeze against.

Sexual dysfunction, in some cases, can also be improved with the help of biofeedback sessions. The most likely women to improve are those with spasm of the pelvic-floor muscles, or the condition of vaginismus discussed in chapter 11.

It's not always necessary to jump into a biofeedback program without first trying simple pelvic-floor exercises on your own. A recent overview of the existing research on biofeedback found that doing Kegels alone usually fares quite well compared to pelvic-floor exercises accompanied by biofeedback. On the other hand, if you've failed Kegel exercises on your own, keep in mind that you might still find success using biofeedback.

ANGELA: AN INSPIRATIONAL TALE OF BIOFEEDBACK SUCCESS

Angela was a thirty-four-year-old mother of two-year-old twin girls. To balance her 24/7 duties at home, she'd vowed to preserve her sanity and fitness by hiring a baby-sitter one afternoon each week. On her own, she'd head out to enjoy her so-called selfish vices—a full-hour aerobics class, a power walk around town, capped by a long cup of coffee with a very junky spy novel.

But on her first few afternoons away, Angela realized that she had a problem. Unlike before her babies were born, her aerobics class was presenting a challenge beyond the exertion itself: leakage. Caught unprepared that first day, she tied her sweatshirt around her waist to cover the ring that had formed at the bottom of her workout pants. The next week, she wore a pad, but her sense of disappointment remained over losing this important part of her life that she'd vowed to preserve.

For six months, she tried Kegel exercises at home, twice each day, to no avail. She had no desire for surgery at this stage in life, and she felt too young for devices. Eventually, Angela went to her doctor. When she squeezed her best Kegel, Angel's gynecologist saw that she was hardly contracting her pelvic-floor muscles at all; what she thought was a squeeze was actually more of a push. Her exercise routine, in other words, had been all wrong.

So she decided to try biofeedback. After two sessions, she'd already improved, with better tone, less leakage, even fewer pads. After the fourth visit, her pelvic-floor muscle strength was close to 100 percent. She was back to aerobics, power walking, and whatever other "selfish vices" this hardworking mom could find the time for.

VAGINAL CONES: ADDING WEIGHTS TO YOUR WORKOUT

As with lifting weights (but guaranteed never to become an Olympic sport), the pelvic muscles can be firmed and strengthened with the help of weighted vaginal cones. These tamponlike devices are inserted into the vagina and can be held inside while you're standing with a Kegel-type contraction; the correct muscles *must* be contracted in order to hold a vaginal cone inside. Vaginal cones are usually made in one size but vary from twenty to over a hundred grams. Your initial goal should be to hold it inside for up to fifteen minutes, always while standing. If the cone falls out, move to a lighter weight. When you're using the correct muscles, you should be able to feel, with the tip of your finger, the cone pulled up into the vagina during your squeeze. If you feel the cone pushing out, then you're using the wrong muscle groups. When the lightest cone is no longer a challenge, perhaps you can graduate to the next higher weight in the set after a week or two. Challenge yourself by trying to hold the cone inside during light activities, such as climbing stairs or walking. As with a regular Kegel exercise, avoid flexing your thighs or buttocks.

Vaginal cones require more privacy than a simple pelvic-floor workout and should not be used during pregnancy. But they can provide an

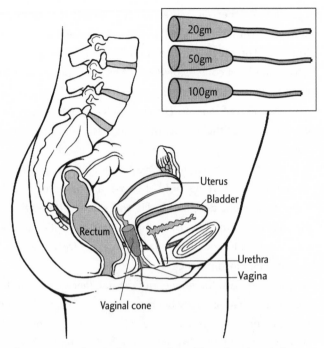

Appearance of vaginal cone, and position when inserted

ideal kick-start for building your pelvic-floor strength and reaping the full range of benefits that can result from a long-term Kegel exercise routine—including improved urinary continence, fecal control, and even sexual function.

THE CUTTING EDGE AND PURELY CAMPY: OTHER FASCINATING PELVIC-FLOOR FACTS, GADGETS, AND UROGYNECOLOGIC GIZMOS

Unlike the Chia Pet or the Clapper, you won't learn about these items by watching late-night infomercials, because they're just too strange. And they're certainly not holiday stocking stuffers that you'll want to share with the whole family. But during your search for another option to manage your postreproductive symptoms, you may come across one of these:

- *Kegelmaster.* A spring-loaded device for insertion into the vagina, with adjustable settings that create progressive resistance between the vaginal walls. By squeezing the two arms of the device together, the Kegel muscles may be trained.

- *GyneFlex.* Another vaginal resistance device that's inserted and then squeezed with the pelvic-floor muscles until the two arms close together. The only device to proudly trademark the VTP system—which stands, of course, for vaginal tightening program. Tell me, does health-care marketing get any funkier than this?

- *Kegelcisor, Kegel-Enhansor.* These weighted stainless-steel devices are like barbells for the vagina. Made to insert and hold, like a vaginal cone.

- *V-brace.* Although its name may sound like an extremely weird women's pro-wrestling hold, the V-brace is actually a feminine-support garment designed to lift and support the vaginal and perineal area with the help of multiple layers of elastic attached over a cotton panty. Intended to relieve symptoms for women with genital prolapse and incontinence.

- *Belly dancing.* Yes, the effects of Oriental dance on pelvic-floor muscle function have actually been studied—in Finland. Women familiar with this pelvic-centered dance style had a superior ability to flex their pelvic-floor muscles, over non–belly dancers. Based on these results, could it be long before doctors are recommending the hustle or the electric slide?

Voiding and Symptom Diary

Postreproductive symptoms occur in very confusing areas of your body. You might sense that everything's different or that nothing feels quite right, but your symptoms often stop short of revealing their specific origin. Pinpointing the basic qualities of your urinary, bowel, sexual, or other postreproductive symptoms—what these symptoms are, where they're arising from, and when they're bothering you—is the first step toward finding relief.

Consider the bladder. Though at first it may seem that your symptoms are random or chaotic, with a symptom diary, you may discover that among a grab bag of symptoms, common patterns and underlying causes exist. How often do you void during the daytime and at night? Are your trips to the bathroom always prompted by an urge, or do you go by sheer habit sometimes? When are you most prone to leak or feel discomfort, and what usually triggers your accidents or pelvic symptoms? Do you lose control silently, or with an urge? Do you have difficulty starting your urine stream or bowel movements, or do you feel the need to strain? Is there pain or burning? Are your symptoms triggered by intercourse, the sound or feel of running water, the rush to open your front door when returning home, or after certain foods or beverages? Do your bladder and bowel symptoms seem to be related? These are some of the symptom patterns that may signal a postreproductive change: perhaps a cystocele or rectocele, a floppy urethra, a very overactive bladder. With the Voiding and Symptom Diary, you can play detective and make some sense of your problem even before seeing the doctor.

Starting Your Diary

The chart on page 334 is a twenty-four-hour diary that you can use for yourself. Copy this diary and use it to record your symptoms for three to seven days.

In the first two columns on the left, record what you drink and eat throughout the day. Columns three to five allow you to record each time you intentionally empty your bladder and the amount you empty. You can measure your urine in a regular measuring cup, or just about any disposable container marked with lines indicating the number of cups, ounces, or milliliters. Columns six to eight allow you to record each time you leak and what you were doing or what you felt at the time of leakage. Whether you were on the StairMaster, washing the dishes, bending over in the garden, or lifting the baby seat, write it down if leakage or any other symptom occurred along with that activity. Was there an urge, or was the leakage silent? Beneath the hour-by-hour grid, your medications can be recorded along with the time of day they were taken. Use the "Other Symptoms" area to track any other unexpected events. Did you have an episode of painful intercourse? Loss of bowel control?

Recalling your symptoms at the day's end can often be inaccurate, so be sure to fill in your diary throughout the day, rather than piecing it together from memory later on.

INTERPRETING YOUR DIARY: DETECTIVE COLUMBO MEETS THE PELVIC FLOOR

Now, after you've completed your own diary, take a look and compare your voiding to the following normal daily habits:

- ✓ Urinating every three to six hours (no more than eight times every twenty-four hours)

✓ Total urine output over twenty-four hours between 1,500 cc and 2,000 cc (70 fluid ounces); over two to three quarts is above the normal range

✓ Not waking with a bladder urge more than once at night

✓ Not feeling fullness right after you've emptied

✓ Able to move your bowels without heavy straining

✓ No accidental leakage of urine, stool, or gas on a regular basis

✓ Intercourse not painful

✓ Never avoiding activities or social situations for fear of accidents

✓ A life without pads!

SEARCHING FOR PATTERNS

Look a bit closer and see if you're able to find a pattern to your symptoms.

- How does the daytime compare with the night? Are your symptoms at their worst in the early morning then gradually improve throughout the day, or is the opposite true?

- Are you at risk to leak only after drinking a cola, coffee, or other food or drink?

- If you've been bothered by bowel symptoms or sexual discomfort, are you able to track when these episodes occur and whether there is a particular trigger?

- Do you leak suddenly with physical stress (stress incontinence), or is it a problem when you're holding back a strong urge (urge incontinence)? Is your leakage triggered by both strong urges and physical stress (mixed incontinence)?

- Is your daily urine output excessive, indicating that your problem with urinary frequency might be cured by laying off that water bottle a bit? Or does your frequency appear to reflect a low bladder capacity? Is your overall urine volume below normal because you're reluctant to drink for fear of accidents?

- Is your urinary stream less forceful than you can remember it being before?

- Compare the pattern of your symptoms to the most common

VOIDING & SYMPTOM DIARY

TIME	FOODS	DRINKS		URINATED		LEAKED URINE				WHAT WERE YOU DOING AT THE TIME?
		What Kind?	How Much?	# of Times This Hour	Amount (ounces)	# of Times This Hour	Amount (S/M/L)	With Urge?	With Stress?	
(Sample)	Bagel	Tea	½ cup	1	8	2	M	Yes	No	Washing Dishes
6–7 A.M.										
7–8 A.M.										
8–9 A.M.										
9–10 A.M.										
10–11 A.M.										
11–12 A.M.										
12–1 P.M.										
1–2 P.M.										
2–3 P.M.										
3–4 P.M.										
4–5 P.M.										
5–6 P.M.										
6–7 P.M.										
7–8 P.M.										
8–9 P.M.										
9–10 P.M.										
10–11 P.M.										
11–12 P.M.										
12–1 A.M.										
1–2 A.M.										
2–3 A.M.										
3–4 A.M.										
4–5 A.M.										
5–6 A.M.										

* Stress: Physical exertion or sudden straining (for example, coughing, sneezing, exercising, lifting, or bending)
* Urge: Sudden strong desire to empty your bladder ("I've gotta go!")

postreproductive problems you've learned about: the overactive bladder, stress incontinence, mixed incontinence, and pelvic prolapse.

Your diary might seem a bit low-tech, but don't be fooled by its appearance. Just as Detective Columbo always solved strange mysteries by taking a closer look at the facts right before him, your diary may reveal surprising clues and even hidden solutions to you and your doctor.

IT HAPPENS EACH MONTH: UNDERSTANDING WHY INCONTINENCE AND OTHER PELVIC SYMPTOMS CAN VARY WITH YOUR MENSTRUAL CYCLE

If you're premenopausal and still have regular menstrual cycles, you may have noticed that certain postreproductive symptoms (such as incontinence or even the pressure resulting from prolapse) become worse at certain times of the month. This pattern highlights the role of the female hormones (estrogen and progesterone) in the urethra, bladder, vagina, and whole pelvic area. Stress incontinence is one such example. As the estrogen supply temporarily falls during the premenstrual week, the estrogen-receptor-rich bladder neck and urethra may temporarily become a bit weaker, leaving you more prone to leakage if the pressure inside the bladder suddenly rises. As a new cycle begins, this estrogen-related symptom should improve. Try increasing the intensity of your Kegel routine, or consider asking your doctor about a continence device to use during these high-risk parts of the month (see chapter 8). In urogynecology, the *uro* and *gyn* are often closely connected.

APPENDIX C

Organizations, Resources, and References

*Remember that pelvic-floor symptoms can sometimes relate to impor-
tant medical conditions that shouldn't be neglected. Your doctor is
the only one who can provide you with the most accurate information
specific to your problem.*

Organizations and Websites

UROGYNECOLOGY AND UROLOGY

American Foundation for Urologic Disease
1128 N. Charles Street
Baltimore, MD 21201
(877) 846–3222
www.afud.org
Website includes information on overactive bladder.

American Urogynecology Society (AUGS)
2025 M Street, NW, Suite 800
Washington, D.C. 20036
(202) 367–1167
www.augs.org

The foremost organization of urogynecologists in the United States. Web-site includes locate-a-physician features for finding a specialist in your area.

American Urological Association
(877) DRY–LIFE
www.drylife.org

Canadian Continence Foundation
P.O. Box 30, Victoria Branch
Westmount, Quebec H3Z 2V4
(800) 265–9575
www.continence-fdn.ca

International Urogynecology Association
1000 Central Street, Suite 730
Evanston, IL 60201
(847) 570–2750
www.iuga.org
Specialists in urinary and pelvic floor dysfunction from more than forty countries.

National Association for Continence
P.O. Box 8310
Spartanburg, SC 29305
(800) BLADDER or (864) 579–7900
www.nafc.org
A highly recommended site, with resources including tapes and manuals for learning pelvic-floor exercises, and a catalog for locating incontinence-related products. The resource guide contains an extensive listing of incontinence products, manufacturers, and distributors.

National Kidney and Urologic Diseases Information Clearinghouse
3 Information Way
Bethesda, MD 20892
(800) 891–5388
www.niddk.nih.gov
E-mail: nkudic@aerie.com

The Simon Foundation for Continence
P.O. Box 835
Wilmette, IL 60091
(800) 23-SIMON
www.simonfoundation.org

Provides newsletters, educational materials, and videos.

OBSTETRICS, GYNECOLOGY, AND WOMEN'S HEALTH

American Association of Gynecologic Laparoscopists
13021 East Florence Avenue
Santa Fe Springs, CA 90670
(562) 946-8774
www.aagl.com

American College of Obstetricians and Gynecologists
409 12th Street, SW
Washington, D.C. 20024
www.acog.org

American College of Nurse-Midwives
(202) 728-9860
www.midwife.org

Hysterectomy Educational Resources and Services
422 Brynn Mawr Avenue
Bala-Cynwyd, PA 19004
(215) 667-7757

International Foundation for Functional Gastrointestinal Disorders
P.O. Box 170864
Milwaukee, WI 53217-8076
(888) 964-2001
www.iffgd.org

International Women's Health Coalition
24 East 21st Street
New York, NY 10010
(212) 979-8500
www.iwhc.org

National Women's Health Resource Center
2440 M Street, NW, Suite 325
Washington, D.C. 20037
(202) 293–6045
www.healthywomen.org
Nonprofit educational organization.

General Search Tools

www.medlineplus.com
Site of the National Library of Medicine. Research the medical literature for any topic or author, using keywords.

www.cochrane.de
International library of clinical trials on various medical topics, including childbirth and pelvic-floor disorders.

Commercial Websites

www.ivillage.com
Numerous bulletin boards and links on women's-health topics.

www.childbirth.org
Focused on natural-delivery information.

www.babycenter.com
"Birth and Labor" section with information and links.

www.babyzone.com
"Birth and Labor" section with information and links.

www.thepregnancycentre.com
Australian site emphasizing physiotherapy.

www.obgyn.net
Large ob/gyn site with chat and message board, including mothers-to-be and doctors.

Companies and Products

The following selected references are included because their products are mentioned in the preceding chapters—not as a specific endorsement.

American Medical Systems, Inc
(800) 328–3881
www.visitams.com
Information on two female-incontinence procedures, including SPARC.

As We Change
(800) 203–5585
www.aswechange.com
Catalog of products for midlife women, including several pelvic-floor training devices.

Boston Scientific Corporation
(800) 225–3226
www.bsci.com
Products and devices for incontinence and pelvic-floor disorders.

Bruce Medical
(800) 225–8446
www.brucemedical.com
Incontinence products by mail.

Carbon Medical Technologies, Inc.
(877) 277–1788
www.carbonmed.com
Information on Durasphere injectable bulking agent.

C. R. Bard, Inc.
(800) 526–2687
www.bardcontigen.com
Contigen periurethral injections for stress incontinence.

Deschutes Medical Products, Inc.
(800) 383–2588

www.deschutesmed.com
Urinary incontinence products, including a handheld Kegel training device.

Endocare
(800) 438–8592
Vaginal cones.

Eli Lilly and Company
(800) 545–5979
www.lilly.com
Women's-health pharmaceuticals, including a medication in development for stress urinary incontinence.

Empi, Inc.
(888) FOR–EMPI
www.empi.com
Products for pelvic-floor stimulation and related devices.

Fembrace, Inc.
(877) 535–6800
www.fembrace.com
Makers of the V-Brace support device.

FemiScan
(781) 259–0489
Portable pelvic-floor exercise and biofeedback system for home use.

Gynecare (Division of Ethicon, Inc., Johnson & Johnson)
(888) GYNECARE
www.ethicon.com or www.gynecare.com
Information on the TVT incontinence procedure.

Hollister, Inc.
(800) 323–4060
www.hollister.com
Pelvic-floor biofeedback and electrical-stimulation devices. Website contains educational resources.

Kegelmaster 2000, Ltd.
(877) 796–8267
www.kegelmaster.com
Progressive-resistance vaginal exerciser.

Kimberly Clark
(800) 558–6423
www.depend.com
Depends and other absorbent products.

Medtronic, Inc.
(800) 328–2518
www.medtronic.com
The Interstim (pelvic pacemaker) for urinary control.

Mentor Urology, Inc.
(800) 525–8161
www.mentorcorp.com
Pessaries and incontinence-related products, including the SABRE sling.

Milex, Inc.
(773) 736–5500 or (800) 621–1278
www.milexproducts.com
Pessaries and vaginal cones.

Neotonus, Inc.
(800) 717–0714
www.neocontrol.com
The magnetic chair for pelvic-floor stimulation therapy.

Ortho-McNeil
(800) 682–6532
www.ortho-mcneil.com
Pharmaceuticals, including Ditropan XL for overactive bladder.

Pelvic Muscle Therapy (PMTx)
(800) 442–7689
A pelvic-floor training device.

Pharmacia and Upjohn
(888) 768–5501
www.pharmacia.com
Pharmaceuticals, including Detrol LA for overactive bladder.

Rochester Medical
(800) FEM–SOFT
www.rocm.com
The Femsoft urethral insert.

ShopInPrivate.com
(800) 809–0610
Wide range of incontinence and feminine items, ranging from absorbent
products to FemTone vaginal weights.
www.shopinprivate.com

Step-Free Vaginal Cones
(877) 933–9300

SURx, Inc.
(877) ASK–SURX
www.surx.com
Radio-frequency bladder neck suspension device.

Tena, Inc.
(800) 992–9939
www.tena-usa.com
Serenity absorbent products (formerly Promise).

The Coffee Bean and Tea Leaf
(800) TEA–LEAF
www.coffeebean.com
Acid-neutral coffees for diet-sensitive symptoms.

UroSurge, Inc.
(800) 658–5965
www.urosurge.com
Bladder retraining devices and SANS system.

Watson Pharmaceuticals, Inc.
(800) 272–5525
www.watsonpharm.com
Producer of the only existing transdermal (skin-patch) medication for overactive bladder.

Glossary

Anal Incontinence: Loss of control over gas or stool.

Anal Sphincter: Circular muscles that surround the anal opening and maintain control over the bowel contents.

Anal Sphincteroplasty: The surgical repair of a torn anal sphincter muscle; for the treatment of fecal incontinence.

Androgens: Male hormones, of which testosterone is the most important; also present in women in much lower amounts.

Anorectal Manometry: A test that measures pressure, strength, and sensation within the anus and rectum. Sometimes used during the evaluation of anal incontinence.

Anterior Colporrhaphy: A vaginal operation to repair certain types of cystoceles.

Anticholinergics: Medications commonly used to treat overactive-bladder symptoms.

Anus: The lowest part of the gastrointestinal tract, between the rectum and anal sphincter.

Atrophy (Urogenital, Vaginal, Vulvar): Thinning of the tissues of the urinary and genital tract, most commonly resulting from a lack of estrogen. A common cause of irritation, infections, and discomfort with intercourse.

Autonomic Nervous System: Nerves that control involuntary systems in the body; for example, heartbeat, breathing, and bladder function.

Bacterial Vaginosis: An overgrowth of certain vaginal bacteria causing discharge and irritation.

Biofeedback: A technique providing feedback—in the form of a visual or audio signal—when pelvic-floor exercises are performed correctly. Used to improve pelvic muscle strength, enhance control over the bladder and bowels, and alleviate certain other pelvic symptoms.

Bladder: The muscular organ that stores urine.

Bladder Drills: A technique for retraining an overactive bladder to improve urinary symptoms and urge incontinence. The time between voids is increased gradually and systematically, improving the bladder's ability to tolerate increasing fullness.

Bladder Spasm: A sudden and involuntary contraction of the bladder muscle, causing an urge to urinate (see Overactive Bladder).

Burch Urethropexy (Retropubic Bladder-Neck Suspension): An operation for certain types of urinary stress incontinence, performed through an abdominal incision or sometimes laparoscopically.

Candidiasis: The most common type of vaginal yeast infection, caused by an overgrowth of candida yeast.

Catheter: A flexible tube inserted into the bladder to drain urine.

Cervix: The narrow bottom portion of the uterus.

Cystitis: Inflammation of the bladder's inner lining, most commonly resulting from a bacterial infection but with a variety of other noninfectious causes.

Cystocele: Dropping of the bladder, due to weakening of the upper vaginal wall.

Cystometry: A test measuring pressure within the bladder while it is filled with fluid. Often used to diagnose an overactive bladder.

Cystoscopy: Inspection of the inner bladder surface through a small telescopic camera.

Cystourethrography: A specialized X-ray picture of the bladder and urethra.

Defecography: A specialized X ray of the anus and rectum, performed during straining and defecation.

Detrusor: The muscular wall of the bladder.

Diuretic: A substance (water pill) that causes the kidneys to excrete water and salt from the body.

Diverticulum: An outpouching from the wall of the bladder or urethra; can lead to irritation and infection.

Dysuria: An uncomfortable burning sensation during urination.

Endoanal Ultrasound: A specialized ultrasound used to identify hidden injuries in the anal sphincter. Sometimes used during the evaluation of anal incontinence.

Eneuresis (Nocturnal Eneuresis): Involuntary leakage of urine at night (bed-wetting).

Enterocele: A prolapse bulge caused by the small intestines bulging into the top of the vagina.

Episiotomy: A cut made into the perineum during childbirth, creating more space for delivery.

Estrogen: The main female hormone produced by the ovaries. Also available as medication.

Fibroids: Benign muscular growths (tumors) within the wall of the uterus.

Fistula: An abnormal hole or passage between the vagina and an adjacent structure, such as bladder, rectum, intestine, or uterus.

Frequency: Voiding at an abnormally frequent interval (going too often).

Hematuria: Blood in the urine.

Hemorrhoids: Swollen tender areas around the anus or rectum, resulting from engorged veins.

Hesitancy: Difficulty initiating the urinary stream.

Hormone Replacement Therapy (HRT): Female hormones (estrogen, progestins) taken in the form of pills or patches as a substitute for natural ovarian hormones after they are no longer produced.

Hysterectomy: Surgical removal of the uterus.

Interstitial Cystitis: An inflammatory condition in the bladder causing frequent urination, nighttime voiding, and pain.

Intravenous Pyelogram: A specialized X-ray picture of the kidneys and upper urinary system above the bladder.

Intrinsic Sphincter Deficiency (ISD): A type of stress urinary incontinence characterized by thin and weak urethral walls; also called the low-pressure urethra.

Kegel Exercise: See "Pelvic-Floor Exercises."

Lactobacillus Acidophilus: A good bacteria found naturally in the vagina; helps to reduce the odds of bad bacteria causing infections. Also contained in certain foods, such as yogurt, and available in over-the-counter supplements.

Laparoscopic Assisted Vaginal Hysterectomy (LAVH): Removal of the uterus using a combination of laparoscopic and vaginal techniques.

Laparoscopy: Abdominal surgery performed through minimally invasive keyhole incisions using telescopic operating devices and fiber-optic lighting.

Laparotomy: An open surgical incision on the abdomen.

Libido: Sex drive.

Macrosomia: A large newborn, usually defined as greater than 4,000 to 4,500 grams.

Magnetic Innervation Therapy: A chair equipped with an electromagnetic stimulating device; used for treating urinary incontinence.

Marshall-Marchetti-Kranz (MMK) Procedure: An operation for urinary stress incontinence, performed through an open abdominal incision.

Menopause: The permanent cessation of menstrual cycles and ovarian hormone production.

Mixed Incontinence: Having a combination of two or more incontinence types: stress, urge, and overflow.

Needle Suspension (Stamey or Raz Procedures): Operations for urinary stress incontinence that stabilize the urethra, using small incisions and specialized needle devices. They have been largely replaced by newer, minimally invasive techniques.

Neuromodulation: An implantable pacemaker used to treat overactive-bladder symptoms and certain forms of pelvic pain and urinary retention. The device is surgically inserted beneath the skin of the lower back.

Nocturia: Waking frequently at night to urinate.

Overactive Bladder: A condition caused by involuntary bladder contractions, leading to urinary frequency, strong bladder urges, nighttime voiding, and urge incontinence.

Osteoporosis: Loss of bone density (thinning) associated with an increased risk of fractures.

Overflow Incontinence: Urine leakage resulting from a bladder that fails to empty and spills when the urine amount exceeds its capacity.

Paravaginal Defect: A type of cystocele that occurs when the upper vaginal wall detaches from its areas of fixation along the sides of the pelvis.

Paravaginal Repair: Surgical correction of a paravaginal defect.

Pelvic Floor: A complex layer of muscles beneath the abdominal and pelvic organs that supports and helps control the bladder, urethra, vagina, uterus, and rectum.

Pelvic-Floor Electrical Stimulation: Stimulation of the pelvic-floor muscles and nerves with a gentle electrical current. Used for the treatment of incontinence, overactive bladder, and certain types of pelvic or sexual pain.

Pelvic-Floor (Kegel) Exercises: Exercises that strengthen the levator muscles; used to treat certain types of urinary incontinence, anal incontinence, and sexual dysfunction.

Pelvic Organ Prolapse: Dropping or bulging of a pelvic organ, such as the uterus, vaginal walls, bladder, rectum, or bowels (see Cystocele, Enterocele, Rectocele, Uterine Prolapse, Vaginal Vault Prolapse).

Pelvimetry: Measurements of the pelvic bones, with special focus on the areas most important for vaginal birth.

Pelvis: The bones surrounding the pelvic cavity and its organs.

Perineal Massage: A technique used during pregnancy and childbirth to soften the perineal tissues, preparing them for delivery.

Perineometer: A device that measures the strength of pelvic-floor (Kegel) squeezes.

Perineorrhaphy: Surgical reconstruction of a loose perineum and vaginal opening.

Perineum: The anatomic area between the genital and anal openings.

Periurethral Injections: Bulking up the urethra by injecting material (collagen, Durasphere, Teflon) into its walls. An office-based therapy for urinary stress incontinence.

Pessary: An object usually made of silicone or rubber, available in various shapes and sizes; worn like a diaphragm in the vagina to support pelvic prolapse.

Pyelonephritis: Infection in one or both kidneys.

Phytoestrogens: Natural estrogenlike substances found in various foods, such as soy products.

Posterior Colporrhaphy (Posterior Repair): A vaginal operation to repair a rectocele.

Progesterone: A female hormone abundant during pregnancy and present in smaller quantities during the normal menstrual cycle.

Progestin: Synthetic progesterone.

Prolapse: Weakening of pelvic supports leading to dropping or bulging of the pelvic organs (see: Cystocele, Enterocele, Rectocele, Uterine Prolapse, Vaginal Vault Prolapse).

Pudendal Nerve: A nerve providing sensation and normal muscle tone to much of the pelvic floor, including the levator muscles, perineal area, bladder, and anal sphincter.

Rectocele: The rectum bulging up into a weakened lower vaginal wall.

Rectum: The lowest portion of the digestive tract, storing the bowel contents right before defecation; located right above the anal canal.

Retention (Urinary Retention): An abnormal amount of urine remaining in the bladder after voiding. Indicates an inability to fully empty the bladder.

Sacral Colpopexy: Surgically attaching the top of the vagina to the sacrum, a bone at the back of the pelvis. Performed either through an open abdominal incision or by laparoscopy.

Sacral Nerve Stimulation (Neuromodulation, Interstim): A pacemaker for the pelvis, implanted near the tailbone and sacral nerves, used to treat a variety of bladder and pelvic symptoms.

Sacrospinous Vaginal Vault Suspension: A vaginal operation that secures a prolapsed vaginal vault to the sacrospinous ligament, located deep within the pelvis.

Salpingo-oophrectomy: Removal of the tubes (salpingo) and ovaries (oophoron).

Sensory Urgency: Frequent strong bladder urges, resulting from irritation or sensitivity within the bladder or urethral lining.

Sphincter: Muscle that surrounds the opening of an organ (including the anus and urethra), controlling the outflow of waste products.

Splinting: Supporting the lower vaginal wall, usually with a finger, in order to help stool empty from a rectocele bulge.

Stress Urinary Incontinence: Involuntary loss of urine during moments of increased physical stress (lifting, coughing, laughing, sneezing).

Suburethral Sling (Bladder Sling): A stress incontinence procedure that places a strip of synthetic or natural material beneath the bladder neck and/or urethra.

Suprapubic Catheter: A catheter inserted into the bladder through a tiny incision in the abdomen.

Tension-free Sling (TVT, SPARC, SABRE, and others): Minimally invasive operations that place a loose synthetic mesh beneath the urethra; a highly effective and increasingly popular treatment for several types of stress urinary incontinence.

Ureters: The pair of long narrow tubes connecting the kidneys to the bladder.

Urethra: The anatomic tube leading from the bladder to the outside of the body.

Urethral Hypermobility: A floppy urethra caused by a loss of underlying vaginal support; often found in association with urinary stress incontinence.

Urethritis: Inflammation of the urethra.

Urethrolysis: A procedure intended to loosen the urethral support after a previous incontinence operation, if voiding problems occur and persist after surgery.

Urge Incontinence: Involuntary loss of urine triggered by an urge to urinate; most often resulting from an overactive bladder.

Urgency: A strong and often sudden desire to urinate.

Urinalysis: A test of the urine that can immediately identify chemicals suggestive of infection or other urinary conditions.

Urinary Incontinence: Any involuntary leakage of urine.

Urine Culture: A test for bacterial growth in the urine, requiring incubation for up to several days.

Urodynamics: A test used to diagnose the specific underlying causes of incontinence symptoms and voiding problems.

Uroflowmetry: A test that calculates the rate of urine flow during urination.

Urogynecologist: A subspecialist devoted to the diagnosis and treatments of disorders related to the female pelvic floor and lower urinary tract. Urogynecologists are trained in obstetrics and gynecology, then receive additional subspecialty training.

Urologist: Physician specializing in both male and female urinary systems. Subspecialists in female urology devote additional training to the female urinary and genital systems.

Uterine Prolapse: A dropped uterus caused by weakening of the surrounding pelvic ligaments that secure it to the bony pelvis.

Uterosacral Ligament Suspension: Reinforcing the top (apex) of the vagina to the uterosacral ligaments on the pelvic walls. Performed with vaginal, abdominal, or laparoscopic techniques.

Uterus: The pear-shaped muscular organ that consists of a main portion (body) and a narrowed lower part (cervix) opening into the top of the vagina.

Vagina: The canal between the uterus and outer genital area.

Vaginal Hysterectomy: Removal of the uterus through the vagina, with no abdominal incision.

Vaginal Vault Prolapse: Bulging of the upper vagina after it detaches from its pelvic supports, in a woman with a previous hysterectomy.

Vaginal Vault Suspension: An operation suspending the top (apex) of the vagina to pelvic ligaments.

Vaginitis: Inflammation of the vagina with a number of potential causes, including infection, chemical irritants, or a lack of estrogen (atrophic vaginitis).

VBAC: Vaginal birth after a previous cesarean section.

Voiding and Symptom Diary: A log for recording urinary patterns, incontinence episodes, and other pelvic-floor symptoms.

Vulva: The outer female genitalia.

Bibliography

URINARY INCONTINENCE AND BLADDER PROBLEMS

Arya, L.A., Jackson, N.D., Myers, D.L., and Verma, A. "Risk of New-Onset Urinary Incontinence After Forceps and Vacuum Delivery in Primiparous Women." *American Journal of Obstetrics and Gynecology* 185(6)(2001):1318–23.

Beck, R.P., and Hsu, N. "Pregnancy, Childbirth and the Menopause Related to the Development of Stress Incontinence." *American Journal of Obstetrics and Gynecology* 91(1965):820–23.

Black, N.A., Bowling, A., Griffiths, J.M., Pope, C., and Abel, P.D. "Impact of Surgery for Stress Incontinence on the Social Lives of Women." *British Journal of Obstetrics and Gynaecology* 105(1998):605–12.

Bo, K., Talseth, T., and Holme, I. "Single Blind, Randomized Controlled Trial of Pelvic Floor Exercises, Electrical Stimulation, Vaginal Cones and No Treatment in Management of Genuine Stress Incontinence in Women." *British Medical Journal* 318(1999):487–93.

Brubaker, L., Benson, J.T., Bent, A., Clark, A., and Shott, S. "Transvaginal Electrical Stimulation for Female Urinary Incontinence." *American Journal of Obstetrics and Gynecology* 177(1997):536–40.

Burgio, K.L., Robinson, J.C., and Engel, B.T. "The Role of Biofeedback in Kegel Exercise Training for Stress Urinary Incontinence." *American Journal of Obstetrics and Gynecology* 154(1986):58–64.

Burgio, K.L., Matthews, K.A., and Engel, B.T. "Prevalence, Incidence and Correlates of Urinary Incontinence in Healthy, Middle-Aged Women." *Journal of Urology* 146(1991):1255–59.

Cardozo, L.D., and Kelleher, C.J. "Sex Hormones, the Menopause, and Urinary Problems." *Gynecologic Endocrinology* 9(1995):75–84.

Chiarelli, P., and Cockburn, J. "Promoting Urinary Continence in Women After Delivery: Randomized Controlled Trial." *British Medical Journal* 324(2002):1241.

Diokno, A.C. "Epidemiology and Psychosocial Aspects of Incontinence." *Urologic Clinics of North America* 22(3)(1995):481–85.

Farrell, S.A., Allen, V.M., and Baskett, T.F. "Parturition and Urinary Incontinence in Primiparas." *Obstetrics and Gynecology* 97(3)(2001):350–56.

Francis, W.J.A. "The Onset of Stress Incontinence." *Journal of Obstetrics and Gynaecology of the British Empire* 67(1960):899–903.

Hannah, M.E., Hannah, W.J., et al., Term Breech Trial 3-Month Follow-Up Collaborative Group. "Outcomes at 3 Months After Planned Cesarean vs. Planned Vaginal Delivery for Breech Presentation at Term: The International Randomized Term Breech Trial." *Journal of the American Medical Association* 287(14)(2002):1822–31.

Hassouna, M.M., Siegel, S.W., Nyeholt, A.A.B., et al. "Sacral Neuromodulation in the Treatment of Urgency-Frequency Symptoms: A Multicenter Study on Efficacy and Safety." *Journal of Urology* 163(6)(2000):1849–54.

Kegel, A.H. "Progressive Resistance Exercise in the Functional Restoration of the Perineal Muscles." *American Journal of Obstetrics and Gynecology* 56(1948):238–48.

Mason, L., Glenn, S., Walton, I., and Hughes, C. "Women's Reluctance to Seek Help for Stress Incontinence During Pregnancy and Following Childbirth." *Midwifery* 17(3)(2001):212–21.

Meyer, S., Hohlfeld, P., Achtari, C., and De Grandi, P. "Pelvic Floor Education After Vaginal Delivery." *Obstetrics and Gynecology* 97(2001): 673–77.

Morkved, S., and Bo, K. "Effect of Postpartum Pelvic Floor Muscle Training in Prevention and Treatment of Urinary Incontinence: A One-Year Follow-up." *British Journal of Obstetrics and Gynecology* 107(2000):1022–28.

Nygaard, I., DeLancey, J.O.L., Arnsdorf, L., Murphy, E. "Exercise and Incontinence." *Obstetrics and Gynecology* 75(1990):848–51.

Persson, J., Wolner-Hanssen, P.A.L., and Rydhstroem, H. "Obstetric Risk Factors for Stress Urinary Incontinence: A Population-Based Study." *Obstetrics and Gynecology* 96(2000):440–45.

Peschers, U., Schaer, G., Anthuber, C., Delancey, J.O.L., and Schuessler, B. "Changes in Vesical Neck Mobility Following Vaginal Delivery." *Obstetrics and Gynecology* 88(1996):1001–6.

Reilly, E.T., Freeman, R.M., Waterfield, M.R., Waterfield, A.E., Steggles, P., and Pedlar, F. "Prevention of Postpartum Stress Incontinence in Primigravidae with Increased Bladder Neck Mobility: a Randomised Controlled Trial of Antenatal Pelvic Floor Exercises." *British Journal of Obstetrics and Gynaecology* 109(1)(2002):68–76.

Sampselle, C.M., Miller, J.M., Mims, B.L., DeLancey, J.O.L., Ashton-Miller, J.A., and Antonakos, C.L. "Effect of Pelvic Muscle Exercise on Transient Incontinence During Pregnancy and After Childbirth." *Obstetrics and Gynecology* 91(1998):406–12.

Sand, P.K., Richardson, D.A., Staskin, D.R., Swift, S.E., Appell, R.A., Whitmore, K.E., and Ostergard, D.A. "Pelvic Floor Electrical Stimulation in the Treatment of Genuine Stress Incontinence: A Multi-Center Placebo-Controlled Trial." *American Journal of Obstetrics and Gynecology* 173(1995):72–79.

Steele, A.C., Kohli, N., Mallipeddi, P., and Karram, M. "Pharmacologic Causes of Female Incontinence." *International Urogynecol Journal* 10(1999):106–10.

Stewart, W., Herzog, R., Wein, A., et al. "The Prevalence and Impact of Overactive Bladder in the U.S.: Results from the NOBLE Program." *Neurourology and Urodynamics* 20(2001):406–8.

Subak, L.L., Quesenberry, C.P., Posner, S.F., Cattolica, E., and Soghikian K. "The Effect of Behavioral Therapy on Urinary Incontinence: A Randomized Controlled Trial." *Obstetrics and Gynecology* 100(2002):72–78.

Thorp, J.M., Norton, P.A., Wall, L.L., Kuller, J.A., Eucker, B., and Wells, E. "Urinary Incontinence in Pregnancy and the Puerperium: A Prospective Study." *American Journal of Obstetrics and Gynecology* 181(1999):266–73.

Viktrup, L., Lose, G., Rolff, M., and Barfoed, K. "The Symptom of Stress Incontinence Caused by Pregnancy or Delivery in Primiparas." *Obstetrics and Gynecology* 79(1992):945–49.

Viktrup, L., and Lose, G. "The Risk of Stress Incontinence 5 Years After First Delivery." *American Journal of Obstetrics and Gynecology* 185(2001):82–87.

Wilson, P.D., Herbison, R.M., and Herbison, G.P. "Obstetric Practice and the Prevalence of Urinary Incontinence Three Months After Delivery." *British Journal of Obstetrics and Gynaecology* 103(2)(1996):154–61.

ANAL INCONTINENCE

Bek, K.M., and Laurberg, S. "Risks of Anal Incontinence from Subsequent Vaginal Delivery After a Complete Obstetric Anal Sphincter Tear." *British Journal of Obstetrics and Gynaecology* 99(1992):724–26.

Crawford, L.A., Quint, E.H., Pearl, M.L., DeLancey, J.O.L. "Incontinence Following Rupture of the Anal Sphincter During Delivery." *Obstetrics and Gynecology* 82(1993):527–31.

Donnely, V., Fynes, M., Campbell, D., Johnson, H., O'Connell, P.R., and O'Herlihy, C. "Obstetric Events Leading to Anal Sphincter Damage." *Obstetrics and Gynecology* 92(1998):955–61.

Eason, E., Labrecque, M., Marcoux, S., and Monder, M. "Anal Incontinence After Childbirth." *Canadian Medical Association Journal* 166(3)(2002):326–30. Available: www.cma.ca/cmaj/vol-166/issue-3/0326.asp.

Fynes, M., Donnelly, V.S., O'Connell, P.R., and O'Herlihy, C. "Cesarean Delivery and Anal Sphincter Injury." *Obstetrics and Gynecology* 92(1998):496–500.

Fynes, M., et al. "Effect of a Second Vaginal Delivery on Anorectal Physiology and Faecal Incontinence: A Prospective Study." *Lancet* 354(1995):983–86.

Kammerer-Doak, D.N., Wesol, A.B., Rogers, R.B., Dominguez, C.E., and Dovin, M.H. "A Prospective Cohort Study of Women After Primary Repair of Obstetric Anal Sphincter Laceration." *American Journal of Obstetrics and Gynecology* 181(6)(1999):1317–22.

Malouf, A.J., Norton, C.S., Engel, A.F., Nicholls, R.J., Kamm, M.A. "Long-term Results of Overlapping Anal Sphincter Repair for Obstetrical Trauma." *Lancet* 355(2000):260–65.

Norton, C., Hosker, G., and Brazzelli, M. "Effectiveness of Biofeedback and/or Sphincter Exercises for the Treatment of Faecal Incontinence in Adults." *Cochrane Database of Systematic Reviews* 2(2000): CD002111.

Rieger, N., Schloithe, A., Saccone, G., and Wattchow, D. "The Effect of a Normal Vaginal Delivery on Anal Function." *Obstetrics and Gynecology* 53(1998)345–46.

Sultan, A.H., Kamm, M.A., Hudson, C.N., and Bartam, C.L. "Anal Sphincter Disruption During Vaginal Delivery." *New England Journal of Medicine* 329(1993):1905–11.

Swash, M. "Fecal Incontinence: Childbirth Is Responsible for Most Cases." *British Medical Journal* 307(1993):636–37.

SEXUAL DYSFUNCTION

Clark, A., and Romm, J. "Effect of Urinary Incontinence on Sexual Activity in Women." *Journal of Reproductive Medicine* 38(1993):679–83.

Glazener, C.M. "Sexual Function After Childbirth: Women's Experiences, Persistent Morbidity, and Lack of Professional Recognition." *British Journal of Obstetrics and Gynaecology* 104(1997):330–35.

Kelleher, C., Cardozo, L., Wise, B., et al. "The Impact of Urinary Incontinence on Sexual Function." *Neurology and Urodynamics* 11(1992):359–60.

Rogers, R.G. "Sexual Function in Women with Pelvic Floor Disorders." *American Urogynecologic Society Quarterly Report* XXI(2002):1–3.

Signorello, L.B., Harlow, B.L., Chekos, A.K., and Repke, J.T. "Postpartum Sexual Functioning and Its Relationship to Perineal Trauma: A Retrospective Cohort Study of Primiparous Women." *American Journal of Obstetrics and Gynecology* 184(2001):881–88.

Sutherherst, J.R. "Sexual Dysfunction and Urinary Incontinence." *British Journal of Obstetrics and Gynaecology* 86(1979):387–88.

Weber, A.M., Walters, M.D., and Piedmote, M.R. "Sexual Function and Vaginal Anatomy in Women Before and After Surgery for Pelvic Organ Prolapse and Urinary Incontinence." *American Journal of Obstetrics and Gynecology* 182(2000):1610–15.

PELVIC-FLOOR INJURY

Allen, R.E., Hosker, G.L., Smith, A.R.B., Warrell, D.W. "Pelvic Floor Damage and Childbirth: A Neurophysiological Study." *British Journal of Obstetrics and Gynaecology* 97(1990):770–79.

Angioli, R., Gomez-Martin, O., and Cantuaria, G. "Severe Perineal Lacerations During Vaginal Delivery: The University of Miami Experience." *American Journal of Obstetrics and Gynecology* 182(5)(2000):1083–85.

DeLeeuw, J.W., Struijk, P.C., Vierhout, M.E., and Wallenberg, H.C. "Risk Factors for Third Degree Perineal Ruptures During Delivery." *British Journal of Obstetrics and Gynaecology* 108(4)(2001):383–87.

Mallett, V., Hosker, G., Smith, A.R.B., and Warrell, D. "Pelvic Floor Damage and Childbirth: A Neurophysiologic Follow-up Study." *Neurourology and Urodynamics* 13(1994):357–58.

Martin, S., Labreque, M., Marcoux, S., Berube, S., and Pinault, J.J. "The Association Between Perineal Trauma and Spontaneous Perineal Tear." *Journal of Family Practice* 50(4)(2001):333–37.

Meyer, S., Schreyer, A., DeGrandi, P., and Hohfeld, P. "The Effects of Birth on Urinary Continence Mechanisms and Other Pelvic-Floor Characteristics." *Obstetrics and Gynecology* 92(1998):613–18.

Olsen, A.L., Smith, V.J., Bergstrom, J.O., Colling, J.C., Clark, A.L. "Epidemiology of Surgically Managed Pelvic Organ Prolapse and Urinary Incontinence." *Obstetrics and Gynecology* 89(1997):501–6.

Peschers, U.M., Schaer, G.N., DeLancey, J.O.L., and Schuessler, B. "Levator Function Before and After Childbirth." *British Journal of Obstetrics and Gynaecology* 104(1997):1004–8.

Smith, A.R.B., Hosker, G.L., and Warrell, D.W. "The Role of Pudendal Nerve Damage in the Aetiology of Genuine Stress Incontinence in Women." *British Journal of Obstetrics and Gynaecology* 96(1989): 29–32.

Snooks, S.J., Swash, M., Setchell, M., and Henry, M.M. "Injury to Innervation of Pelvic Floor Sphincter Musculature in Childbirth." *Lancet* 2(1984):546–50.

Snooks, S.J., Swash, M., Mathers, S.E., and Henry, M.M. "Effect of Vaginal Delivery on the Pelvic Floor: A Five-Year Follow-up. *British Journal of Surgery* 77(1990):1358–60.

Sultan, A.H., Kamm, M.A., and Hudson, C.N. "Pudendal Nerve Damage During Labor: Prospective Study Before and After Outcome of Primary Repair." *British Medical Journal* 101(1994):22–28.

OBSTETRICAL PRACTICE, POSTPARTUM STRATEGIES, AND THE PELVIC FLOOR

ACOG Committee Opinion. "Exercise During Pregnancy and the Postpartum Period." *Obstetrics and Gynecology* 99(1)(2002):171–73.

Al-Mufti, R., McCarthy, A., and Fisk, N.M. "Obstetricians' Personal Choice and Mode of Delivery." *Lancet* 347(1996):544.

Argentine Episiotomy Trial Collaborative Group. "Routine Versus Selective Episiotomy: A Randomized Controlled Trial." *Lancet* 342(1993): 1517–18.

Barros, F.C., Vaughan, J.P., Victora, C.G., and Huttly, S.R.A. "Epidemic of Cesarean Sections in Brazil." *Lancet* 338(1991):167–69.

Bomfim-Hyppolito, S. "Influence of the Position of the Mother at Delivery Over Some Maternal and Neonatal Outcomes." *International Journal of Gynaecology and Obstetrics* 63(1998):67–73.

Brown, S., and Lumley, J. "Maternal Health After Childbirth: Results of an

Australian-Based Population Survey." *British Journal of Obstetrics and Gynaecology* 105(1998):156–61.

Carroli, G., and Belizan, J. "Episiotomy for Vaginal Birth." *Cochrane Database Systematic Reviews* (2)2000:CD000081.

De Jong, P.R., Johanson, R.B., Baxen, P., Adrians, V.D., Van Der Westhuisen, S., and Jones P.W. "Randomised Trial Comparing the Upright and Supine Positions for the Second Stage of Labour." *British Journal of Obstetrics and Gynaecology* 104(5)(1997):567–71.

DeMello, E., and Souza, C. "Cesarean Sections as Ideal Births: The Cultural Constructions of Beneficence and Patients' Rights in Brazil." *Cambridge Quarterly Health Ethics* 3(1994):358–66.

Eason, E.L., Labrecque, M., Well, G., and Feldman, P. "Preventing Perineal Trauma During Childbirth: A Systematic Review." *Obstetrics and Gynecology* 95(2000):464–71.

Farrell, S.A. "Cesarean Section Versus Forceps-Assisted Vaginal Birth: It's Time to Include Pelvic Injury in the Risk-Benefit Equation." *Canadian Medical Association Journal* 166(3)(2002):337–38.

Flynn, P., Franiek, J., Janssen, P., Hannah, W.J., and Klein, M.C. "How Can Second-Stage Management Prevent Perineal Trauma?" *Canadian Family Physician* 43(1997)73–84.

Fraser, W.D., et al. "Multicenter Randomized Controlled Trial of Delayed Pushing for Multiparous Women in the Second Stage of Labor with Continuous Lumbar Epidural Anesthesia." *American Journal of Obstetrics and Gynecology* 182(2000):1168.

Fynes, M., Donnelly, V.S., O'Connell, P.R., and O'Herlihy, C. "Cesarean Delivery and Anal Sphincter Injury." *Obstetrics and Gynecology* 92(1998):496–500.

Graham, W.J., Hundley, V., McCheyne, A.L., Hall, M.H., Gurney, E., and Milne, J. "An Investigation of Women's Involvement in the Decision to Deliver by Cesarean Section." *British Journal of Obstetrics and Gynaecology* 106(1999):213–20.

Handa, V.L., Harris, T.A., Ostergard, D.R. "Protecting the Pelvic Floor: Obstetric Management to Prevent Incontinence and Pelvic Organ Prolapse." *Obstetrics and Gynecology* 88(1996):470–78.

Hanlon, T. *Fit for Two: The Official YMCA Prenatal Exercise Guide.* Human Kinetics Publishers, 1995.

Hansen, S.L., Clark, S.L., Foster, J.C. "Active Pushing Versus Passive Fetal Descent in the Second Stage of Labor: A Randomized Controlled Trial." *Obstetrics and Gynecology* 99(2002):29–34.

Jovine, V. *The Girlfriend's Guide to Surviving the First Year of Motherhood.* Berkley Publishing Group, 1997.

Johanson, R.B., and Menon, B.K.V. "Vacuum Extraction Versus Forceps for Assisted Vaginal Delivery." *Cochrane Review* 4(1999):

Klein, M.C., Gauthier, R.T., et al. "Relationship of Episiotomy to Perineal Trauma and Morbidity, Sexual Dysfunction, and Pelvic Floor Relaxation." *American Journal of Obstetrics and Gynecology* 171(3)(1994):591–98.

Labrecque, M., Eason, E., Marcoux, S., Lemieux, F., Pinault, J.J., Feldman, P., and Laperriere, L. "Randomized Controlled Trial of Prevention of Perineal Trauma by Perineal Massage During Pregnancy." *American Journal of Obstetrics and Gynecology* 180(1999):593–600.

Lydon-Rochelle, M., Holt, V.L., Easterling, T.R., and Martin, D.P. "Cesarean Delivery and Postpartum Mortality Among Primiparas in Washington State, 1987–1996." *Obstetrics and Gynecology* 97(2001):169–74.

McMahon, M.J., Luther, E.R., Bowes, W.A., Olshan, A.F. "Comparison of a Trial of Labour with an Elective Second Cesarean Section." *New England Journal of Medicine* 335(1996):689–95.

Mould, T.A.J., Chong, S., Spencer, J.A.D., and Gallivan, S. "Women's Involvement with the Decision Preceding Their Cesarean Section and Their Degree of Satisfaction." *British Journal of Obstetrics and Gynaecology* 103(1996):1074–77.

O'Boyle, A.L., Davis, G., Calhoun, B.C. "Informed Consent and Birth: Protecting the Pelvic Floor and Ourselves." *American Journal of Obstetrics and Gynecology* 187(2002):981–83.

Paterson-Brown, S. "Should Doctors Perform an Elective Cesarean Section on Request? Yes, as long as the Woman Is Fully Informed." *British Medical Journal* 317(1998):462–63.

Payne, T.N., Carey, J.C., and Rayburn, W.F. "Prior Third- or Fourth-Degree Perineal Tears and Recurrence Risks." *International Journal of Gynaecology and Obstetrics* 64(1)(1999):55–7.

Pearl, M.L., Roberts, J.M., Laros, R.K., and Hurd, W.W. "Vaginal Delivery from the Persistent Occiput Posterior Position: Influence on Maternal and Neonatal Morbidity." *Journal of Reproductive Medicine* 38(12)(1993): 955–61.

Robinson, J.N., Norwitz, E.R., Cohen, A.P., McElrath, T.F., Lieberman, E.S. "Epidural Analgesia and Third- or Fourth-Degree Lacerations in Nulliparas." *Obstetrics and Gynecology* 94(1999):261.

Rowe, J.W. "NIH Consensus Development Panel: Urinary Incontinence in

Adults." *Journal of the American Medical Association* 261(1989): 2685–90.

Sachs, B.P., Kobelin, C., Castro, M.A., and Frigoletto, E. "The Risk of Lowering the Cesarean Delivery Rate." *New England Journal of Medicine* 340(1999):54–57.

Shorten, A., Donsante, J., and Shorten, B. "Birth Position, Accroucheur and Perineal Outcomes: Informing Women About Choices for Vaginal Birth." *Birth* 29(2002):18–27.

Stamp, G., Fruzins, G., and Crowther, C. "Perineal Massage in Labour and Prevention of Perineal Trauma: Randomized Controlled Trial." *British Medical Journal* 322(2001):1277–80.

Sultan, A.H., Johanson, R.B., and Carter, J.E. "Occult Anal Sphincter Trauma Following Randomized Forceps and Vacuum Delivery. *International Journal of Gynaecology and Obstetrics* 61(2)(1998):113–19.

Sultan, A.H., and Stanton, S.L. "Preserving the Pelvic Floor and Perineum During Vaginal Childbirth—Elective Cesarean Section?" *British Journal of Obstetrics and Gynaecology* 103(1996):731–34.

Teasdill, W. *Step-by-Step Yoga for Pregnancy: Essential Exercises for the Childbearing Year.* McGraw-Hill, 2000.

Walker, M.P.R., Farine, D., Rolbin, S.H., and Ritchie, J.W.K. "Epidural Anesthesia, Episiotomy, and Obstetric Laceration." *Obstetrics and Gynecology* 77(1991):668–71.

Wall, L.L. "Birth Trauma and the Pelvic Floor: Lessons from the Developing World." *Journal of Women's Health* 8(1999):149–55.

Wall, L.L., Norton, P.A., Delancey, J.O.L. *Practical Urogynecology.* Baltimore, MD: Williams and Wilkins, 1993.

POST-REPRODUCTIVE WOMEN'S HEALTH

Corio, L.E. *The Change Before the Change.* New York: Bantam, 2000.

Love, S. *Dr. Susan Love's Menopause Book.* New York: Crown Publishing, 2003.

Reichman, J. *I'm Too Young to Get Old.* New York: Crown Publishers, 1998.

Sabel, M. *The Soy Solution.* New York: Fireside, 2003.

Shandler, N. *Estrogen the Natural Way.* New York: Villard, 1997.

Stewart, E. *The V-Book.* New York: Bantam, 2002.

Index

ABOUT THE AUTHOR

DR. ROGER GOLDBERG practices urogynecology and reconstructive pelvic surgery in the Chicago area, at the Evanston Continence Center and the Continence Center at Lincoln Park. He is also a clinical instructor in obstetrics and gynecology at Northwestern University Medical School. He received his B.A. from Cornell University, his M.D. from Northwestern University, and a master's of public health degree from Johns Hopkins University prior to his residency at Harvard University's Beth Israel Hospital. His areas of special interest include the minimally invasive surgical and nonsurgical treatment of pelvic prolapse and incontinence, and the obstetrical risk factors leading to these disorders. Dr. Goldberg received the Society of Gynecologic Surgeons President's Award in 2001 for outstanding research in gynecologic surgery; the 2002–2003 American College of Obstetricians and Gynecologists/Pharmacia Award for overactive bladder research; and the 2002 Central Association of Obstetricians and Gynecologists Young Investigator's Award for the study of pelvic-floor disorders after multiple childbirth. He and his wife, Elena, live in Evanston, Illinois.